Hospital Statistics™

2003 Edition

AHA Institutional Members $145
Nonmembers $235
AHA Catalog NUMBER 082003
Telephone ORDERS 1-800-AHA-2626

ISSN 0090-6662
ISBN 0-87258-783-5

Printed in the U.S.A.

Contents

Acknowledgements & Advisements

Acknowledgments

The 2003 edition of Hospital Statistics is published by Health Forum an affiliate of the American Hospital Association, Richard J. Davidson, President.

Advisements

The data published here should be used with the following advisements: The data are based on replies to an annual survey that seeks a variety of information, not all of which is published in this book. The information gathered by the survey includes specific services, but not all of each hospital's services. Therefore, the data do not reflect an exhaustive list of all services offered by all hospitals. For information on the availability of additional data, please contact Health Forum, (800) 821-2039.

Health Forum does not assume responsibility for the accuracy of information voluntarily reported by the individual institutions surveyed. The purpose of this publication is to provide basic data reflecting the delivery of health care in the United States and associated areas, and is not to serve an official and all-inclusive list of services offered by individual hospitals.

Introduction

For more than five decades, *Hospital Statistics*™ has reported aggregate hospital data derived from the AHA Annual Survey and is the definitive source when doing trend analysis with data by bed size category, U.S. Census Divisions, States, and Metropolitan Statistical Areas (MSAs). As the health care delivery system changes, so have the data tracked by the survey and presented in this report. Recent additions include:

- **Community health indicators** that offer readers a connection to the community for their analysis and planning: the data are broken down into beds, admissions, inpatient days, ER outpatient visits, and other indicators per 1000 population, as well as expense per capita.

- **Utilization, personnel and finance** by all MSAs in the United States.

- **Five-year trend data** on physician models, insurance products, and managed care contracts enable you to identify changes in relationships between hospitals and other health care systems and providers.

- **Tables 3 through 6 have been organized** to show breakdowns between inpatient and outpatient care to better reflect market shifts toward outpatient-centered care. Additional clarity is gained by the breakdown between total facility data (which includes nursing home type units under the control of the hospital) and hospital units (which exclude the nursing home data).

TABLE 6 Your State

U.S. Registered Community Hospitals
(Nonfederal, short-term general and other special hospitals)

Overview 1997-2001

	2001	2000	1999	1998	1997
Physician Models					
Independent Practice Association	14	17	17	17	14
Group Practice without Walls	4	5	5	8	4
Open Physician-Hospital Organization	20	21	24	23	18
Closed Physician-Hospital Organization	21	17	18	17	11
Management Service Organization	14	18	20	14	9
Integrated Salary Model	35	29	30	26	24
Equity Model	4	3	4	6	3
Foundation	9	8	23	21	19
Insurance Products					
Health Maintenance Organization	20	22	23	24	19
Preferred Provider Organization	39	47	52	53	37
Indemnity Fee for Service	7	12	14	12	6
Managed Care Contracts					
Health Maintenance Organization	64	67	62	49	42
Preferred Provider Organization	97	93	92	87	72

Example of five-year trend data

- **Facilities and Services information** on more than 90 categories of hospital facilities and services in Table 7. At a glance, you can determine the number and percentage of hospitals offering a specific service such as Oncology, Angioplasty, Palliative Care Program, Complementary Medicine, Women's Health Services and Tobacco Cessation.

- **Plus, System and Network involvement along with Group Purchasing Organizations** that demonstrate ways in which organizations are linked.

The survey instrument and the glossary

A good place to begin your analysis is the AHA Annual Survey instrument. Found on page 197, it includes the instructions, questions, and terms that were used to gather the data for fiscal year 2001. This can be extremely valuable for a clearer understanding of the data we collect and the tables presented in *Hospital Statistics*.

Please also review the glossary in the back of the book. The glossary contains complete definitions for specific terms used in the tables and text of *Hospital Statistics*. These definitions will clarify how terminology is being used.

As mentioned above, it is important to note that the primary focus of the most detailed data contained in *Hospital Statistics* is community hospitals. As defined, community hospitals are all non-federal, short-term general and special hospitals whose facilities and services are available to the public. If the majority of a hospital's patients are admitted to units where the average length of stay is 30 days or less, a hospital may still be classified as short-term even if it includes a nursing- home-type unit. (For a more complete definition of community hospitals, please see the glossary definition, located on page 187.)

Getting the most out of *Hospital Statistics*

This section of the book provides an introduction for getting the most out of your *Hospital Statistics* 2003 edition. Here, you'll find a guide to the book, with insights into each table.

Equity model: An arrangement that allows established practitioners to become shareholders in a professional corporation in exchange for tangible and intangible assets of their existing practices.

Expenses: Includes all expenses for the reporting period including payroll, non-payroll, bad debt, and all nonoperating expenses. *Payroll expenses* include all salaries and wages. *Non-payroll expenses* are all professional fees and those salary expenditures excluded from payroll. *Labor related expenses* are defined as payroll expenses plus employee benefits. *Non-labor related expenses* are all other non-payroll expenses. *Bad debt* has been reclassified from a "reduction in revenue" to an expense in accordance with the revised AICPA Audit Guide. However, for purposes of historical consistency, the expense total that appears throughout *Hospital Statistics does not include "bad debt" as an expense item.* Note: Financial data may not add due to rounding.

Extracorporeal shock wave lithotripter (ESWL): A medical device used for treating stones in the kidney or ureter. The device disintegrates kidney stones noninvasively through the transmission of acoustic shock waves directed at the stones.

Fitness center: Provides exercise, testing, or evaluation programs and fitness activities to the community and hospital employees.

Example of Glossary definitions.

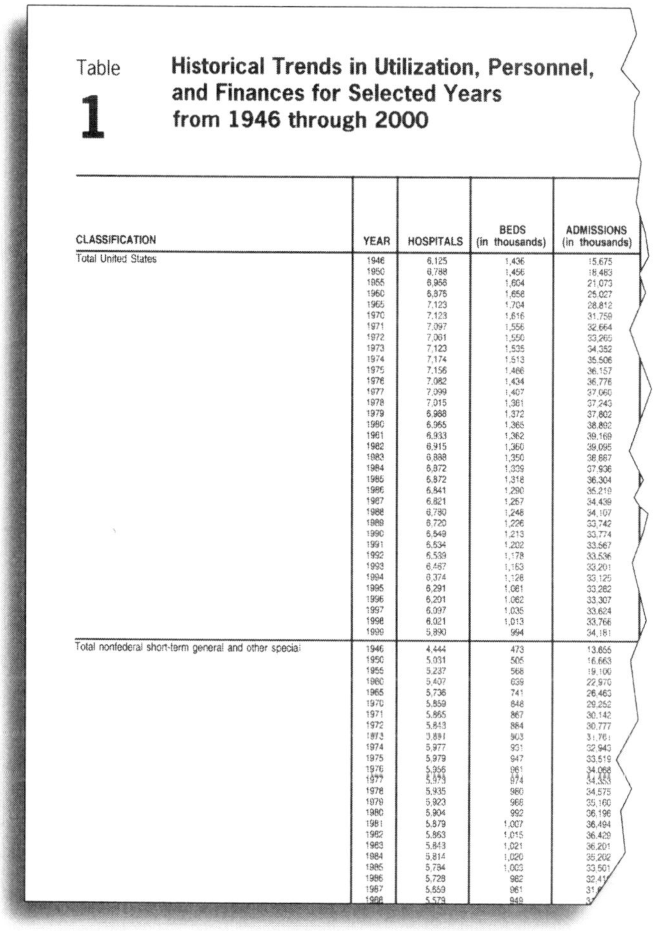

Table **1** **Historical Trends in Utilization, Personnel, and Finances for Selected Years from 1946 through 2000**

CLASSIFICATION	YEAR	HOSPITALS	BEDS (in thousands)	ADMISSIONS (in thousands)
Total United States	1946	6,125	1,436	15,675
	1950	6,788	1,456	18,483
	1955	6,956	1,604	21,073
	1960	6,876	1,658	25,027
	1965	7,123	1,704	28,812
	1970	7,123	1,616	31,759
	1971	7,097	1,556	32,664
	1972	7,061	1,550	33,265
	1973	7,123	1,535	34,352
	1974	7,174	1,513	35,506
	1975	7,156	1,466	36,157
	1976	7,082	1,434	36,776
	1977	7,099	1,407	37,060
	1978	7,015	1,381	37,243
	1979	6,988	1,372	37,802
	1980	6,965	1,365	38,892
	1981	6,933	1,362	39,169
	1982	6,915	1,360	39,095
	1983	6,888	1,350	38,887
	1984	6,872	1,339	37,936
	1985	6,872	1,318	36,304
	1986	6,841	1,290	35,219
	1987	6,821	1,257	34,439
	1988	6,780	1,248	34,107
	1989	6,720	1,226	33,742
	1990	6,649	1,213	33,774
	1991	6,634	1,202	33,567
	1992	6,539	1,178	33,536
	1993	6,467	1,163	33,201
	1994	6,374	1,128	33,125
	1995	6,291	1,081	33,282
	1996	6,201	1,062	33,307
	1997	6,097	1,035	33,624
	1998	6,021	1,013	33,766
	1999	5,890	994	34,181
Total nonfederal short-term general and other special	1946	4,444	473	13,655
	1950	5,031	505	16,663
	1955	5,237	568	19,100
	1960	5,407	639	22,970
	1965	5,736	741	26,463
	1970	5,859	848	29,252
	1971	5,865	867	30,142
	1972	5,843	884	30,777
	1973	5,891	903	31,761
	1974	5,977	931	32,943
	1975	5,979	947	33,519
	1976	5,956	961	34,068
	1977	5,973	974	34,353
	1978	5,935	980	34,575
	1979	5,923	988	35,160
	1980	5,904	992	36,198
	1981	5,879	1,007	36,494
	1982	5,863	1,015	36,429
	1983	5,843	1,021	36,201
	1984	5,814	1,020	35,202
	1985	5,784	1,003	33,501
	1986	5,728	962	32,41
	1987	5,659	961	31,
	1988	5,579	949	[illegible]

Example of Table 1

Table 1 — Historical Trends in Utilization, Personnel and Finances for Selected Years from 1946 through 2001

Table 1 at a Glance

This table is used to evaluate historical data and allows you to examine long-term trends in health care with data dating back more than fifty years. Table 1 reports on all AHA registered hospitals in the United States. One important note: To be considered an AHA-registered hospital, a hospital does not need to be an AHA member. Rather, the hospital must meet particular certification or satisfy a number of requirements. These Registration Requirements immediately follow this section and begin on page xiv.

This table segments the data into various organizational structure categories. Here's a brief look at these different classifications:

- Total United States Hospitals.
- Total Non-Federal Short-term and other special hospitals.
- Community hospitals
- Non-government not-for-profit community hospitals
- Investor-owned (for-profit) community hospitals
- State and local government community hospitals

Table 1 also provides input on nationwide utilization, personnel and finance trends. You'll find answers to questions such as: *Over the past 25 years, what trends do I see comparing the average length of stay at government and non-government not-for-profit community hospitals and investor-owned for-profit community hospitals?* or *What has been the trend in outpatient visits?*

Table 2 — 2001 U.S. Registered Hospitals: Utilization, Personnel and Finances

Table 2 at a Glance

This table takes a closer look at U.S. Registered Hospitals for 2001. It offers a snapshot of utilization, personnel and finance statistics, and breaks down this information for specialty hospitals. In addition, this is the only table that outlines data on federal hospitals. You'll be able to use this table to better understand the number of beds set-up and staffed, how many personnel and trainees are on the payroll, and what the financial implications of these may be.

TABLE 3

TOTAL UNITED STATES

U.S. Registered Community Hospitals
(Nonfederal, short-term general and other special hospitals)

Utilization, Personnel, Revenue and Expenses, Community Health Indicators 1997-2001

	2001	2000	1999	1998	1997
TOTAL FACILITY (Includes Hospital and Nursing Home Units)					
Utilization - Inpatient					
Beds	839,988	853,287	862,352	872,736	902,061
Admissions	31,811,673	31,576,960	31,098,959	30,945,357	30,718,136
Inpatient Days	191,430,450	192,504,015	193,747,004	199,876,367	207,180,278
Average Length of Stay	6.0	6.1	6.2	6.5	6.7
Inpatient Surgeries	9,735,705	9,509,081	9,545,612	9,700,613	9,833,938
Births	3,726,233	3,742,191	3,723,871	3,764,698	3,809,367
HOSPITAL UNIT (Excludes Separate Nursing Home Units)					
Utilization - Inpatient					
Beds	758,186	769,505	782,504	794,502	824,969
Admissions	31,265,867	31,047,930	30,652,820	30,577,564	30,403,766
Inpatient Days	165,644,176	165,605,620	168,189,130	174,898,504	182,702,882
Average Length of Stay	5.3	5.3	5.5	5.7	6.0
Personnel					
Total Full Time	3,235,153	3,183,730	3,154,603	3,166,729	3,147,922
Total Part Time	1,213,426	1,214,232	1,153,790	1,146,082	1,122,957
Revenue and Expenses - Totals (Includes Inpatient and Outpatient)					
Total Net Revenue	$333,054,828,642	$322,459,942,930	$310,513,291,998	$298,519,717,355	$285,858,018,951
Total Expenses	314,709,758,455	301,905,101,393	290,128,641,153	282,372,557,487	272,840,121,437

Example of Table 3. Helps contrast acute and long-term care

Table 3 — Total United States

Table 3 at a Glance
This table provides a look at all U .S. Registered Community Hospitals, in terms of general overview with utilization by inpatient and outpatient, personnel, revenue, expenses and community health indicators. It provides a snapshot of the past five years, allowing you to track emerging trends.

This national information can be compared to local or regional trends, for benchmarking

- Both inpatient and outpatient information is included, for better evaluation of data.
- Reporting by total facility *Includes hospital and Nursing Home Units* and hospital unit only *Excludes Separate Nursing Home Units* helps contrast acute and long-term care.
- Community health indicators can help uncover trends and help determine future facility needs

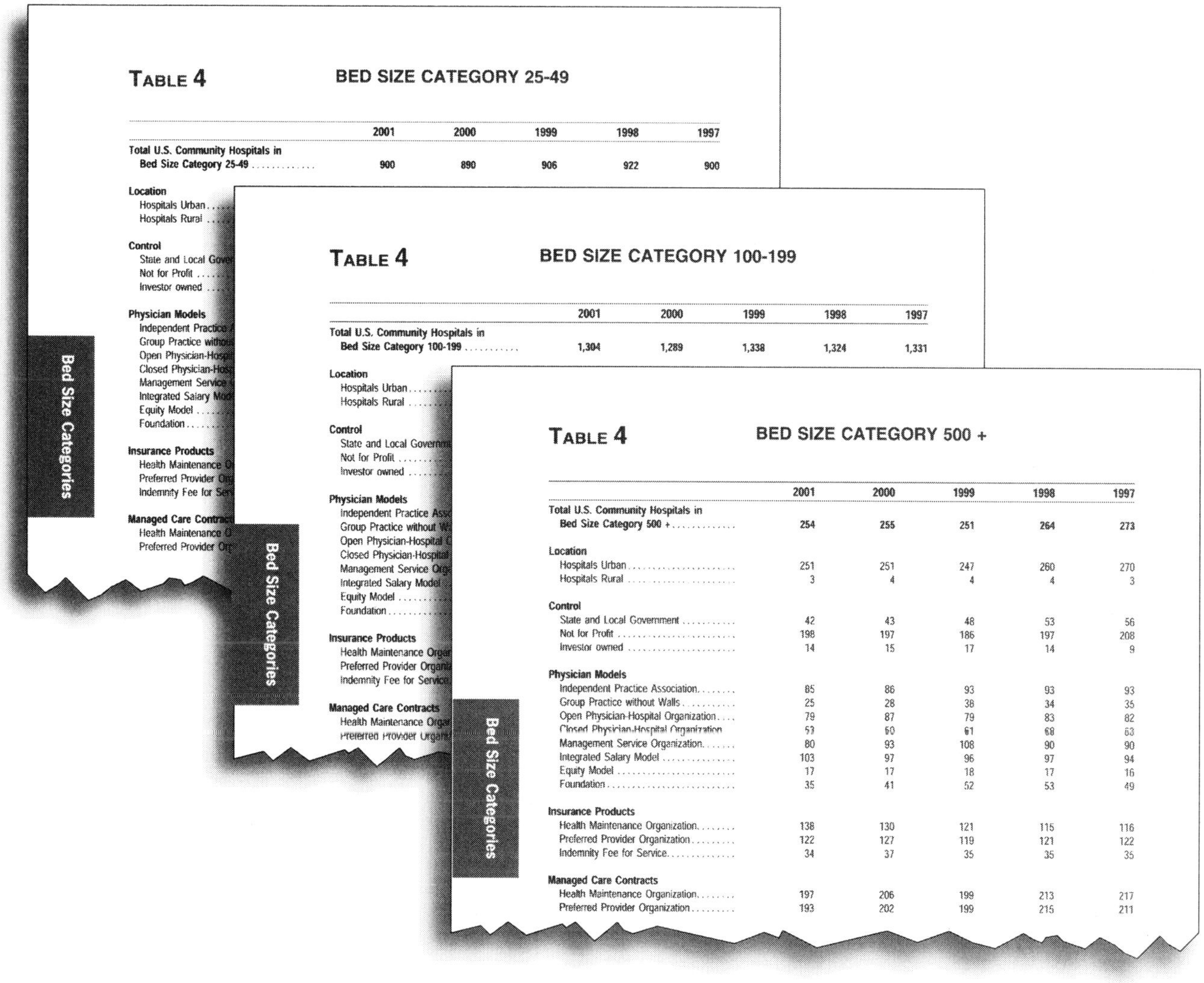

TABLE 4 BED SIZE CATEGORY 25-49

	2001	2000	1999	1998	1997
Total U.S. Community Hospitals in Bed Size Category 25-49	900	890	906	922	900

TABLE 4 BED SIZE CATEGORY 100-199

	2001	2000	1999	1998	1997
Total U.S. Community Hospitals in Bed Size Category 100-199	1,304	1,289	1,338	1,324	1,331

TABLE 4 BED SIZE CATEGORY 500 +

	2001	2000	1999	1998	1997
Total U.S. Community Hospitals in Bed Size Category 500 +	254	255	251	264	273
Location					
Hospitals Urban	251	251	247	260	270
Hospitals Rural	3	4	4	4	3
Control					
State and Local Government	42	43	48	53	56
Not for Profit	198	197	186	197	208
Investor owned	14	15	17	14	9
Physician Models					
Independent Practice Association	85	86	93	93	93
Group Practice without Walls	25	28	38	34	35
Open Physician-Hospital Organization	79	87	79	83	82
Closed Physician-Hospital Organization	53	60	61	68	63
Management Service Organization	80	93	108	90	90
Integrated Salary Model	103	97	96	97	94
Equity Model	17	17	18	17	16
Foundation	35	41	52	53	49
Insurance Products					
Health Maintenance Organization	138	130	121	115	116
Preferred Provider Organization	122	127	119	121	122
Indemnity Fee for Service	34	37	35	35	35
Managed Care Contracts					
Health Maintenance Organization	197	206	199	213	217
Preferred Provider Organization	193	202	199	215	211

Example of Table 4. Compares facilities with peers.

Table 4 — Bed Size Categories

Table 4 at a Glance

This table provides a look at all U.S. Registered Community Hospitals, broken down by bed size. The table includes general overview, utilization, personnel, and revenue and expense information. These categories of bed sizes were developed by the AHA, and have become an industry standard. By categorizing each facility into a peer group, this table provides a snapshot of the past five years allowing you to compare facilities with their peers.

TABLE 5

U.S. CENSUS DIVISION 2: MIDDLE ATLANTIC

U.S. Registered Community Hospitals
(Nonfederal, short-term general and other special hospitals)

Utilization, Personnel, Revenue and Expenses, Community Health Indicators 1997-2001

	2001	2000	1999	1998	1997
COMMUNITY HEALTH INDICATORS PER 1000 POPULATION					
Total Population (in thousands)	38,292	38,216	38,184	38,147	38,108
Inpatient					
Beds	3.6	3.8	3.9	4.0	4.1
Admissions	135.8	136.7	136.2	138.3	137.4
Inpatient Days	963.5	988.8	1,019.0	1,093.8	1,145.0
Inpatient Surgeries	42.2	41.4	41.2	42.7	43.6
Births	13.0	13.2	13.6	13.7	14.3
Outpatient					
Emergency Outpatient Visits	367.7	362.0	363.4	379.5	360.1
Other Outpatient Visits	1,970.9	1,802.3	1,767.7	1,680.3	1,573.9
Total Outpatient Visits	2,338.6	2,164.3	2,131.1	2,059.8	1,934.0
Outpatient Surgeries	67.8	62.4	59.9	55.4	53.5
Expense per Capita (per person)	$1,494.9	$1,462.7	$1,428.6	$1,429.8	$1,369.2

Example of Table 5. Uncovers trends to determine future facility needs.

Table 5 — U.S. Census Divisions

Table 5 at a Glance
This table provides a look at all U.S. Registered Community Hospitals, broken down by Census Division. The table includes general overview, utilization, personnel, and expenses, and community health indicator information. It provides a snapshot of the past five years, allowing you to track trends on a regional level. In addition, this allows you to compare this data to other population based health indicators, offering a more comprehensive look than the survey data alone. Community health indicators can help uncover trends and help determine future facility needs.

Table 6 — States

Table 6 at a Glance
This table provides a look at all U.S. Registered Community Hospitals, broken down by State. The table includes general overview, utilization, personnel, revenue and expenses, and community health indicator information. It provides a snapshot of the past five years, allowing you to track trends on a state level.

Note:
You can use the information in tables 3,4,5 and 6 to make accurate comparisons across Total U.S., Bed Size Category, Census Division and State.

Table 7 — 2001 Facilities and Services in the U.S. Census Divisions and States

Table 7 at a Glance
This table examines facilities and services by both Census Division and State. A comprehensive alphabetical guide helps make each facility or service easy to find. This table will allow you to better understand what service lines are emerging and how many facilities offer a particular service in a discrete state or region.

This collection of facilities and services information data is unique to *Hospital Statistics* and the list is continually growing. Recent additions include:

- Pain Management Programs
- Complementary Medicine (i.e. Alternative Medicine)
- Chiropractic Services
- Acute Long Term Care
- Auxiliary
- Ambulance Services
- Enabling Services
- Palliative Care Program
- Enrollment Assistance Services
- Hemodialysis
- Sleep Center
- Tobacco Treatment/Cessation Program

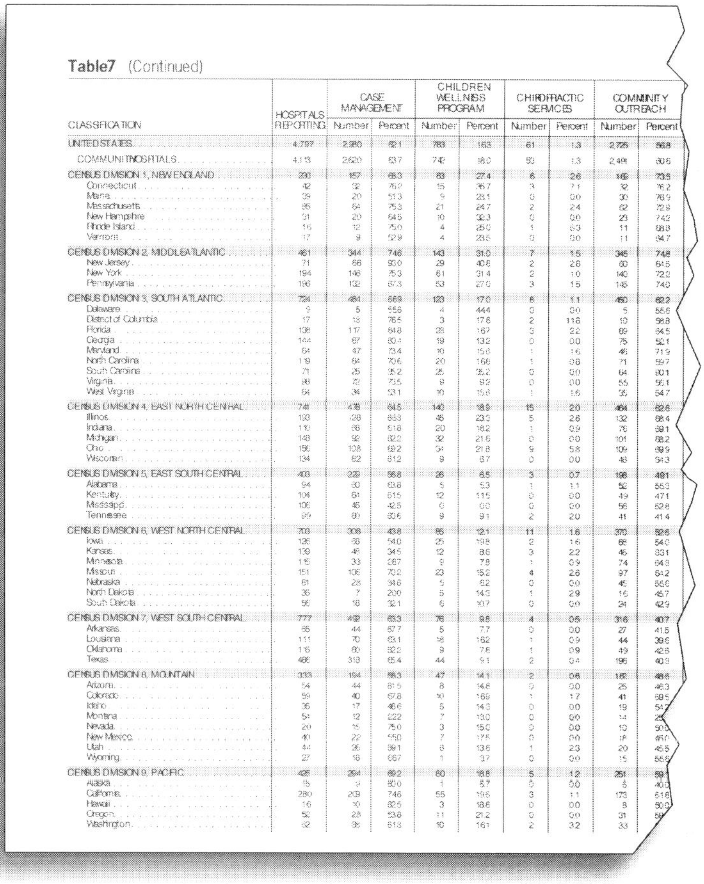

Table7 (Continued)

CLASSIFICATION	HOSPITALS REPORTING	CASE MANAGEMENT		CHILDREN WELLNESS PROGRAM		CHIROPRACTIC SERVICES		COMMUNITY OUTREACH	
		Number	Percent	Number	Percent	Number	Percent	Number	Percent
UNITED STATES	4,797	2,980	62.1	783	16.3	61	1.3	2,725	56.8
COMMUNITY HOSPITALS	4,113	2,620	63.7	742	18.0	53	1.3	2,491	60.6
CENSUS DIVISION 1, NEW ENGLAND	230	157	68.3	63	27.4	6	2.6	169	73.5
Connecticut	42	32	76.2	15	35.7	3	7.1	32	76.2
Maine	39	20	51.3	9	23.1	0	0.0	30	76.9
Massachusetts	85	64	75.3	21	24.7	2	2.4	62	72.9
New Hampshire	31	20	64.5	10	32.3	0	0.0	23	74.2
Rhode Island	16	12	75.0	4	25.0	1	6.3	11	68.8
Vermont	17	9	52.9	4	23.5	0	0.0	11	64.7
CENSUS DIVISION 2, MIDDLE ATLANTIC	461	344	74.6	143	31.0	7	1.5	345	74.8
New Jersey	71	66	93.0	29	40.8	2	2.8	60	84.5
New York	194	146	75.3	61	31.4	2	1.0	140	72.2
Pennsylvania	196	132	67.3	53	27.0	3	1.5	145	74.0
CENSUS DIVISION 3, SOUTH ATLANTIC	724	484	66.9	123	17.0	8	1.1	450	62.2
Delaware	9	5	55.6	4	44.4	0	0.0	5	55.6
District of Columbia	17	13	76.5	3	17.6	2	11.8	10	58.8
Florida	138	117	84.8	23	16.7	3	2.2	89	64.5
Georgia	144	87	60.4	19	13.2	0	0.0	75	52.1
Maryland	64	47	73.4	10	15.6	1	1.6	46	71.9
North Carolina	119	84	70.6	20	16.8	1	0.8	71	59.7
South Carolina	71	25	35.2	25	35.2	0	0.0	64	90.1
Virginia	98	72	73.5	9	9.2	0	0.0	55	56.1
West Virginia	64	34	53.1	10	15.6	1	1.6	35	54.7
CENSUS DIVISION 4, EAST NORTH CENTRAL	741	478	64.5	140	18.9	15	2.0	464	62.6
Illinois	193	128	66.3	45	23.3	5	2.6	132	68.4
Indiana	110	68	61.8	20	18.2	1	0.9	76	69.1
Michigan	148	92	62.2	32	21.6	0	0.0	101	68.2
Ohio	156	108	69.2	34	21.8	9	5.8	109	69.9
Wisconsin	134	82	61.2	9	6.7	0	0.0	46	34.3
CENSUS DIVISION 5, EAST SOUTH CENTRAL	403	229	56.8	26	6.5	3	0.7	198	49.1
Alabama	94	60	63.8	5	5.3	1	1.1	52	55.3
Kentucky	104	64	61.5	12	11.5	0	0.0	49	47.1
Mississippi	106	45	42.5	0	0.0	0	0.0	56	52.8
Tennessee	99	60	60.6	9	9.1	2	2.0	41	41.4
CENSUS DIVISION 6, WEST NORTH CENTRAL	703	308	43.8	85	12.1	11	1.6	370	52.6
Iowa	126	68	54.0	25	19.8	2	1.6	68	54.0
Kansas	139	48	34.5	12	8.6	3	2.2	46	33.1
Minnesota	115	33	28.7	9	7.8	1	0.9	74	64.3
Missouri	151	106	70.2	23	15.2	4	2.6	97	64.2
Nebraska	81	28	34.6	5	6.2	0	0.0	45	55.6
North Dakota	35	7	20.0	5	14.3	1	2.9	16	45.7
South Dakota	56	18	32.1	6	10.7	0	0.0	24	42.9
CENSUS DIVISION 7, WEST SOUTH CENTRAL	777	492	63.3	76	9.8	4	0.5	316	40.7
Arkansas	65	44	67.7	5	7.7	0	0.0	27	41.5
Louisiana	111	70	63.1	18	16.2	1	0.9	44	39.6
Oklahoma	115	60	52.2	9	7.8	1	0.9	49	42.6
Texas	486	318	65.4	44	9.1	2	0.4	196	40.3
CENSUS DIVISION 8, MOUNTAIN	333	194	58.3	47	14.1	2	0.6	162	48.6
Arizona	54	44	81.5	8	14.8	0	0.0	25	46.3
Colorado	59	40	67.8	10	16.9	1	1.7	41	69.5
Idaho	35	17	48.6	5	14.3	0	0.0	19	54.[illegible]
Montana	54	12	22.2	7	13.0	0	0.0	14	2[illegible]
Nevada	20	15	75.0	3	15.0	0	0.0	10	50.[illegible]
New Mexico	40	22	55.0	7	17.5	0	0.0	18	45.[illegible]
Utah	44	26	59.1	6	13.6	1	2.3	20	45.5
Wyoming	27	18	66.7	1	3.7	0	0.0	15	55.6
CENSUS DIVISION 9, PACIFIC	425	294	69.2	80	18.8	5	1.2	251	59.[illegible]
Alaska	15	9	60.0	1	6.7	0	0.0	6	40.0
California	280	209	74.6	55	19.6	3	1.1	173	61.8
Hawaii	16	10	62.5	3	18.8	0	0.0	8	50.0
Oregon	52	28	53.8	11	21.2	0	0.0	31	59.[illegible]
Washington	62	38	61.3	10	16.1	2	3.2	33	[illegible]

Example of Table 7.

These new categories reflect the trends as hospitals expand their service lines to reflect the needs of their patients. For example, services such as acupuncture or massage therapy are now accounted for in the Complementary Medicine service item.

This table can answer questions such as: *What percentage of hospitals in the United States offer complementary medicine or chiropractic services?* or *How are these new services distributed by state?*

Table 8 — Utilization, Personnel and Finances in Community Hospitals by MSAs for 2001.

Table 8 at a Glance
This table provides a look at all U.S. Registered Community Hospitals, broken down by Metropolitan Statistical Area (MSA). The table includes general overview, utilization, personnel, and finance information. It provides a snapshot of the past year.

Additional Resources
Again, in the back of the book you will find the comprehensive glossary and the 2001 annual survey questionnaire. The survey itself can be a valuable resource to understanding what was asked in order to gather the data in the book. This survey is also used to produce the *AHA Guide®* and AHA Annual Survey Database™.

Registration Requirements for Hospitals

AHA-Registered Hospitals

Any institution that can be classified as a hospital according to the requirements may be registered if it so desires. Membership in the American Hospital Association is not a prerequisite.

The American Hospital Association may, at the sole discretion of the Executive Committee of the Board of Trustees, grant, deny, or withdraw the registration of an institution.

An institution may be registered by the American Hospital Association as a hospital if it is accredited as a hospital by the Joint Commission on Accreditation of Healthcare Organizations or is certified as a provider of acute services under Title 18 of the Social Security Act and has provided the Association with documents verifying the accreditation or certification.

In lieu of the preceding accreditation or certification, an institution licensed as a hospital by the appropriate state agency may be registered by AHA as a hospital by meeting the following alternative requirements:

Function: The primary function of the institution is to provide patient services, diagnostic and therapeutic, for particular or general medical conditions.

1. The institution shall maintain at least six inpatient beds, which shall be continuously available for the care of patients who are nonrelated and who stay on the average in excess of 24 hours per admission.

2. The institution shall be constructed, equipped, and maintained to ensure the health and safety of patients and to provide uncrowded, sanitary facilities for the treatment of patients.

3. There shall be an identifiable governing authority legally and morally responsible for the conduct of the hospital.

4. There shall be a chief executive to whom the governing authority delegates the continuous responsibility for the operation of the hospital in accordance with establish policy.

5. There shall be an organized medical staff of fully licensed physicians* that may include other licensed individuals permitted by law and by the hospital to provide patient care services independently in the hospital. The medical staff shall be accountable to the governing authority for maintaining proper standards of medical care, and it shall be governed by bylaws adopted by said staff and approved by the governing authority.

6. Each patient shall be admitted on the authority of a member of the medical staff who has been granted the privilege to admit patients to inpatient services in accordance with state law and criteria for standards of medical care established by the individual medical staff. Each patient's general medical condition is the responsibility of a qualified physician member of the medical staff. When nonphysician members of the medical staff are granted privileges to admit patients, provision is made for prompt medical evaluation of these patients by a qualified physician. Any graduate of a foreign medical school who is permitted to assume responsibilities for patient care shall possess a valid license to practice medicine, or shall be certified by the Educational Commission for Foreign Medical Graduates, or shall have qualified for and have successfully completed an academic year of supervised clinical training under the direction of a medical school approved by the Liaison Committee on GAT Medical Education.

7. Registered nurse supervision and other nursing services are continuous.

8. A current and complete‡ medical record shall be maintained by the institution for each patient and shall be available for reference.

9. Pharmacy service shall be maintained in the institution and shall be supervised by a registered pharmacist.

10. The institution shall provide patients with food service that meets their nutritional and therapeutic requirements; special diets shall also be available.

Types of Hospitals

In addition to meeting these 10 general registration requirements, hospitals are registered as one of four types of hospitals: general, special, rehabilitation and chronic disease, or psychiatric. The following type of hospital and special requirements for registration are employed:

General

The primary function of the institution is to provide patient services, diagnostic and therapeutic, for a variety of medical conditions. A general hospital also shall provide:

- diagnostic x-ray services with facilities and staff for a variety of procedures
- clinical laboratory service with facilities and staff for a variety of procedures and with anatomical pathology services regularly and conveniently available
- operating room service with facilities and staff.

Special

The primary function of the institution is to provide diagnostic and treatment services for patients who have specified medical conditions, both surgical and nonsurgical. A special hospital also shall provide:

- such diagnostic and treatment services as may be determined by the Executive Committee of the Board of Trustees of the American Hospital Association to be appropriate for the specified medical conditions for which medical services are provided shall be maintained in the institution with suitable facilities and staff. If such conditions do not normally require diagnostic x-ray service, laboratory service, or operating room service, and if any such services are therefore not maintained in the institution, there shall be written arrangements to make them available to patients requiring them.
- clinical laboratory services capable of providing tissue diagnosis when offering pregnancy termination services.

Rehabilitation and Chronic Disease

The primary function of the institution is to provide diagnostic and treatment services to handicapped or disabled individuals requiring restorative and adjustive services. A rehabilitation and chronic disease hospital also shall provide:

- arrangements for diagnostic x-ray services, as required, on a regular and conveniently available basis
- arrangements for clinical laboratory service, as required on a regular and conveniently available basis
- arrangements for operating room service, as required, on a regular and conveniently available basis
- a physical therapy service with suitable facilities and staff in the institution
- an occupational therapy service with suitable facilities and staff in the institution
- arrangements for psychological and social work services on a regular and conveniently available basis

* Physician–Term used to describe an individual with an M.D. or D.O. degree who is fully licensed to practice medicine in all its phases.

‡ The completed records in general shall contain at least the following: the patient's identifying data and consent forms, medical history, record of physical examination, physicians' progress notes, operative notes, nurses' notes, routine x-ray and laboratory reports, doctors' orders, and final diagnosis.

- arrangements for educational and vocational services on a regular and conveniently available basis
- written arrangements with a general hospital for the transfer of patients who require medical, obstetrical, or surgical services not available in the institution.

Psychiatric

The primary function of the institution is to provide diagnostic and treatment services for patients who have psychiatric-related illnesses. A psychiatric hospital also shall provide:

- arrangements for clinical laboratory service, as required, on a regular and conveniently available basis
- arrangements for diagnostic x-ray services, as required on a regular and conveniently available basis
- psychiatric, psychological, and social work service with facilities and staff in the institution
- arrangements for electroencephalograph services, as required, on a regular and conveniently available basis.
- written arrangements with a general hospital for the transfer of patients who require medical, obstetrical, or surgical services not available in the institution.

The American Hospital Association may, at the sole discretion of the Executive Committee of the Board of Trustees, grant, deny, or withdraw the registration of an institution.

AOHA-Listed Hospitals

The list of osteopathic hospitals includes both members and nonmembers of the American Osteopathic Healthcare Association.

Data Comparability

The economic climate, demographic characteristics, personnel issues, and health care financing and payment policies differ by region, state, and city across the country. *Differences in these factors must be taken into account when using the data.* In addition, the profiles of hospitals across comparison groups vary. For example, states will differ in terms of the number and percentage of hospitals by size, ownership, services provided, types of patients treated, and so forth. *Differences in these variables must also be taken into consideration when doing a comparative analysis.*

Notes on the Survey

The 2003 edition of *Hospital Statistics*™ draws its data from the 2001 AHA Annual Survey of Hospitals. It is the statistical complement to the 2002-2003 edition of the *AHA Guide*®, which contains selected data about individual hospitals.

The AHA Survey was mailed to all hospitals, both AHA-registered and nonregistered, in the U.S. and its associated areas: American Samoa, Guam, the Marshall Islands, Puerto Rico, and the Virgin Island. U.S. government hospitals located outside the U.S. were not included. Overall, the average response rate over the past five years has been approximately 83 percent.

Reporting Period

In completing the survey, hospitals were requested to report data for a full year, in accord with their fiscal year, ending in 2001. The statistical table present data reported or estimated for a 12-month period, except for data on personnel, which represent situations as they existed at the end of the reporting period.

Respondents

Data for Tables 1 and 2 include 5,801 AHA-registered hospitals in the U.S. Data on community hospitals (nonfederal, short-term general and other special hospitals) only are presented in Tables 3-6, and Table 8.

It is important to note that the AHA-registered hospitals included in *Hospital Statistics* are not necessarily identical to those included in *AHA Guide*. The institutions listed in the 2002-2003 edition of *AHA Guide* include all of those institutions registered as of April 2001. Tables 1-6 in *Hospital Statistics* present data for AHA-registered hospitals that were in operation during the 12-month reporting period ending 2001.

Estimates

Estimates were made of data for nonreporting hospitals and for reporting hospitals that submitted incomplete AHA Annual Survey questionnaires. Estimates were not made for beds, bassinets and facilities and services. Data for beds and bassinets of nonreporting hospitals were based on the most recent information from those hospitals. (Note that in all statistical tables, whenever bed-size categories are listed, all eight categories appear, whether or not there are hospitals in every category.)

Missing revenue, expenses, admissions, births, inpatient days, surgical operations, outpatient visits, and full-time-equivalent personnel values are estimates from regression models. For all other variables the estimates were based on ratios such as per bed averages derived from data reported by hospitals similar in size, control, major service provided, length of stay, and geographical characteristics to the hospitals that did not report this information.

Tables 1–2

Table **1**

Historical Trends in Utilization, Personnel, and Finances for Selected Years from 1946 through 2001

Data are for all AHA-registered hospitals in the United States. Data are estimated for nonreporting hospitals with the exception of newborn and outpatient data before 1972. Personnel data exclude residents, interns, and students from 1952 on; personnel data include full-time personnel and full-time equivalents for part-time personnel from 1954 on. As a result of the AHA Annual Survey validation process, the New York state expense data from 1976 were revised after the 1977 edition was published. The revised figures are included below. In order to provide trend data on a consistent basis, the 1970 and 1971 psychiatric and long-term data have been slightly modified. The 1982 FTE figures have updated to provide the most accurate data possible.

									NEWBORNS		FTE PERSONNEL		TOTAL EXPENSES		
CLASSIFICATION	YEAR	HOSPITALS	BEDS (in thousands)	ADMISSIONS (in thousands)	AVERAGE DAILY CENSUS (in thousands)	ADJUSTED AVERAGE DAILY CENSUS (in thousands)	AVERAGE STAY (days)	OUTPATIENT VISITS (in thousands)	Bassinets	Births	Number (in thousands)	Per 100 Adjusted Census	Amount (In Millions of dollars)	Adjusted per Inpatient Stay (dollars)	Adjusted per Inpatient Day (dollars)
Total United States	1946	6,125	1,436	15,675	1,142	—	—	—	85,585	2,135,327	830	—	$1,963	—	—
	1950	6,788	1,456	18,483	1,253	—	—	—	90,101	2,742,780	1,058	—	$3,651	—	—
	1955	6,956	1,604	21,073	1,363	—	—	—	98,823	3,476,753	1,301	—	$5,594	—	—
	1960	6,876	1,658	25,027	1,402	—	—	—	102,764	3,835,735	1,598	—	$8,421	—	—
	1965	7,123	1,704	28,812	1,403	—	—	125,793	101,287	3,565,344	1,952	—	$12,948	—	—
	1970	7,123	1,616	31,759	1,298	—	—	181,370	97,128	3,537,000	2,537	—	$25,556	—	—
	1971	7,097	1,556	32,664	1,237	—	—	199,725	94,344	3,464,513	2,589	—	$28,812	—	—
	1972	7,061	1,550	33,265	1,209	—	—	219,182	92,960	3,231,875	2,671	—	$32,667	—	—
	1973	7,123	1,535	34,352	1,189	—	—	233,555	90,071	3,087,210	2,769	—	$36,290	—	—
	1974	7,174	1,513	35,506	1,167	—	—	250,481	88,269	3,043,386	2,919	—	$41,406	—	—
	1975	7,156	1,466	36,157	1,125	—	—	254,844	86,875	3,091,629	3,023	—	$48,706	—	—
	1976	7,082	1,434	36,776	1,090	—	—	270,951	85,284	3,067,063	3,108	—	$56,005	—	—
	1977	7,099	1,407	37,060	1,066	—	—	263,775	83,193	3,223,699	3,213	—	$63,630	—	—
	1978	7,015	1,381	37,243	1,042	—	—	263,606	80,650	3,250,373	3,280	—	$70,927	—	—
	1979	6,988	1,372	37,802	1,043	—	—	262,009	79,720	3,376,467	3,382	—	$79,796	—	—
	1980	6,965	1,365	38,892	1,060	—	—	262,951	79,842	3,500,043	3,492	—	$91,886	—	—
	1981	6,933	1,362	39,169	1,061	—	—	265,332	78,823	3,558,274	3,661	—	$107,146	—	—
	1982	6,915	1,360	39,095	1,053	—	—	313,667	77,998	3,615,751	3,746	—	$123,219	—	—
	1983	6,888	1,350	38,887	1,028	—	—	273,168	77,837	3,596,146	3,707	—	$136,315	—	—
	1984	6,872	1,339	37,938	970	—	—	276,566	77,845	3,563,106	3,630	—	$144,114	—	—
	1985	6,872	1,318	36,304	910	—	—	282,140	77,202	3,630,961	3,625	—	$153,327	—	—
	1986	6,841	1,290	35,219	883	—	—	294,634	76,002	3,680,178	3,647	—	$165,194	—	—
	1987	6,821	1,267	34,439	873	—	—	310,707	74,770	3,698,294	3,742	—	$178,662	—	—
	1988	6,780	1,248	34,107	863	—	—	336,208	72,568	3,794,369	3,839	—	$196,704	—	—
	1989	6,720	1,226	33,742	853	—	—	352,248	71,491	3,920,384	3,937	—	$214,886	—	—
	1990	6,649	1,213	33,774	844	—	—	368,184	70,539	4,046,704	4,063	—	$234,870	—	—
	1991	6,634	1,202	33,567	827	—	—	387,675	69,464	4,047,504	4,165	—	$258,508	—	—
	1992	6,539	1,178	33,536	807	—	—	417,874	69,052	4,007,179	4,236	—	$282,531	—	—
	1993	6,467	1,163	33,201	783	—	—	435,619	67,911	3,949,788	4,289	—	$301,538	—	—
	1994	6,374	1,128	33,125	745	—	—	453,584	67,311	3,886,667	4,270	—	$310,834	—	—
	1995	6,291	1,081	33,282	710	—	—	483,195	66,256	3,833,132	4,273	—	$320,252	—	—
	1996	6,201	1,062	33,307	685	—	—	505,455	65,138	3,790,678	4,276	—	$330,531	—	—
	1997	6,097	1,035	33,624	673	—	—	520,600	64,649	3,811,522	4,333	—	$342,334	—	—
	1998	6,021	1,013	33,766	662	—	—	545,481	63,485	3,795,212	4,407	—	$355,450	—	—
	1999	5,890	994	34,181	657	—	—	573,461	62,714	3,829,881	4,369	—	$372,933	—	—
	2000	5,810	984	34,891	650	—	—	592,673	61,915	3,940,017	4,454	—	$395,391	—	—
	2001	5,801	987	35,644	658	—	—	612,276	61,527	3,929,733	4,535	—	$426,849	—	—

Table 1 (Continued)

CLASSIFICATION	YEAR	HOSPITALS	BEDS (in thousands)	ADMISSIONS (in thousands)	AVERAGE DAILY CENSUS (in thousands)	ADJUSTED AVERAGE DAILY CENSUS (in thousands)	AVERAGE LENGTH OF STAY (days)	OUTPATIENT VISITS (in thousands)	NEWBORNS		FTE PERSONNEL		EXPENSES		
									Bassinets	Births	Number (in thousands)	Per 100 Adjusted Census	Amount (In Millions of dollars)	Adjusted per Inpatient Stay (dollars)	Adjusted per Inpatient Day (dollars)
Total nonfederal short-term general and other special	1946	4,444	473	13,655	341	—	9.1	—	80,987	2,087,503	505	—	$1,169	—	—
	1950	5,031	505	16,663	372	—	8.1	—	86,019	2,660,982	662	—	$2,120	—	—
	1955	5,237	568	19,100	407	—	7.8	—	93,868	3,304,451	826	—	$3,434	—	—
	1960	5,407	639	22,970	477	—	7.6	—	98,127	3,678,051	1,080	—	$5,617	—	—
	1965	5,736	741	26,463	563	620	7.8	92,631	96,782	3,413,370	1,386	224	$9,147	$316.37	$40.56
	1970	5,859	848	29,252	662	727	8.2	133,545	93,079	3,403,064	1,929	265	$19,560	$604.59	$73.73
	1971	5,865	867	30,142	665	736	8.0	148,423	90,444	3,337,605	1,999	272	$22,400	$667.44	$83.43
	1972	5,843	884	30,777	664	739	7.9	166,983	89,315	3,119,446	2,056	278	$25,549	$747.42	$94.61
	1973	5,891	903	31,761	681	768	7.8	178,939	86,851	2,987,089	2,149	280	$28,496	$793.88	$101.78
	1974	5,977	931	32,943	701	793	7.8	194,838	85,208	2,947,342	2,289	289	$32,751	$883.04	$113.21
	1975	5,979	947	33,519	708	806	7.7	196,311	83,834	2,998,590	2,399	298	$39,110	$1,024.72	$133.08
	1976	5,956	961	34,068	715	816	7.7	207,725	82,307	2,962,305	2,483	304	$45,402	$1,172.25	$152.24
	1977	5,973	974	34,353	717	820	7.6	204,238	80,228	3,117,756	2,581	315	$51,832	$1,316.70	$173.25
	1978	5,935	980	34,575	720	841	7.6	204,461	78,090	3,156,570	2,662	323	$58,348	$1,470.13	$193.81
	1979	5,923	988	35,160	729	841	7.6	203,873	77,277	3,287,157	2,762	328	$66,184	$1,631.16	$215.75
	1980	5,904	992	36,198	748	861	7.6	206,752	77,539	3,408,699	2,879	334	$76,970	$1,844.19	$244.44
	1981	5,879	1,007	36,494	764	876	7.6	206,729	76,567	3,465,683	3,039	347	$90,739	$2,167.70	$283.94
	1982	5,863	1,015	36,429	763	882	7.6	250,888	75,739	3,514,761	3,110	353	$105,094	$2,493.09	$326.68
	1983	5,843	1,021	36,201	750	869	7.6	213,995	75,471	3,490,629	3,102	357	$116,632	$2,775.55	$368.01
	1984	5,814	1,020	35,202	703	824	7.3	216,474	75,587	3,456,467	3,023	367	$123,550	$2,984.00	$409.85
	1985	5,784	1,003	33,501	650	780	7.1	222,773	74,899	3,521,296	3,003	385	$130,700	$3,238.94	$459.57
	1986	5,728	982	32,410	631	774	7.1	234,270	73,688	3,584,530	3,032	392	$140,907	$3,529.60	$499.19
	1987	5,659	961	31,633	624	780	7.2	247,704	72,516	3,602,416	3,120	400	$152,909	$3,848.79	$536.96
	1988	5,579	949	31,480	622	795	7.2	271,436	70,361	3,706,748	3,209	404	$168,941	$4,194.39	$581.08
	1989	5,497	936	31,141	619	805	7.3	287,909	69,436	3,831,051	3,307	411	$185,204	$4,572.23	$630.59
	1990	5,420	929	31,203	620	820	7.3	302,691	68,443	3,958,646	3,423	417	$203,927	$4,929.93	$681.52
	1991	5,370	926	31,084	612	828	7.2	323,202	67,440	3,965,489	3,539	427	$225,230	$5,345.63	$745.37
	1992	5,321	923	31,053	606	832	7.1	349,397	67,095	3,925,024	3,624	436	$248,318	$5,788.52	$815.99
	1993	5,289	921	30,770	593	834	7.0	368,358	66,060	3,870,392	3,681	441	$266,382	$6,120.94	$874.98
	1994	5,256	904	30,739	569	814	6.8	384,880	65,728	3,809,367	3,697	454	$276,148	$6,230.33	$929.65
	1995	5,220	874	30,966	549	811	6.5	415,710	64,742	3,764,756	3,718	458	$286,073	$6,220.54	$966.79
	1996	5,160	864	31,116	531	800	6.2	440,845	63,646	3,723,907	3,728	466	$293,920	$6,225.95	$1,005.45
	1997	5,082	855	31,595	529	813	6.1	450,907	63,247	3,742,240	3,794	467	$306,088	$6,266.24	$1,031.68
	1998	5,039	842	31,830	527	821	6.0	474,366	62,162	3,726,234	3,835	467	$319,035	$6,387.53	$1,064.93
	1999	4,977	831	32,377	527	835	5.9	495,850	61,534	3,760,295	3,840	460	$335,405	$6,512.44	$1,101.47
	2000	4,934	825	33,102	527	850	5.8	522,970	60,845	3,880,166	3,916	461	$356,757	$6,650.68	$1,147.99
	2001	4,927	828	33,834	534	866	5.8	539,316	60,454	3,873,395	3,990	461	$383,911	$6,979.29	$1,216.04

Table 1 (Continued)

CLASSIFICATION	YEAR	HOSPITALS	BEDS (in thousands)	ADMISSIONS (in thousands)	AVERAGE DAILY CENSUS (in thousands)	ADJUSTED AVERAGE DAILY CENSUS (in thousands)	AVERAGE LENGTH OF STAY (days)	OUTPATIENT VISITS (in thousands)	NEWBORNS		FTE PERSONNEL		EXPENSES		
									Bassinets	Births	Number (in thousands)	Per 100 Adjusted Census	Amount (In Millions of dollars)	Adjusted per Inpatient Stay (dollars)	Adjusted per Inpatient Day (dollars)
Total community hospitals	1975	5,875	942	33,435	706	798	7.7	190,672	83,829	2,998,552	2,392	300	$38,962	$1,030.34	$133.81
	1976	5,857	956	33,979	713	810	7.7	201,247	82,296	2,962,216	2,475	306	$45,240	$1,176.25	$152.76
	1979	5,842	984	35,099	727	833	7.6	198,778	77,266	3,287,012	2,756	331	$66,004	$1,641.67	$217.34
	1980	5,830	988	36,143	747	857	7.6	202,310	77,522	3,408,482	2,873	335	$76,851	$1,851.04	$245.12
	1981	5,813	1,003	36,438	763	873	7.6	202,768	76,561	3,465,401	3,033	347	$90,572	$2,171.20	$284.33
	1982	5,801	1,012	36,379	762	878	7.6	248,124	75,733	3,514,457	3,103	353	$104,876	$2,500.52	$327.37
	1983	5,783	1,018	36,152	749	864	7.6	210,044	75,465	3,490,254	3,096	358	$116,438	$2,789.18	$369.49
	1984	5,759	1,017	35,155	702	820	7.3	211,961	75,581	3,456,308	3,017	368	$123,336	$2,995.38	$411.10
	1985	5,732	1,001	33,449	649	777	7.1	218,716	74,893	3,521,135	2,997	386	$130,499	$3,244.74	$460.19
	1986	5,678	978	32,379	629	770	7.1	231,912	73,682	3,584,408	3,025	393	$140,654	$3,532.51	$500.81
	1987	5,611	958	31,601	622	776	7.2	245,524	72,510	3,602,296	3,114	401	$152,585	$3,850.16	$538.96
	1988	5,533	947	31,453	620	787	7.2	269,129	70,325	3,706,402	3,205	407	$168,722	$4,206.73	$586.33
	1989	5,455	933	31,116	618	796	7.2	285,712	69,405	3,830,615	3,303	415	$184,898	$4,587.87	$636.96
	1990	5,384	927	31,181	619	813	7.2	301,329	68,412	3,958,263	3,420	421	$203,693	$4,946.68	$686.83
	1991	5,342	924	31,064	611	820	7.2	322,048	67,434	3,965,396	3,535	431	$225,023	$5,359.56	$752.10
	1992	5,292	921	31,034	604	827	7.1	348,522	67,089	3,924,944	3,620	437	$248,095	$5,794.43	$819.83
	1993	5,261	919	30,748	592	828	7.0	366,885	66,054	3,870,376	3,677	444	$266,089	$6,132.06	$880.52
	1994	5,229	902	30,718	568	812	6.7	382,924	65,722	3,809,367	3,692	455	$275,779	$6,229.83	$930.71
	1995	5,194	873	30,945	548	809	6.5	414,345	64,736	3,764,698	3,714	459	$285,588	$6,215.51	$967.69
	1996	5,134	862	31,099	531	799	6.2	439,863	63,640	3,723,871	3,725	466	$293,755	$6,224.94	$1,006.14
	1997	5,057	853	31,577	528	811	6.1	450,140	63,241	3,742,191	3,790	467	$305,763	$6,261.93	$1,032.70
	1998	5,015	840	31,812	525	819	6.0	474,193	62,156	3,726,233	3,831	468	$318,834	$6,385.99	$1,066.96
	1999	4,956	830	32,359	526	833	5.9	495,346	61,528	3,760,295	3,838	461	$335,246	$6,511.72	$1,102.61
	2000	4,915	824	33,089	526	849	5.8	521,404	60,839	3,880,166	3,911	461	$356,564	$6,648.82	$1,149.40
	2001	4,908	826	33,814	533	865	5.7	538,480	60,448	3,873,395	3,987	461	$383,735	$6,979.53	$1,217.27
Nongovernment not-for-profit community hospitals	1975	3,339	658	23,722	510	574	7.8	131,435	57,496	2,131,057	1,712	298	$27,938	$1,040.21	$133.36
	1976	3,345	670	24,082	517	586	7.9	140,914	56,442	2,100,917	1,791	306	$32,764	$1,208.23	$152.94
	1979	3,330	690	24,874	528	603	7.7	139,565	52,859	2,308,548	1,999	332	$47,937	$1,684.40	$218.06
	1980	3,322	692	25,566	542	621	7.7	142,156	52,659	2,389,478	2,086	336	$55,780	$1,901.64	$245.74
	1981	3,340	706	25,945	555	636	7.8	143,380	52,302	2,455,033	2,213	399	$66,267	$2,225.17	$285.64
	1982	3,338	712	25,898	553	637	7.8	176,245	51,566	2,483,345	2,265	355	$76,806	$2,572.93	$330.41
	1983	3,347	718	25,827	544	629	7.7	150,839	51,649	2,465,604	2,270	362	$85,637	$2,868.80	$373.78
	1984	3,351	716	25,236	512	598	7.4	153,281	51,491	2,446,540	2,222	372	$90,814	$3,072.51	$415.04
	1985	3,349	707	24,179	476	569	7.2	158,953	51,424	2,507,288	2,216	389	$96,150	$3,307.41	$462.69
	1986	3,323	689	23,483	460	563	7.2	167,633	50,885	2,547,170	2,241	398	$103,524	$3,589.64	$503.64
	1987	3,274	673	22,937	455	566	7.2	177,413	50,133	2,557,294	2,298	406	$112,325	$3,914.23	$543.67
	1988	3,242	668	22,939	456	577	7.3	195,363	48,828	2,653,794	2,373	412	$124,703	$4,272.95	$591.13
	1989	3,220	661	22,792	455	584	7.3	209,191	48,305	2,751,426	2,454	420	$136,889	$4,649.22	$642.45
	1990	3,191	657	22,878	455	596	7.3	221,073	47,441	2,833,204	2,533	424	$150,673	$5,001.24	$692.36
	1991	3,175	656	22,964	451	603	7.2	238,204	47,229	2,845,995	2,624	435	$166,806	$5,393.30	$758.21
	1992	3,173	656	23,056	445	606	7.1	257,887	47,185	2,846,386	2,692	443	$183,793	$5,808.80	$828.44
	1993	3,154	651	22,749	432	602	6.9	270,138	46,214	2,802,164	2,711	451	$197,187	$6,177.69	$897.70
	1994	3,139	637	22,704	413	589	6.6	282,653	46,381	2,792,116	2,719	462	$204,219	$6,256.72	$950.31
	1995	3,092	610	22,557	393	578	6.4	303,851	45,198	2,725,641	2,702	468	$209,614	$6,279.17	$994.39
	1996	3,045	598	22,542	379	567	6.1	320,746	44,650	2,683,750	2,711	478	$215,950	$6,344.05	$1,042.04
	1997	3,000	591	22,905	376	575	6.0	330,215	44,484	2,698,086	2,765	481	$225,287	$6,392.74	$1,074.26
	1998	3,026	588	23,282	377	587	5.9	352,114	44,087	2,715,958	2,834	483	$237,978	$6,525.68	$1,110.50
	1999	3,012	587	23,871	381	605	5.8	370,784	44,172	2,746,453	2,862	473	$251,534	$6,607.51	$1,139.89
	2000	3,003	583	24,452	382	618	5.7	393,168	43,655	2,833,615	2,919	472	$267,051	$6,717.48	$1,182.32
	2001	2,998	585	24,983	385	628	5.6	404,901	43,640	2,829,691	2,971	473	$287,250	$7,051.76	$1,255.25

Table 1 (Continued)

CLASSIFICATION	YEAR	HOSPITALS	BEDS (in thousands)	ADMISSIONS (in thousands)	AVERAGE DAILY CENSUS (in thousands)	ADJUSTED AVERAGE DAILY CENSUS (in thousands)	AVERAGE LENGTH OF STAY (days)	OUTPATIENT VISITS (in thousands)	NEWBORNS		FTE PERSONNEL		EXPENSES		
									Bassinets	Births	Number (in thousands)	Per 100 Adjusted Census	Amount (In Millions of dollars)	Adjusted per Inpatient Stay (dollars)	Adjusted per Inpatient Day (dollars)
Investor-owned (for-profit) community hospitals	1975	775	73	2,646	48	53	6.6	7,713	4,062	141,392	139	263	$2,561	$876.48	$132.80
	1976	732	76	2,734	50	54	6.6	8,048	4,044	144,751	147	272	$3,085	$1,031.91	$156.35
	1979	727	83	2,963	53	59	6.6	9,289	4,110	174,843	174	300	$4,820	$1,476.42	$225.87
	1980	730	87	3,165	57	62	6.5	9,696	4,439	199,722	189	304	$5,847	$1,675.85	$257.12
	1981	729	88	3,239	58	63	6.5	9,961	4,523	207,405	203	322	$6,856	$1,952.56	$299.02
	1982	748	91	3,316	60	66	6.6	13,193	4,736	219,675	212	320	$8,177	$2,224.75	$340.03
	1983	757	94	3,299	59	66	6.5	10,389	5,039	228,883	213	323	$9,208	$2,517.53	$385.42
	1984	786	100	3,314	57	64	6.3	11,090	5,807	242,088	214	335	$10,251	$2,748.51	$438.30
	1985	805	104	3,242	54	63	6.1	12,378	6,117	266,839	221	350	$11,486	$3,033.06	$500.48
	1986	834	107	3,231	54	65	6.1	14,896	6,305	291,112	229	354	$12,987	$3,341.79	$552.40
	1987	828	106	3,157	54	66	6.2	16,566	6,391	306,492	242	367	$14,067	$3,617.19	$585.01
	1988	790	104	3,090	53	66	6.2	17,926	6,254	308,828	249	379	$15,545	$4,022.77	$649.33
	1989	769	102	3,071	53	67	6.3	19,341	6,354	325,711	261	390	$17,240	$4,406.20	$707.90
	1990	749	101	3,066	54	69	6.4	20,110	6,261	340,555	273	396	$18,822	$4,727.27	$751.55
	1991	738	100	3,016	52	69	6.3	21,174	6,358	359,115	281	409	$20,516	$5,133.53	$820.19
	1992	723	99	2,969	51	69	6.3	22,900	6,519	357,776	285	412	$22,496	$5,548.24	$888.73
	1993	717	99	2,946	51	69	6.2	24,936	6,395	363,358	289	417	$23,077	$5,643.21	$914.39
	1994	719	101	3,035	50	70	6.1	26,443	6,329	354,477	302	434	$23,445	$5,528.91	$923.90
	1995	752	106	3,428	55	77	5.8	31,940	7,164	408,339	343	443	$26,653	$5,425.20	$946.99
	1996	759	109	3,684	56	82	5.6	37,347	7,441	444,697	359	437	$28,385	$5,207.44	$945.49
	1997	797	115	3,953	60	89	5.5	40,919	8,026	465,919	385	433	$31,179	$5,218.69	$961.96
	1998	771	113	3,971	60	90	5.5	42,072	7,895	466,025	383	425	$31,732	$5,262.44	$968.00
	1999	747	107	3,905	58	86	5.5	39,896	7,486	467,585	362	422	$31,179	$5,350.07	$999.03
	2000	749	110	4,141	61	90	5.4	43,378	7,792	503,497	378	418	$34,969	$5,642.18	$1,057.32
	2001	754	109	4,197	63	92	5.4	44,706	7,413	494,669	379	413	$37,348	$5,971.81	$1,121.31
State and local government community hospitals	1975	1,761	210	7,067	148	171	7.6	51,525	22,271	726,103	540	316	$8,463	$1,030.86	$135.64
	1976	1,760	210	7,163	146	170	7.5	52,286	21,810	716,548	537	315	$9,391	$1,132.50	$151.00
	1979	1,785	211	7,262	146	171	7.4	49,924	20,297	803,621	583	341	$13,247	$1,561.04	$211.89
	1980	1,778	209	7,413	149	174	7.3	50,459	20,424	819,282	598	343	$15,204	$1,750.13	$238.63
	1981	1,744	210	7,255	150	174	7.6	49,427	19,736	802,963	618	354	$17,449	$2,071.57	$274.25
	1982	1,7[illegible]5	210	7,165	149	175	7.6	58,685	19,431	811,437	627	320	$19,893	$2,364.09	$311.56
	1983	1,679	207	7,025	145	170	7.6	48,816	18,777	795,767	613	360	$21,593	$2,621.28	$347.56
	1984	1,622	201	6,606	133	158	7.3	47,590	18,283	767,680	581	368	$22,271	$2,823.13	$385.17
	1985	1,578	189	6,028	119	145	7.2	47,386	17,352	747,008	561	387	$22,863	$3,106.14	$432.84
	1986	1,521	182	5,665	114	142	7.4	49,383	16,492	746,126	555	391	$24,143	$3,404.69	$466.17
	1987	1,509	180	5,507	113	144	7.5	51,544	15,986	738,510	573	399	$26,192	$3,717.77	$499.33
	1988	1,501	175	5,424	112	145	7.6	55,840	15,243	743,780	583	403	$28,474	$4,033.67	$538.63
	1989	1,466	170	5,253	110	145	7.7	57,179	14,746	753,478	589	406	$30,769	$4,430.12	$582.15
	1990	1,444	169	5,236	111	148	7.7	60,146	14,710	784,504	614	415	$34,198	$4,837.76	$634.45
	1991	1,429	168	5,084	108	148	7.8	62,670	13,847	760,286	630	424	$37,701	$5,339.75	$695.89
	1992	1,396	166	5,008	108	152	7.9	67,734	13,385	720,782	643	424	$41,806	$5,870.76	$753.92
	1993	1,390	169	5,054	109	157	7.8	71,811	13,445	704,854	676	430	$45,825	$6,205.52	$799.73
	1994	1,371	164	4,979	104	154	7.6	73,828	13,012	662,774	672	438	$48,115	$6,513.39	$858.62
	1995	1,350	157	4,961	100	154	7.4	78,554	12,374	630,718	670	435	$49,322	$6,445.18	$877.85
	1996	1,330	155	4,873	96	150	7.2	81,770	11,549	595,424	654	437	$49,420	$6,418.65	$903.41
	1997	1,260	148	4,720	92	148	7.1	79,007	10,731	578,186	640	433	$49,298	$6,475.07	$913.62
	1998	1,218	139	4,559	87	142	7.0	80,008	10,174	544,250	614	433	$49,123	$6,612.23	$949.36
	1999	1,197	136	4,583	86	143	6.9	84,667	9,870	546,257	614	430	$52,534	$6,923.35	$1,006.91
	2000	1,163	131	4,496	83	140	6.7	84,858	9,392	543,054	614	438	$54,544	$7,106.05	$1,063.75
	2001	1,156	132	4,634	85	145	6.7	88,873	9,395	549,035	637	438	$59,137	$7,400.01	$1,113.79

Table
2

2001 U.S. Registered Hospitals: Utilization, Personnel, and Finances

Excludes U.S.-Associated Areas, Puerto Rico, and nonregistered hospitals.

CLASSIFICATION	HOSPITALS	BEDS	ADMISSIONS	INPATIENT DAYS	ADJUSTED PATIENT DAYS	AVERAGE DAILY CENSUS	ADJUSTED AVERAGE DAILY CENSUS	AVERAGE STAY (days)	SURGICAL OPERATIONS	OUTPATIENT VISITS		NEWBORNS	
										Emergency	Total	Bassinets	Births
UNITED STATES	5,801	987,440	35,644,440	240,012,878	—	658,410	—	—	27,210,829	109,838,319	612,276,444	61,527	3,929,733
6-24 Beds	332	5,830	160,247	723,593	—	1,989	—	—	155,819	1,040,908	7,333,037	523	12,482
25-49	1,033	37,401	1,110,142	6,047,975	—	16,590	—	—	981,066	5,873,074	32,642,614	2,877	92,470
50-99	1,352	97,251	2,841,815	20,621,213	—	56,825	—	—	2,234,449	12,061,365	65,539,544	6,713	284,846
100-199	1,420	202,392	7,231,132	46,440,604	—	127,371	—	—	5,983,595	26,358,001	130,016,858	14,320	813,736
200-299	725	176,137	6,879,694	43,401,974	—	118,904	—	—	5,296,582	20,795,431	110,199,850	12,192	742,280
300-399	398	137,097	5,488,426	34,063,032	—	93,557	—	—	4,053,604	15,662,351	81,148,256	8,734	636,156
400-499	220	97,750	3,859,488	25,338,036	—	69,422	—	—	2,809,689	9,399,876	64,328,563	5,544	462,372
500 or more	321	233,582	8,073,496	63,376,451	—	173,752	—	—	5,696,025	18,647,313	121,067,722	10,624	885,391
Psychiatric	503	93,366	767,453	28,216,713	—	77,252	—	—	12,410	161,581	8,719,455	0	0
Hospitals	491	87,034	767,080	26,527,818	—	72,624	—	—	12,410	161,581	8,718,941	0	0
Institutions for mentally retarded	12	6,332	373	1,688,895	—	4,628	—	—	0	0	514	0	0
General	4,880	849,168	34,183,200	199,666,906	—	547,904	—	—	26,764,644	108,901,784	588,086,712	60,898	3,884,753
Hospitals	4,858	846,608	34,161,773	199,046,675	—	546,205	—	—	26,752,624	108,837,823	587,043,190	60,892	3,884,753
Hospital units of institutions	22	2,560	21,427	620,231	—	1,699	—	—	12,020	63,961	1,043,522	6	0
TB and other respiratory diseases	4	259	836	46,302	—	126	—	—	0	0	2,892	6	0
Obstetrics and gynecology	11	1,481	74,681	328,496	—	900	—	—	51,577	104,308	782,379	434	38,601
Eye, ear, nose and throat	8	282	6,707	19,295	—	53	—	—	65,481	28,851	499,703	17	815
Rehabilitation	180	15,325	235,957	4,195,752	—	11,505	—	—	7,609	9,644	6,176,698	11	247
Orthopedic	24	1,462	47,791	257,779	—	707	—	—	78,387	69,578	637,626	0	0
Chronic Disease	20	7,291	22,981	2,242,105	—	6,142	—	—	3,879	24,469	343,827	0	0
All other	171	18,806	304,834	5,039,530	—	13,821	—	—	226,842	538,104	7,027,152	161	5,317
Federal	243	51,900	1,000,882	13,229,616	—	36,248	—	—	710,568	3,595,973	64,034,584	1,046	56,209
Psychiatric	12	4,604	25,579	1,449,289	—	3,971	—	—	3,199	0	1,347,988	0	0
General and other special	231	47,296	975,303	11,780,327	—	32,277	—	—	707,369	3,595,973	62,686,596	1,046	56,209
Nonfederal	5,558	935,540	34,643,558	226,783,262	—	622,162	—	—	26,500,261	106,242,346	548,241,860	60,481	3,873,524
Psychiatric	491	88,762	741,874	26,767,424	—	73,281	—	—	9,211	161,581	7,371,467	0	0
Hospitals	479	82,430	741,501	25,078,529	—	68,653	—	—	9,211	161,581	7,370,953	0	0
Institutions for mentally retarded	12	6,332	373	1,688,895	—	4,628	—	—	0	0	514	0	0
TB and other respiratory diseases	4	259	836	46,302	—	126	—	—	0	0	2,892	6	0
Long-term general and other special	136	18,750	67,020	5,415,144	—	14,850	—	—	15,717	81,861	1,551,272	21	129
Short-term general and other special	4,927	827,769	33,833,828	194,554,392	—	533,905	—	—	26,475,333	105,998,904	539,316,229	60,454	3,873,395
Hospital units of institutions	19	1,803	20,239	448,076	—	1,227	—	—	11,024	41,126	835,851	6	0
Community Hospitals	4,908	825,966	33,813,589	194,106,316	315,240,946	532,678	865,053	5.7	26,464,309	105,957,778	538,480,378	60,448	3,873,395
6-24 Beds	281	4,964	140,467	566,345	1,581,530	1,556	4,351	4.0	144,438	796,297	4,555,782	423	9,300
25-49	916	33,263	1,030,375	5,159,467	12,542,601	14,147	34,401	5.0	953,232	5,346,064	27,940,635	2,712	87,770
50-99	1,070	76,924	2,421,938	15,461,340	30,578,198	42,692	84,355	6.4	2,074,128	11,093,357	51,331,347	6,278	262,605
100-199	1,218	174,024	6,777,542	38,508,731	68,152,415	105,684	187,000	5.7	5,804,978	25,605,993	114,920,517	14,093	804,377
200-299	635	154,420	6,630,307	36,923,111	58,704,111	101,154	160,833	5.6	5,175,944	20,309,391	99,596,191	12,081	733,456
300-399	348	119,753	5,328,441	28,949,110	44,119,663	79,549	121,171	5.4	3,973,661	15,412,370	75,242,019	8,693	628,124
400-499	191	84,745	3,778,746	21,312,743	31,727,186	58,393	86,921	5.6	2,786,509	9,345,972	59,579,645	5,544	462,372
500 or more	249	177,873	7,705,773	47,225,469	67,835,242	129,503	186,021	6.1	5,551,419	18,048,334	105,314,242	10,624	885,391
Nongovernment not-for-profit	2,998	585,070	24,982,640	140,395,071	228,838,770	385,155	627,711	5.6	19,883,427	76,001,295	404,901,061	43,640	2,829,691
Investor-owned (for profit)	754	108,718	4,196,744	22,785,445	33,307,292	62,801	91,856	5.4	3,300,521	12,681,022	44,706,095	7,413	494,669
State and Local Government	1,156	132,178	4,634,205	30,925,800	53,094,884	84,722	145,486	6.7	3,280,361	17,275,461	88,873,222	9,395	549,035

Table 2 (Continued)

CLASSIFICATION	FULL-TIME EQUIVALENT PERSONNEL					FULL-TIME EQUIVALENT TRAINEES			EXPENSES: LABOR				EXPENSES: TOTAL		
	Physicians and Dentists	Registered Nurses	Licensed Practical Nurses	Other Salaried Personnel	Total Personnel	Medical and Dental Residents	Other Trainees	Total Trainees	Payroll (in thousands)	Employee Benefits (in thousands)	Total (in thousands)	Percent of Total	Amount (in thousands)	Adjusted per Admission	Adjusted per Inpatient Day
UNITED STATES	97,501	1,045,501	153,800	3,238,260	4,535,062	87,548	10,022	97,570	$184,041,395	$40,167,271	$224,208,666	52.5	$426,849,488	—	—
6-24 Beds	978	5,899	2,084	23,034	31,995	9	256	265	$980,120	$191,132	$1,171,252	52.3	$2,239,905	—	—
25-49	3,958	32,179	9,862	119,735	165,734	255	128	383	$5,513,985	$1,155,482	$6,669,466	52.4	$12,732,145	—	—
50-99	7,317	77,491	20,036	281,266	386,110	1,548	1,388	2,936	$13,433,778	$3,023,650	$16,457,428	54.5	$30,215,880	—	—
100-199	15,932	194,271	34,609	614,313	859,125	6,292	785	7,077	$33,003,274	$7,195,702	$40,198,976	53.6	$75,050,932	—	—
200-299	14,209	190,320	26,520	567,196	798,245	8,203	1,838	10,041	$32,732,881	$7,092,654	$39,825,535	52.6	$75,779,724	—	—
300-399	14,951	160,109	19,833	469,876	664,769	10,911	1,092	12,003	$26,724,948	$5,902,255	$32,627,203	51.5	$63,327,624	—	—
400-499	8,852	117,584	12,796	347,490	486,722	14,535	1,836	16,371	$21,120,911	$4,765,475	$25,886,386	52.0	$49,783,280	—	—
500 or more	31,304	267,648	28,060	815,350	1,142,362	45,795	2,699	48,494	$50,531,498	$10,840,922	$61,372,420	52.1	$117,719,996	—	—
Psychiatric	5,591	28,709	10,002	168,450	212,752	514	805	1,319	$7,588,823	$2,021,129	$9,609,952	72.7	$13,224,892	—	—
Hospitals	5,492	28,383	9,631	155,926	199,432	514	802	1,316	$7,127,995	$1,902,693	$9,030,688	72.1	$12,518,757	—	—
Institutions for mentally retarded	99	326	371	12,524	13,320	0	3	3	$460,828	$118,436	$579,264	82.0	$706,135	—	—
General	86,420	985,126	136,874	2,938,520	4,146,940	85,336	8,063	93,399	$169,507,636	$36,571,169	$206,078,805	51.8	$397,702,070	—	—
Hospitals	86,208	984,467	136,426	2,935,406	4,142,507	85,330	8,040	93,370	$169,361,597	$36,537,102	$205,898,699	51.8	$397,399,280	—	—
Hospital units of institutions	212	659	448	3,114	4,433	6	23	29	$146,039	$34,067	$180,106	59.5	$302,790	—	—
TB and other respiratory diseases	0	135	77	542	754	0	0	0	$20,924	$6,319	$27,244	60.4	$45,121	—	—
Obstetrics and gynecology	131	1,914	173	6,114	8,332	41	2	43	$368,709	$71,009	$439,718	55.0	$800,050	—	—
Eye, ear, nose and throat	124	451	42	1,903	2,520	99	29	128	$89,360	$17,699	$107,058	42.1	$254,459	—	—
Rehabilitation	625	9,264	2,555	42,818	55,262	160	54	214	$1,930,806	$380,137	$2,310,943	57.0	$4,053,424	—	—
Orthopedic	387	1,685	233	6,072	8,377	67	4	71	$369,999	$79,625	$449,625	49.5	$909,182	—	—
Chronic Disease	235	1,645	933	9,571	12,384	15	17	32	$527,569	$163,595	$691,164	71.9	$961,926	—	—
All other	3,988	16,572	2,911	64,270	87,741	1,316	1,048	2,364	$3,637,569	$856,589	$4,494,158	50.5	$8,898,364	—	—
Federal	21,199	53,733	15,215	209,325	299,472	9,226	3,207	12,433	$13,234,724	$3,148,971	$16,383,695	59.6	$27,471,316	—	—
Psychiatric	460	1,817	846	8,309	11,432	26	32	58	$589,348	$140,511	$729,859	68.6	$1,064,412	—	—
General and other special	20,739	51,916	14,369	201,016	288,040	9,200	3,175	12,375	$12,645,376	$3,008,460	$15,653,836	59.3	$26,406,903	—	—
Nonfederal	76,302	991,768	138,585	3,028,935	4,235,590	78,322	6,815	85,137	$170,806,671	$37,018,300	$207,824,971	52.0	$399,378,172	—	—
Psychiatric	5,131	26,892	9,156	160,141	201,320	488	773	1,261	$6,999,475	$1,880,618	$8,880,093	73.0	$12,160,480	—	—
Hospitals	5,032	26,566	8,785	147,617	188,000	488	770	1,258	$6,538,647	$1,762,182	$8,300,829	72.5	$11,454,345	—	—
Institutions for mentally retarded	99	326	371	12,524	13,320	0	3	3	$460,828	$118,436	$579,264	82.0	$706,135	—	—
TB and other respiratory diseases	0	135	77	542	754	0	0	0	$20,924	$6,319	$27,244	60.4	$45,121	—	—
Long-term general and other special	693	6,165	2,702	34,222	43,782	97	282	379	$1,701,436	$416,431	$2,117,867	64.9	$3,261,956	—	—
Short-term general and other special	70,478	958,576	126,650	2,834,030	3,989,734	77,737	5,760	83,497	$162,084,836	$34,714,932	$196,799,768	51.3	$383,910,615	—	—
Hospital units of institutions	154	550	398	1,358	2,460	6	0	6	$74,429	$17,694	$92,123	52.4	$175,858	—	—
Community Hospitals	70,324	958,026	126,252	2,832,672	3,987,274	77,731	5,760	83,491	$162,010,407	$34,697,237	$196,707,644	51.3	$383,734,757	$6,979.53	$1,217.27
6-24 Beds	395	4,733	1,808	16,582	23,518	5	35	40	$701,733	$147,651	$849,384	52.6	$1,613,937	$3,825.80	$1,020.49
25-49	2,890	28,862	8,959	105,835	146,546	178	73	251	$4,906,879	$1,023,111	$5,929,990	52.1	$11,381,539	$4,556.94	$907.43
50-99	3,232	63,945	15,830	215,028	298,035	280	842	1,122	$10,502,329	$2,338,478	$12,840,807	53.4	$24,030,936	$4,942.68	$785.88
100-199	10,477	175,131	29,298	529,372	744,278	3,713	347	4,060	$28,525,557	$6,131,884	$34,657,441	52.2	$66,360,396	$5,594.82	$973.71
200-299	9,294	176,754	22,414	509,045	717,507	5,869	407	6,276	$29,262,107	$6,230,093	$35,492,200	51.5	$68,913,526	$6,589.73	$1,173.91
300-399	12,037	151,530	17,106	429,196	609,869	9,973	581	10,554	$24,570,829	$5,280,490	$29,851,320	50.6	$59,027,238	$7,239.62	$1,337.89
400-499	7,366	112,335	11,007	321,739	452,447	14,256	1,722	15,978	$19,723,289	$4,359,752	$24,083,041	50.9	$47,321,476	$8,435.45	$1,491.51
500 or more	24,633	244,736	19,830	705,875	995,074	43,457	1,753	45,210	$43,817,683	$9,185,778	$53,003,462	50.4	$105,085,709	$9,453.00	$1,549.13
Nongovernment not-for-profit	57,579	710,857	80,778	2,122,203	2,971,417	57,083	4,244	61,327	$122,561,924	$25,937,671	$148,499,596	51.7	$287,250,461	$7,051.76	$1,255.25
Investor-owned (for profit)	1,799	101,755	19,370	256,350	379,274	885	92	977	$14,589,751	$2,901,377	$17,491,128	46.8	$37,347,701	$5,971.81	$1,121.31
State and Local Government	10,946	145,414	26,104	454,119	636,583	19,763	1,424	21,187	$24,858,732	$5,858,189	$30,716,921	51.9	$59,136,596	$7,400.01	$1,113.79

Tables 3–6

TABLE 3

TOTAL UNITED STATES

U.S. Registered Community Hospitals
(Nonfederal, short-term general and other special hospitals)

Overview 1997–2001

	2001	2000	1999	1998	1997
TOTAL U.S. Community Hospitals	**4,908**	**4,915**	**4,956**	**5,015**	**5,057**
Bed Size Category					
6-24	281	288	299	293	281
25-49	916	910	887	900	890
50-99	1,070	1,055	1,082	1,085	1,111
100-199	1,218	1,236	1,266	1,304	1,289
200-299	635	656	642	644	679
300-399	348	341	365	352	367
400-499	191	182	161	183	185
500 +	249	247	254	254	255
Location					
Hospitals Urban	2,741	2,740	2,767	2,816	2,852
Hospitals Rural	2,167	2,175	2,189	2,199	2,205
Control					
State and Local Government	1,156	1,163	1,197	1,218	1,260
Not for Profit	2,998	3,003	3,012	3,026	3,000
Investor owned	754	749	747	771	797
Physician Models					
Independent Practice Association	824	831	874	966	1,056
Group Practice without Walls	250	211	198	232	285
Open Physician-Hospital Organization	849	939	975	1,055	1,077
Closed Physician-Hospital Organization	316	360	414	451	485
Management Service Organization	545	655	770	866	964
Integrated Salary Model	1,122	1,126	1,106	1,039	1,016
Equity Model	58	91	103	121	125
Foundation	212	252	290	349	416
Insurance Products					
Health Maintenance Organization	715	870	1,009	1,099	1,166
Preferred Provider Organization	873	1,028	1,156	1,303	1,543
Indemnity Fee for Service	247	286	303	387	493
Managed Care Contracts					
Health Maintenance Organization	2,738	2,804	2,916	2,933	3,095
Preferred Provider Organization	3,217	3,233	3,310	3,291	3,534
Affiliations					
Hospitals in a System	2,260	2,217	2,238	2,176	2,226
Hospitals in a Network	1,341	1,327	1,310	1,380	1,492
Hospitals in a Group Purchasing Organization	3,495	3,344	3,080	2,778	—

TABLE 3

TOTAL UNITED STATES

U.S. Registered Community Hospitals
(Nonfederal, short-term general and other special hospitals)

Utilization, Personnel, Revenue and Expenses, Community Health Indicators 1997–2001

	2001	2000	1999	1998	1997
TOTAL FACILITY (Includes Hospital and Nursing Home Units)					
Utilization - Inpatient					
Beds	825,966	823,560	829,575	839,988	853,287
Admissions	33,813,589	33,089,467	32,359,042	31,811,673	31,576,960
Inpatient Days	194,106,316	192,420,368	191,884,270	191,430,450	192,504,015
Average Length of Stay	5.7	5.8	5.9	6.0	6.1
Inpatient Surgeries	9,779,583	9,729,336	9,539,593	9,735,705	9,509,081
Births	3,873,395	3,890,166	3,760,295	3,726,233	3,742,191
Utilization - Outpatient					
Emergency Outpatient Visits	105,957,778	103,144,030	99,484,462	94,771,405	92,819,892
Other Outpatient Visits	432,522,600	418,260,946	395,861,824	379,422,063	357,320,118
Total Outpatient Visits	538,480,378	521,404,976	495,346,286	474,193,468	450,140,010
Outpatient Surgeries	16,684,726	16,383,374	15,845,492	15,593,614	14,678,290
Personnel					
Full Time RNs	751,095	745,113	739,086	733,365	708,245
Full Time LPNs	104,534	101,683	106,739	109,882	112,517
Part Time RNs	413,832	424,801	397,950	392,622	385,909
Part Time LPNs	43,446	45,011	45,561	47,191	49,489
Total Full Time	3,428,159	3,332,232	3,297,689	3,294,274	3,248,861
Total Part Time	1,285,207	1,320,696	1,246,661	1,242,121	1,246,592
Revenue - Inpatient					
Gross Inpatient Revenue	$544,088,000,000	$481,754,000,000	$436,803,000,000	$407,650,000,000	$380,625,000,000
Revenue - Outpatient					
Gross Outpatient Revenue	$289,606,000,000	$255,130,000,000	$224,677,000,000	$201,951,000,000	$183,804,000,000
Revenue and Expenses - Totals (Includes Inpatient and Outpatient)					
Total Gross Revenue	$833,693,000,000	$736,884,000,000	$661,440,000,000	$609,602,000,000	$564,429,000,000
Deductions from Revenue	463,168,000,000	394,635,000,000	340,074,000,000	299,969,000,000	263,849,000,000
Net Patient Revenue	370,525,000,000	342,249,000,000	321,366,000,000	309,633,000,000	300,580,000,000
Other Operating Revenue	23,816,314,195	21,691,829,666	20,954,555,617	19,347,513,120	18,063,654,341
Other Nonoperating Revenue	6,353,280,081	9,649,649,680	9,207,219,318	9,322,323,105	8,995,500,053
Total Net Revenue	400,695,000,000	373,590,000,000	351,528,000,000	338,302,000,000	327,639,000,000
Total Expenses	383,735,000,000	356,564,000,000	335,197,000,000	318,834,000,000	305,763,000,000
HOSPITAL UNIT (Excludes Separate Nursing Home Units)					
Utilization - Inpatient					
Beds	753,592	746,918	746,638	758,186	769,505
Admissions	33,408,199	32,639,620	31,814,468	31,265,867	31,047,930
Inpatient Days	171,049,431	168,133,112	165,919,000	165,644,176	165,605,620
Average Length of Stay	5.1	5.2	5.2	5.3	5.3
Personnel					
Total Full Time	3,376,958	3,274,082	3,239,743	3,235,153	3,183,730
Total Part Time	1,259,927	1,291,840	1,218,813	1,213,426	1,214,232
Revenue and Expenses - Totals (Includes Inpatient and Outpatient)					
Total Net Revenue	$396,134,000,000	$368,509,000,000	$346,323,000,000	$333,055,000,000	$322,460,000,000
Total Expenses	380,087,000,000	353,071,000,000	331,218,000,000	314,710,000,000	301,905,000,000
COMMUNITY HEALTH INDICATORS PER 1000 POPULATION					
Total Population (in thousands)	284,797	281,422	272,691	270,248	267,784
Inpatient					
Beds	2.9	2.9	3.0	3.1	3.2
Admissions	118.7	117.6	118.7	117.7	117.9
Inpatient Days	681.6	683.7	703.7	708.4	718.9
Inpatient Surgeries	34.3	34.6	35.0	36.0	35.5
Births	13.6	13.8	13.8	13.8	14.0
Outpatient					
Emergency Outpatient Visits	372.0	366.5	364.8	350.7	346.6
Other Outpatient Visits	1,518.7	1,486.2	1,451.7	1,404.0	1,334.4
Total Outpatient Visits	1,890.8	1,852.8	1,816.5	1,754.7	1,681.0
Outpatient Surgeries	58.6	58.2	58.1	57.7	54.8
Expense per Capita (per person)	$1,347.4	$1,267.0	$1,229.2	$1,179.8	$1,141.8

TABLE 4

BED SIZE CATEGORY 6-24

U.S. Registered Community Hospitals
(Nonfederal, short-term general and other special hospitals)

Overview 1997–2001

	2001	2000	1999	1998	1997
Total U.S. Community Hospitals in Bed Size Category 6-24	**281**	**288**	**299**	**293**	**281**
Location					
Hospitals Urban	56	57	64	59	61
Hospitals Rural	225	231	235	234	220
Control					
State and Local Government	135	143	151	155	155
Not for Profit	122	126	127	123	110
Investor owned	24	19	21	15	16
Physician Models					
Independent Practice Association	38	31	25	26	28
Group Practice without Walls	12	12	9	12	12
Open Physician-Hospital Organization	17	20	21	30	26
Closed Physician-Hospital Organization	9	6	8	9	9
Management Service Organization	14	12	15	19	11
Integrated Salary Model	73	64	65	73	59
Equity Model	3	3	5	4	4
Foundation	9	7	13	16	13
Insurance Products					
Health Maintenance Organization	30	34	30	37	37
Preferred Provider Organization	35	42	40	48	59
Indemnity Fee for Service	11	10	5	12	20
Managed Care Contracts					
Health Maintenance Organization	100	101	120	127	127
Preferred Provider Organization	160	164	175	174	172
Affiliations					
Hospitals in a System	73	72	64	67	59
Hospitals in a Network	79	77	67	66	65
Hospitals in a Group Purchasing Organization	192	178	169	162	—

TABLE 4

BED SIZE CATEGORY 6-24

U.S. Registered Community Hospitals
(Nonfederal, short-term general and other special hospitals)

Utilization, Personnel, Revenue and Expenses 1997–2001

	2001	2000	1999	1998	1997
TOTAL FACILITY (Includes Hospital and Nursing Home Units)					
Utilization - Inpatient					
Beds	4,964	5,156	5,442	5,351	5,128
Admissions	140,467	140,735	145,418	138,676	139,253
Inpatient Days	566,345	601,199	651,124	643,241	659,269
Average Length of Stay	4.0	4.3	4.5	4.6	4.7
Inpatient Surgeries	23,655	21,084	22,445	24,994	24,751
Births	9,300	9,836	11,283	9,835	14,371
Utilization - Outpatient					
Emergency Outpatient Visits	796,297	743,260	676,879	720,202	677,713
Other Outpatient Visits	3,759,485	3,812,179	3,973,601	3,558,219	3,241,926
Total Outpatient Visits	4,555,782	4,555,439	4,650,480	4,278,421	3,919,639
Outpatient Surgeries	120,783	111,263	117,592	96,181	107,114
Personnel					
Full Time RNs	3,684	3,744	3,935	3,748	3,661
Full Time LPNs	1,468	1,363	1,469	1,516	1,547
Part Time RNs	2,069	2,443	2,369	2,182	2,478
Part Time LPNs	669	713	752	678	790
Total Full Time	18,993	18,944	20,593	18,869	19,062
Total Part Time	9,128	10,287	10,026	9,728	10,419
Revenue - Inpatient					
Gross Inpatient Revenue	$865,976,268	$785,583,707	$803,992,451	$785,821,717	$680,688,667
Revenue - Outpatient					
Gross Outpatient Revenue	$1,560,963,930	$1,539,812,867	$1,377,204,771	$1,187,401,957	$1,134,227,463
Revenue and Expenses - Totals (Includes Inpatient and Outpatient)					
Total Gross Revenue	$2,426,940,198	$2,325,396,574	$2,181,197,222	$1,973,223,674	$1,814,916,130
Deductions from Revenue	951,093,256	907,556,076	782,264,529	742,459,310	628,816,197
Net Patient Revenue	1,475,846,942	1,417,840,498	1,398,932,693	1,230,764,364	1,186,099,933
Other Operating Revenue	154,437,602	115,552,533	170,916,578	139,388,003	120,115,952
Other Nonoperating Revenue	33,912,311	38,248,611	87,134,276	43,645,742	30,803,338
Total Net Revenue	1,664,196,855	1,571,641,642	1,656,983,547	1,413,798,109	1,337,019,223
Total Expenses	1,613,936,534	1,549,776,034	1,658,451,372	1,382,369,992	1,273,227,832
HOSPITAL UNIT (Excludes Separate Nursing Home Units)					
Utilization - Inpatient					
Beds	4,864	5,063	5,352	5,246	5,002
Admissions	140,181	140,230	144,893	137,990	138,570
Inpatient Days	528,596	568,533	623,695	611,534	627,519
Average Length of Stay	3.8	4.1	4.3	4.4	4.5
Personnel					
Total Full Time	18,929	18,716	20,537	18,808	18,990
Total Part Time	9,066	10,074	9,985	9,684	10,341
Revenue and Expenses - Totals (Includes Inpatient and Outpatient)					
Total Net Revenue	$1,654,040,740	$1,564,960,209	$1,650,222,760	$1,404,198,000	$1,331,848,408
Total Expenses	1,608,501,142	1,543,940,406	1,653,276,803	1,376,587,586	1,267,605,736

TABLE 4

BED SIZE CATEGORY 25-49

U.S. Registered Community Hospitals
(Nonfederal, short-term general and other special hospitals)

Overview 1997–2001

	2001	2000	1999	1998	1997
Total U.S. Community Hospitals in Bed Size Category 25-49	**916**	**910**	**887**	**900**	**890**
Location					
Hospitals Urban	214	201	192	201	192
Hospitals Rural	702	709	695	699	698
Control					
State and Local Government	374	375	374	391	394
Not for Profit	442	440	423	411	408
Investor owned	100	95	90	98	88
Physician Models					
Independent Practice Association	121	106	114	124	120
Group Practice without Walls	45	29	17	30	27
Open Physician-Hospital Organization	83	102	96	118	103
Closed Physician-Hospital Organization	33	39	40	39	40
Management Service Organization	53	62	64	75	67
Integrated Salary Model	200	183	169	139	130
Equity Model	4	10	9	12	9
Foundation	23	26	31	36	37
Insurance Products					
Health Maintenance Organization	87	89	110	115	122
Preferred Provider Organization	133	143	153	173	211
Indemnity Fee for Service	45	45	48	58	54
Managed Care Contracts					
Health Maintenance Organization	416	406	436	439	436
Preferred Provider Organization	557	561	571	569	590
Affiliations					
Hospitals in a System	275	270	274	248	240
Hospitals in a Network	219	216	208	220	223
Hospitals in a Group Purchasing Organization	639	612	584	532	—

Table 4

BED SIZE CATEGORY 25-49

U.S. Registered Community Hospitals
(Nonfederal, short-term general and other special hospitals)

Utilization, Personnel, Revenue and Expenses 1997–2001

	2001	2000	1999	1998	1997
TOTAL FACILITY (Includes Hospital and Nursing Home Units)					
Utilization - Inpatient					
Beds	33,263	33,333	32,816	33,510	33,138
Admissions	1,030,375	994,641	959,482	964,802	932,506
Inpatient Days	5,159,467	5,031,151	4,957,792	5,034,160	4,877,092
Average Length of Stay	5.0	5.1	5.2	5.2	5.2
Inpatient Surgeries	205,619	206,859	197,717	209,849	194,643
Births	87,770	88,275	84,491	91,733	93,186
Utilization - Outpatient					
Emergency Outpatient Visits	5,346,064	5,195,946	5,055,140	4,945,356	4,650,346
Other Outpatient Visits	22,594,571	21,811,383	18,814,467	17,748,273	17,031,445
Total Outpatient Visits	27,940,635	27,007,329	23,869,607	22,693,629	21,681,791
Outpatient Surgeries	747,613	676,172	610,784	608,488	497,430
Personnel					
Full Time RNs	22,343	22,830	21,305	21,992	21,700
Full Time LPNs	7,400	7,333	6,978	7,214	7,205
Part Time RNs	13,038	14,072	13,333	13,828	12,883
Part Time LPNs	3,132	3,424	3,191	3,112	3,144
Total Full Time	120,976	116,462	110,210	110,258	106,892
Total Part Time	51,639	54,820	50,931	53,108	51,223
Revenue - Inpatient					
Gross Inpatient Revenue	$7,883,987,594	$7,196,766,831	$6,561,005,229	$6,129,218,618	$5,790,871,470
Revenue - Outpatient					
Gross Outpatient Revenue	$10,608,878,116	$9,410,834,420	$7,991,583,099	$7,236,681,368	$6,397,469,679
Revenue and Expenses - Totals (Includes Inpatient and Outpatient)					
Total Gross Revenue	$18,492,865,710	$16,607,601,251	$14,552,588,328	$13,365,899,986	$12,188,341,149
Deductions from Revenue	8,222,555,507	7,231,526,571	6,067,585,675	5,164,085,375	4,439,292,370
Net Patient Revenue	10,270,310,203	9,376,074,680	8,485,002,653	8,201,814,611	7,749,048,779
Other Operating Revenue	1,134,586,636	959,276,038	826,240,928	744,101,510	534,466,535
Other Nonoperating Revenue	212,155,156	312,430,036	217,293,330	222,857,115	252,234,249
Total Net Revenue	11,617,051,995	10,647,780,754	9,528,536,911	9,168,773,236	8,535,749,563
Total Expenses	11,381,539,275	10,391,935,057	9,283,978,476	8,835,814,359	8,088,329,513
HOSPITAL UNIT (Excludes Separate Nursing Home Units)					
Utilization - Inpatient					
Beds	31,189	31,299	30,763	31,513	31,376
Admissions	1,023,053	987,780	952,964	957,140	926,760
Inpatient Days	4,511,675	4,419,903	4,319,613	4,416,725	4,338,307
Average Length of Stay	4.4	4.5	4.5	4.6	4.7
Personnel					
Total Full Time	119,566	115,277	109,069	109,094	105,846
Total Part Time	50,898	54,115	50,264	52,363	50,419
Revenue and Expenses - Totals (Includes Inpatient and Outpatient)					
Total Net Revenue	$11,521,210,710	$10,559,902,580	$9,428,841,798	$9,077,370,329	$8,459,409,142
Total Expenses	11,315,045,682	10,335,837,413	9,223,711,698	8,767,241,151	8,038,426,363

TABLE 4

BED SIZE CATEGORY 50-99

U.S. Registered Community Hospitals
(Nonfederal, short-term general and other special hospitals)

Overview 1997–2001

	2001	2000	1999	1998	1997
Total U.S. Community Hospitals in Bed Size Category 50-99	**1,070**	**1,055**	**1,082**	**1,085**	**1,111**
Location					
Hospitals Urban	407	400	414	419	436
Hospitals Rural	663	655	668	666	675
Control					
State and Local Government	278	279	285	281	298
Not for Profit	593	581	584	606	590
Investor owned	199	195	213	198	223
Physician Models					
Independent Practice Association	155	153	158	168	159
Group Practice without Walls	52	38	36	38	39
Open Physician-Hospital Organization	158	168	177	189	182
Closed Physician-Hospital Organization	45	54	61	62	63
Management Service Organization	70	85	114	130	130
Integrated Salary Model	196	191	195	178	171
Equity Model	3	9	14	16	12
Foundation	29	49	50	59	64
Insurance Products					
Health Maintenance Organization	105	121	154	182	192
Preferred Provider Organization	149	178	226	250	283
Indemnity Fee for Service	42	54	61	73	97
Managed Care Contracts					
Health Maintenance Organization	509	511	541	529	574
Preferred Provider Organization	660	644	662	640	717
Affiliations					
Hospitals in a System	435	405	431	414	414
Hospitals in a Network	267	264	269	264	295
Hospitals in a Group Purchasing Organization	751	697	637	559	—

TABLE 4

BED SIZE CATEGORY 50-99

U.S. Registered Community Hospitals
(Nonfederal, short-term general and other special hospitals)

Utilization, Personnel, Revenue and Expenses 1997–2001

	2001	2000	1999	1998	1997
TOTAL FACILITY (Includes Hospital and Nursing Home Units)					
Utilization - Inpatient					
Beds	76,924	75,865	78,121	78,035	79,837
Admissions	2,421,938	2,354,896	2,316,862	2,264,836	2,310,771
Inpatient Days	15,461,340	15,195,600	15,548,467	15,564,337	15,805,358
Average Length of Stay	6.4	6.5	6.7	6.9	6.8
Inpatient Surgeries	588,354	580,886	568,696	655,043	583,483
Births	262,605	276,308	266,469	257,485	267,447
Utilization - Outpatient					
Emergency Outpatient Visits	11,093,357	10,601,048	10,292,153	9,781,573	9,521,443
Other Outpatient Visits	40,237,990	38,783,686	35,863,458	32,379,666	31,360,576
Total Outpatient Visits	51,331,347	49,384,734	46,155,611	42,161,239	40,882,019
Outpatient Surgeries	1,485,774	1,448,514	1,385,596	1,465,553	1,274,859
Personnel					
Full Time RNs	49,209	48,531	48,609	49,048	48,333
Full Time LPNs	12,956	12,749	13,349	12,965	14,194
Part Time RNs	29,477	31,250	30,651	29,470	29,898
Part Time LPNs	5,747	6,141	6,460	6,149	6,859
Total Full Time	244,068	233,169	233,659	233,003	232,870
Total Part Time	110,165	115,307	110,546	107,517	109,731
Revenue - Inpatient					
Gross Inpatient Revenue	$24,513,608,917	$22,750,944,141	$21,097,563,298	$20,094,829,572	$19,217,264,602
Revenue - Outpatient					
Gross Outpatient Revenue	$22,106,129,277	$19,990,370,027	$17,597,291,726	$15,882,964,599	$14,765,948,216
Revenue and Expenses - Totals (Includes Inpatient and Outpatient)					
Total Gross Revenue	$46,619,738,194	$42,741,314,168	$38,694,855,024	$35,977,794,171	$33,983,212,818
Deductions from Revenue	23,028,290,004	21,022,033,394	18,058,805,944	16,276,818,923	14,402,063,365
Net Patient Revenue	23,591,448,190	21,719,280,774	20,636,049,080	19,700,975,248	19,581,149,453
Other Operating Revenue	1,028,923,986	992,807,456	1,007,752,277	1,023,064,020	840,828,367
Other Nonoperating Revenue	683,658,777	657,785,910	448,107,493	496,150,441	492,839,151
Total Net Revenue	25,304,030,953	23,369,874,140	22,091,908,850	21,220,189,709	20,914,816,971
Total Expenses	24,030,935,779	22,322,022,731	20,967,397,999	20,021,471,000	19,489,570,110
HOSPITAL UNIT (Excludes Separate Nursing Home Units)					
Utilization - Inpatient					
Beds	64,717	63,189	65,129	65,288	66,500
Admissions	2,384,021	2,315,942	2,269,013	2,217,188	2,261,834
Inpatient Days	11,602,606	11,205,030	11,512,534	11,522,253	11,490,503
Average Length of Stay	4.9	4.8	5.1	5.2	5.1
Personnel					
Total Full Time	237,000	224,763	226,412	225,267	224,624
Total Part Time	105,562	110,426	106,029	102,640	104,484
Revenue and Expenses - Totals (Includes Inpatient and Outpatient)					
Total Net Revenue	$24,745,283,010	$22,858,172,678	$21,542,991,451	$20,672,497,709	$20,374,223,611
Total Expenses	23,602,034,845	21,923,794,277	20,558,590,538	19,608,707,134	19,095,554,560

Bed Size Categories

Table 4

BED SIZE CATEGORY 100-199

U.S. Registered Community Hospitals
(Nonfederal, short-term general and other special hospitals)

Overview 1997–2001

	2001	2000	1999	1998	1997
Total U.S. Community Hospitals in Bed Size Category 100-199	**1,218**	**1,236**	**1,266**	**1,304**	**1,289**
Location					
Hospitals Urban	783	795	816	848	827
Hospitals Rural	435	441	450	456	462
Control					
State and Local Government	198	196	214	212	217
Not for Profit	757	769	791	807	790
Investor owned	263	271	261	285	282
Physician Models					
Independent Practice Association	218	229	222	268	298
Group Practice without Walls	71	55	50	64	81
Open Physician-Hospital Organization	242	274	294	316	318
Closed Physician-Hospital Organization	82	87	100	130	129
Management Service Organization	143	178	213	260	281
Integrated Salary Model	241	265	269	244	232
Equity Model	16	26	21	36	38
Foundation	46	60	66	90	116
Insurance Products					
Health Maintenance Organization	151	196	243	269	276
Preferred Provider Organization	208	247	286	332	399
Indemnity Fee for Service	51	59	79	104	131
Managed Care Contracts					
Health Maintenance Organization	706	752	776	803	831
Preferred Provider Organization	805	820	849	870	921
Affiliations					
Hospitals in a System	580	591	606	609	609
Hospitals in a Network	325	315	315	349	369
Hospitals in a Group Purchasing Organization	858	850	763	688	—

TABLE 4

BED SIZE CATEGORY 100-199

U.S. Registered Community Hospitals
(Nonfederal, short-term general and other special hospitals)

Utilization, Personnel, Revenue and Expenses 1997–2001

	2001	2000	1999	1998	1997
TOTAL FACILITY (Includes Hospital and Nursing Home Units)					
Utilization - Inpatient					
Beds	174,024	175,778	181,115	186,118	182,284
Admissions	6,777,542	6,734,707	6,683,621	6,656,196	6,415,654
Inpatient Days	38,508,731	38,624,802	39,220,552	39,597,014	38,729,193
Average Length of Stay	5.7	5.7	5.9	5.9	6.0
Inpatient Surgeries	1,907,604	1,857,378	1,855,847	1,934,998	1,806,292
Births	804,377	811,163	799,904	796,861	804,255
Utilization - Outpatient					
Emergency Outpatient Visits	25,605,993	25,135,121	24,700,172	23,518,323	22,729,649
Other Outpatient Visits	89,314,524	89,047,867	85,635,833	84,447,896	78,108,686
Total Outpatient Visits	114,920,517	114,182,988	110,336,005	107,966,219	100,838,335
Outpatient Surgeries	3,897,374	3,921,040	3,798,060	3,752,191	3,460,120
Personnel					
Full Time RNs	132,993	134,882	135,087	138,368	131,908
Full Time LPNs	23,871	23,104	24,310	25,706	26,519
Part Time RNs	84,269	89,261	87,233	87,516	82,931
Part Time LPNs	10,859	11,416	11,576	12,281	12,770
Total Full Time	612,894	601,589	607,315	618,784	591,780
Total Part Time	270,898	285,929	281,113	283,392	268,008
Revenue - Inpatient					
Gross Inpatient Revenue	$88,826,998,928	$81,494,205,969	$73,304,767,289	$69,886,029,365	$64,504,978,628
Revenue - Outpatient					
Gross Outpatient Revenue	$59,081,658,626	$55,132,963,490	$48,727,503,116	$45,110,976,826	$39,807,538,883
Revenue and Expenses - Totals (Includes Inpatient and Outpatient)					
Total Gross Revenue	$147,908,657,554	$136,627,169,459	$122,032,270,405	$114,997,006,191	$104,312,517,511
Deductions from Revenue	81,506,420,194	73,520,588,504	61,736,298,969	55,600,577,182	48,852,379,897
Net Patient Revenue	66,402,237,360	63,106,580,955	60,295,971,436	59,396,429,009	55,460,137,614
Other Operating Revenue	2,813,935,425	2,769,788,344	2,772,654,915	2,473,809,438	2,485,090,772
Other Nonoperating Revenue	1,064,678,719	1,377,282,079	1,366,384,506	1,472,900,513	1,315,210,028
Total Net Revenue	70,280,851,504	67,253,651,378	64,435,010,857	63,343,138,960	59,260,438,414
Total Expenses	66,360,396,087	63,358,364,315	60,794,792,716	59,398,078,592	54,876,789,415
HOSPITAL UNIT (Excludes Separate Nursing Home Units)					
Utilization - Inpatient					
Beds	152,541	153,990	156,820	162,427	159,291
Admissions	6,672,956	6,618,001	6,539,049	6,515,996	6,283,207
Inpatient Days	31,662,149	31,797,892	31,621,341	32,112,825	31,277,088
Average Length of Stay	4.7	4.8	4.8	4.9	5.0
Personnel					
Total Full Time	599,785	587,721	591,911	603,547	575,799
Total Part Time	263,165	277,067	272,228	274,306	258,529
Revenue and Expenses - Totals (Includes Inpatient and Outpatient)					
Total Net Revenue	$69,200,831,169	$66,041,517,516	$63,158,997,513	$62,054,937,859	$58,051,160,954
Total Expenses	65,492,148,426	62,568,627,003	59,804,230,111	58,459,560,010	54,057,363,855

TABLE 4

BED SIZE CATEGORY 200-299

U.S. Registered Community Hospitals
(Nonfederal, short-term general and other special hospitals)

Overview 1997–2001

	2001	2000	1999	1998	1997
Total U.S. Community Hospitals in Bed Size Category 200-299	**635**	**656**	**642**	**644**	**679**
Location					
Hospitals Urban	526	551	534	531	563
Hospitals Rural	109	105	108	113	116
Control					
State and Local Government	69	71	71	75	85
Not for Profit	467	488	480	467	474
Investor owned	99	97	91	102	120
Physician Models					
Independent Practice Association	106	127	136	150	199
Group Practice without Walls	27	31	36	34	55
Open Physician-Hospital Organization	143	171	178	187	204
Closed Physician-Hospital Organization	56	61	71	78	90
Management Service Organization	92	118	152	156	205
Integrated Salary Model	154	167	151	147	163
Equity Model	10	20	23	18	24
Foundation	34	43	49	58	82
Insurance Products					
Health Maintenance Organization	113	151	146	153	192
Preferred Provider Organization	123	154	160	180	235
Indemnity Fee for Service	41	46	42	49	86
Managed Care Contracts					
Health Maintenance Organization	424	454	456	456	504
Preferred Provider Organization	435	460	466	456	507
Affiliations					
Hospitals in a System	356	359	350	336	383
Hospitals in a Network	173	195	189	201	229
Hospitals in a Group Purchasing Organization	459	461	418	357	—

Table 4 — BED SIZE CATEGORY 200-299

U.S. Registered Community Hospitals
(Nonfederal, short-term general and other special hospitals)

Utilization, Personnel, Revenue and Expenses 1997–2001

	2001	2000	1999	1998	1997
TOTAL FACILITY (Includes Hospital and Nursing Home Units)					
Utilization - Inpatient					
Beds	154,420	159,807	155,831	156,978	165,197
Admissions	6,630,307	6,702,478	6,389,172	6,229,541	6,352,478
Inpatient Days	36,923,111	37,942,444	36,493,064	36,054,092	37,255,676
Average Length of Stay	5.6	5.7	5.7	5.8	5.9
Inpatient Surgeries	1,910,132	1,992,966	1,883,032	1,870,471	1,925,039
Births	733,456	788,352	755,274	719,232	719,484
Utilization - Outpatient					
Emergency Outpatient Visits	20,309,391	20,436,782	19,533,629	18,569,295	18,774,418
Other Outpatient Visits	79,286,800	78,811,142	71,343,993	66,924,481	65,051,917
Total Outpatient Visits	99,596,191	99,247,924	90,877,622	85,493,776	83,826,335
Outpatient Surgeries	3,265,812	3,358,516	3,163,861	3,117,508	3,011,857
Personnel					
Full Time RNs	136,338	137,548	132,812	132,749	130,715
Full Time LPNs	18,036	18,703	20,192	19,581	20,974
Part Time RNs	80,856	86,744	80,212	75,972	76,869
Part Time LPNs	8,752	9,181	9,349	8,931	10,346
Total Full Time	600,028	614,344	588,843	578,790	587,269
Total Part Time	247,526	265,162	249,790	238,607	244,868
Revenue - Inpatient					
Gross Inpatient Revenue	$103,904,499,291	$92,657,723,538	$84,461,242,677	$78,694,263,284	$75,411,157,286
Revenue - Outpatient					
Gross Outpatient Revenue	$54,235,790,743	$47,912,514,899	$42,225,301,889	$38,024,413,991	$36,086,513,673
Revenue and Expenses - Totals (Includes Inpatient and Outpatient)					
Total Gross Revenue	$158,140,290,034	$140,570,238,437	$126,686,544,566	$116,718,677,275	$111,497,670,959
Deductions from Revenue	90,371,126,069	75,560,084,371	67,487,466,289	60,181,099,208	54,306,698,232
Net Patient Revenue	67,769,163,965	65,010,154,066	59,199,078,277	56,537,578,067	57,190,972,727
Other Operating Revenue	3,278,654,426	3,511,441,863	3,261,463,827	2,942,181,355	2,663,931,645
Other Nonoperating Revenue	1,301,236,089	1,789,700,386	2,038,058,222	1,778,094,925	1,596,352,347
Total Net Revenue	72,349,054,480	70,311,296,315	64,498,600,326	61,257,854,347	61,451,256,719
Total Expenses	68,913,526,440	67,057,555,091	61,099,993,147	57,117,140,326	57,081,712,776
HOSPITAL UNIT (Excludes Separate Nursing Home Units)					
Utilization - Inpatient					
Beds	141,629	145,501	140,318	142,027	149,453
Admissions	6,530,211	6,592,395	6,261,091	6,094,572	6,212,305
Inpatient Days	32,784,136	33,230,080	31,689,032	31,359,766	32,338,064
Average Length of Stay	5.0	5.0	5.1	5.1	5.2
Personnel					
Total Full Time	591,000	602,872	577,378	587,747	574,000
Total Part Time	242,702	259,423	244,444	233,387	238,518
Revenue and Expenses - Totals (Includes Inpatient and Outpatient)					
Total Net Revenue	$71,458,934,077	$69,473,697,175	$63,481,487,264	$60,166,099,815	$60,322,984,219
Total Expenses	68,260,569,539	66,366,724,426	60,356,593,743	56,355,723,184	56,303,006,305

TABLE 4

BED SIZE CATEGORY 300-399

U.S. Registered Community Hospitals
(Nonfederal, short-term general and other special hospitals)

Overview 1997–2001

	2001	2000	1999	1998	1997
Total U.S. Community Hospitals in Bed Size Category 300-399	**348**	**341**	**365**	**352**	**367**
Location					
Hospitals Urban	324	314	339	330	341
Hospitals Rural	24	27	26	22	26
Control					
State and Local Government	38	38	43	44	41
Not for Profit	269	255	274	262	282
Investor owned	41	48	48	46	44
Physician Models					
Independent Practice Association	76	68	89	87	103
Group Practice without Walls	11	11	15	17	27
Open Physician-Hospital Organization	100	94	96	90	112
Closed Physician-Hospital Organization	40	49	62	48	77
Management Service Organization	72	79	93	93	113
Integrated Salary Model	96	90	103	106	105
Equity Model	9	5	13	10	16
Foundation	29	27	33	30	34
Insurance Products					
Health Maintenance Organization	83	94	128	117	132
Preferred Provider Organization	87	96	121	124	151
Indemnity Fee for Service	24	30	33	38	49
Managed Care Contracts					
Health Maintenance Organization	251	237	261	239	268
Preferred Provider Organization	262	243	262	245	281
Affiliations					
Hospitals in a System	233	218	222	207	219
Hospitals in a Network	118	101	107	105	134
Hospitals in a Group Purchasing Organization	263	235	229	206	—

TABLE 4

BED SIZE CATEGORY 300-399

U.S. Registered Community Hospitals
(Nonfederal, short-term general and other special hospitals)

Utilization, Personnel, Revenue and Expenses 1997–2001

	2001	2000	1999	1998	1997
TOTAL FACILITY (Includes Hospital and Nursing Home Units)					
Utilization - Inpatient					
Beds	119,753	117,220	126,259	120,512	126,307
Admissions	5,328,441	5,135,313	5,419,172	5,021,409	5,099,134
Inpatient Days	28,949,110	28,175,816	30,446,266	28,467,524	29,096,358
Average Length of Stay	5.4	5.5	5.6	5.7	5.7
Inpatient Surgeries	1,575,266	1,548,365	1,633,543	1,563,495	1,576,025
Births	628,124	608,029	635,465	636,698	661,814
Utilization - Outpatient					
Emergency Outpatient Visits	15,412,370	14,679,081	14,883,092	13,300,137	13,096,685
Other Outpatient Visits	59,829,649	58,764,729	60,965,514	53,769,976	51,644,467
Total Outpatient Visits	75,242,019	73,443,810	75,848,606	67,070,113	64,741,152
Outpatient Surgeries	2,398,395	2,380,845	2,453,087	2,236,446	2,294,563
Personnel					
Full Time RNs	119,926	115,123	122,695	114,813	111,382
Full Time LPNs	14,521	12,961	13,849	15,245	14,248
Part Time RNs	63,220	64,123	65,952	64,009	66,713
Part Time LPNs	5,187	5,663	5,658	6,048	6,609
Total Full Time	523,968	501,162	532,328	495,732	493,741
Total Part Time	192,906	195,777	194,111	189,580	204,826
Revenue - Inpatient					
Gross Inpatient Revenue	$90,736,055,640	$79,128,945,312	$76,331,193,232	$67,252,272,100	$62,198,123,811
Revenue - Outpatient					
Gross Outpatient Revenue	$43,966,846,914	$37,931,362,986	$36,396,156,547	$30,498,257,999	$28,346,394,996
Revenue and Expenses - Totals (Includes Inpatient and Outpatient)					
Total Gross Revenue	$134,702,902,554	$117,060,308,298	$112,727,349,779	$97,750,530,099	$90,544,518,807
Deductions from Revenue	77,014,066,878	63,980,293,228	58,693,834,397	49,183,505,560	42,713,174,480
Net Patient Revenue	57,688,835,676	53,080,015,070	54,033,515,382	48,567,024,539	47,831,344,327
Other Operating Revenue	3,334,900,779	2,688,378,669	2,807,882,430	2,741,344,421	2,569,966,892
Other Nonoperating Revenue	858,386,079	1,305,643,872	1,555,611,944	1,466,462,294	1,447,668,666
Total Net Revenue	61,882,122,534	57,074,037,611	58,397,009,756	52,774,831,251	51,848,979,885
Total Expenses	59,027,238,261	54,273,518,296	55,544,241,173	49,618,989,358	48,386,951,574
HOSPITAL UNIT (Excludes Separate Nursing Home Units)					
Utilization - Inpatient					
Beds	112,537	110,180	117,501	113,215	117,635
Admissions	5,269,008	5,074,369	5,343,133	4,955,760	5,017,114
Inpatient Days	26,728,772	25,970,657	27,715,550	26,145,252	26,249,552
Average Length of Stay	5.1	5.1	5.2	5.3	5.2
Personnel					
Total Full Time	517,844	494,730	526,524	480,156	486,000
Total Part Time	190,500	193,029	190,991	186,491	201,558
Revenue and Expenses - Totals (Includes Inpatient and Outpatient)					
Total Net Revenue	$61,250,007,293	$56,555,661,812	$57,738,046,612	$52,200,823,573	$51,200,719,420
Total Expenses	58,607,498,709	53,867,071,704	55,030,932,464	49,147,092,391	47,875,417,837

Bed Size Categories

TABLE 4

BED SIZE CATEGORY 400-499

U.S. Registered Community Hospitals
(Nonfederal, short-term general and other special hospitals)

Overview 1997–2001

	2001	2000	1999	1998	1997
Total U.S. Community Hospitals in Bed Size Category 400-499	**191**	**182**	**161**	**183**	**185**
Location					
Hospitals Urban	186	178	157	177	181
Hospitals Rural	5	4	4	6	4
Control					
State and Local Government	27	25	19	18	27
Not for Profit	153	147	132	152	149
Investor owned	11	10	10	13	9
Physician Models					
Independent Practice Association	40	41	45	58	63
Group Practice without Walls	7	9	11	12	16
Open Physician-Hospital Organization	36	41	38	46	45
Closed Physician-Hospital Organization	20	22	24	32	27
Management Service Organization	37	41	42	53	64
Integrated Salary Model	59	61	53	49	59
Equity Model	3	5	5	8	5
Foundation	17	13	17	25	29
Insurance Products					
Health Maintenance Organization	60	69	70	88	85
Preferred Provider Organization	53	63	55	74	78
Indemnity Fee for Service	11	16	11	19	19
Managed Care Contracts					
Health Maintenance Organization	137	138	121	143	149
Preferred Provider Organization	143	139	125	144	144
Affiliations					
Hospitals in a System	122	118	104	119	123
Hospitals in a Network	66	62	52	71	70
Hospitals in a Group Purchasing Organization	141	131	107	115	—

Table 4

BED SIZE CATEGORY 400-499

U.S. Registered Community Hospitals
(Nonfederal, short-term general and other special hospitals)

Utilization, Personnel, Revenue and Expenses 1997–2001

	2001	2000	1999	1998	1997
TOTAL FACILITY (Includes Hospital and Nursing Home Units)					
Utilization - Inpatient					
Beds	84,745	80,763	71,580	81,247	82,250
Admissions	3,778,746	3,616,530	3,045,448	3,390,232	3,360,171
Inpatient Days	21,312,743	20,509,972	17,853,905	19,958,559	20,406,366
Average Length of Stay	5.6	5.7	5.9	5.9	6.1
Inpatient Surgeries	1,143,813	1,102,058	904,289	1,119,239	1,070,138
Births	462,372	439,821	357,548	402,499	411,905
Utilization - Outpatient					
Emergency Outpatient Visits	9,345,972	9,488,926	7,263,184	7,730,076	8,185,358
Other Outpatient Visits	50,233,673	42,716,283	36,604,300	41,292,412	38,393,526
Total Outpatient Visits	59,579,645	52,205,209	43,867,484	49,022,488	46,578,884
Outpatient Surgeries	1,642,696	1,578,111	1,366,726	1,453,863	1,364,809
Personnel					
Full Time RNs	87,244	82,895	72,380	79,795	78,646
Full Time LPNs	9,335	8,237	8,563	10,051	10,147
Part Time RNs	50,157	49,484	35,968	42,276	39,403
Part Time LPNs	3,334	3,052	3,315	4,452	3,654
Total Full Time	398,066	367,265	320,457	364,877	363,411
Total Part Time	140,706	139,517	106,306	127,806	118,596
Revenue - Inpatient					
Gross Inpatient Revenue	$70,893,560,813	$59,609,190,161	$47,414,569,510	$50,002,475,994	$47,670,053,686
Revenue - Outpatient					
Gross Outpatient Revenue	$32,818,521,002	$28,221,840,088	$20,680,259,396	$21,386,610,279	$19,353,489,887
Revenue and Expenses - Totals (Includes Inpatient and Outpatient)					
Total Gross Revenue	$103,712,081,815	$87,831,030,249	$68,094,828,906	$71,389,086,273	$67,023,543,573
Deductions from Revenue	58,861,160,338	48,605,733,601	36,254,726,963	36,658,972,721	33,251,928,377
Net Patient Revenue	44,850,921,477	39,225,296,648	31,840,101,943	34,730,113,552	33,771,615,196
Other Operating Revenue	3,212,320,490	2,780,992,924	2,533,086,920	2,511,192,215	2,419,994,475
Other Nonoperating Revenue	906,755,338	1,176,559,766	923,857,533	1,223,480,642	1,098,805,781
Total Net Revenue	48,969,997,305	43,182,849,338	35,297,046,396	38,464,786,409	37,290,415,452
Total Expenses	47,321,475,681	41,299,819,174	33,866,308,713	36,442,105,640	34,908,110,223
HOSPITAL UNIT (Excludes Separate Nursing Home Units)					
Utilization - Inpatient					
Beds	79,957	76,238	65,996	75,110	75,407
Admissions	3,739,662	3,573,245	2,995,719	3,341,213	3,307,928
Inpatient Days	19,847,882	19,084,886	16,114,892	18,132,991	18,243,299
Average Length of Stay	5.3	5.3	5.4	5.4	5.5
Personnel					
Total Full Time	394,285	362,720	316,895	358,783	357,216
Total Part Time	139,265	137,566	104,747	125,398	115,423
Revenue and Expenses - Totals (Includes Inpatient and Outpatient)					
Total Net Revenue	$48,644,983,381	$42,890,966,938	$34,714,064,245	$38,014,252,666	$36,705,041,188
Total Expenses	46,998,302,690	41,054,265,159	33,528,138,196	36,064,400,098	34,473,536,206

Bed Size Categories

TABLE 4

BED SIZE CATEGORY 500 +

U.S. Registered Community Hospitals
(Nonfederal, short-term general and other special hospitals)

Overview 1997–2001

	2001	2000	1999	1998	1997
Total U.S. Community Hospitals in Bed Size Category 500 +	**249**	**247**	**254**	**254**	**255**
Location					
Hospitals Urban	245	244	251	251	251
Hospitals Rural	4	3	3	3	4
Control					
State and Local Government	37	36	40	42	43
Not for Profit	195	197	201	198	197
Investor owned	17	14	13	14	15
Physician Models					
Independent Practice Association	70	76	85	85	86
Group Practice without Walls	25	26	24	25	28
Open Physician-Hospital Organization	70	69	75	79	87
Closed Physician-Hospital Organization	31	42	48	53	50
Management Service Organization	64	80	77	80	93
Integrated Salary Model	103	105	101	103	97
Equity Model	10	13	13	17	17
Foundation	25	27	31	35	41
Insurance Products					
Health Maintenance Organization	86	116	128	138	130
Preferred Provider Organization	85	105	115	122	127
Indemnity Fee for Service	22	26	24	34	37
Managed Care Contracts					
Health Maintenance Organization	195	205	205	197	206
Preferred Provider Organization	195	202	200	193	202
Affiliations					
Hospitals in a System	186	184	187	176	179
Hospitals in a Network	94	97	103	104	107
Hospitals in a Group Purchasing Organization	192	180	173	159	—

TABLE 4

BED SIZE CATEGORY 500 +

U.S. Registered Community Hospitals
(Nonfederal, short-term general and other special hospitals)

Utilization, Personnel, Revenue and Expenses 1997–2001

	2001	2000	1999	1998	1997
TOTAL FACILITY (Includes Hospital and Nursing Home Units)					
Utilization - Inpatient					
Beds	177,873	175,638	178,411	178,237	179,146
Admissions	7,705,773	7,410,167	7,399,867	7,145,981	6,966,993
Inpatient Days	47,225,469	46,339,384	46,713,100	46,111,523	45,674,703
Average Length of Stay	6.1	6.3	6.3	6.5	6.6
Inpatient Surgeries	2,425,140	2,419,740	2,474,024	2,357,616	2,328,710
Births	885,391	868,382	849,861	811,890	769,729
Utilization - Outpatient					
Emergency Outpatient Visits	18,048,334	16,863,866	17,080,213	16,206,443	15,184,280
Other Outpatient Visits	87,265,908	84,513,677	82,660,658	79,301,140	72,487,575
Total Outpatient Visits	105,314,242	101,377,543	99,740,871	95,507,583	87,671,855
Outpatient Surgeries	3,126,279	2,908,913	2,949,786	2,863,384	2,667,538
Personnel					
Full Time RNs	199,358	199,560	202,263	192,852	181,900
Full Time LPNs	16,947	17,233	18,029	17,604	17,683
Part Time RNs	90,746	87,424	82,232	77,369	74,734
Part Time LPNs	5,766	5,421	5,260	5,540	5,317
Total Full Time	909,166	879,297	884,284	873,961	853,836
Total Part Time	262,239	253,897	243,838	232,383	238,921
Revenue - Inpatient					
Gross Inpatient Revenue	$156,462,924,653	$138,130,198,562	$126,828,183,226	$114,805,458,621	$105,152,037,442
Revenue - Outpatient					
Gross Outpatient Revenue	$65,226,823,758	$54,990,410,746	$49,682,171,548	$42,624,184,029	$37,912,708,824
Revenue and Expenses - Totals (Includes Inpatient and Outpatient)					
Total Gross Revenue	$221,689,748,411	$193,120,609,308	$176,470,354,774	$157,429,642,650	$143,064,746,266
Deductions from Revenue	123,213,421,530	103,806,905,095	90,993,158,498	76,161,795,283	65,255,061,176
Net Patient Revenue	98,476,326,881	89,313,704,213	85,477,196,276	81,267,847,367	77,809,685,090
Other Operating Revenue	8,858,554,851	7,873,591,839	7,574,557,742	6,772,432,158	6,429,259,703
Other Nonoperating Revenue	1,292,497,612	2,991,999,020	2,570,772,014	2,618,731,433	2,761,586,493
Total Net Revenue	108,627,379,344	100,179,295,072	95,622,526,032	90,659,010,950	87,000,531,280
Total Expenses	105,085,709,086	96,310,798,929	91,982,247,309	86,017,901,252	81,658,795,950
HOSPITAL UNIT (Excludes Separate Nursing Home Units)					
Utilization - Inpatient					
Beds	166,158	161,458	164,759	163,360	164,841
Admissions	7,649,107	7,337,658	7,308,606	7,046,008	6,900,212
Inpatient Days	43,383,615	41,856,131	42,322,343	41,342,830	41,041,288
Average Length of Stay	5.7	5.7	5.8	5.9	5.9
Personnel					
Total Full Time	898,569	867,203	872,217	862,751	841,195
Total Part Time	258,769	250,140	240,125	229,157	234,960
Revenue and Expenses - Totals (Includes Inpatient and Outpatient)					
Total Net Revenue	$107,658,500,091	$98,564,608,494	$94,608,758,058	$89,464,648,691	$86,014,555,988
Total Expenses	104,203,128,358	95,410,392,185	91,062,292,669	84,930,446,901	80,794,190,531

Census Divisions

Census Division 1	**New England** Connecticut, Maine, Massachusetts, New Hampshire, Rhode Island, Vermont
Census Division 2	**Middle Atlantic** New Jersey, New York, Pennsylvania
Census Division 3	**South Atlantic** Delaware, District of Columbia, Florida, Georgia, Maryland, North Carolina, South Carolina, Virginia, West Virginia
Census Division 4	**East North Central** Illinois, Indiana, Michigan, Ohio, Wisconsin
Census Division 5	**East South Central** Alabama, Kentucky, Mississippi, Tennessee
Census Division 6	**West North Central** Iowa, Kansas, Minnesota, Missouri, Nebraska, North Dakota, South Dakota
Census Division 7	**West South Central** Arkansas, Louisiana, Oklahoma, Texas
Census Division 8	**Mountain** Arizona, Colorado, Idaho, Montana, Nevada, New Mexico, Utah, Wyoming
Census Division 9	**Pacific** Alaska, California, Hawaii, Oregon, Washington

TABLE 5

U.S. CENSUS DIVISION 1: NEW ENGLAND

U.S. Registered Community Hospitals
(Nonfederal, short-term general and other special hospitals)

Overview 1997–2001

	2001	2000	1999	1998	1997
Total U.S. Community Hospitals in Census Division 1, New England	**205**	**205**	**204**	**207**	**209**
Bed Size Category					
6-24	3	4	5	5	8
25-49	39	38	35	36	33
50-99	44	44	46	50	49
100-199	60	61	62	62	61
200-299	28	26	25	28	29
300-399	16	17	16	11	16
400-499	2	2	2	3	2
500 +	13	13	13	12	11
Location					
Hospitals Urban	128	128	127	130	134
Hospitals Rural	77	77	77	77	75
Control					
State and Local Government	8	8	9	9	11
Not for Profit	186	185	184	187	186
Investor owned	11	12	11	11	12
Physician Models					
Independent Practice Association	57	52	61	57	64
Group Practice without Walls	18	15	18	18	22
Open Physician-Hospital Organization	71	71	78	76	79
Closed Physician-Hospital Organization	20	21	21	22	20
Management Service Organization	36	36	48	47	42
Integrated Salary Model	71	67	71	64	70
Equity Model	4	4	4	5	8
Foundation	15	13	18	19	23
Insurance Products					
Health Maintenance Organization	28	31	37	49	47
Preferred Provider Organization	19	18	22	37	45
Indemnity Fee for Service	5	5	5	11	18
Managed Care Contracts					
Health Maintenance Organization	163	161	169	170	175
Preferred Provider Organization	149	148	151	153	161
Affiliations					
Hospitals in a System	107	99	109	96	102
Hospitals in a Network	61	66	60	53	57
Hospitals in a Group Purchasing Organization	164	155	153	144	—

TABLE 5

U.S. CENSUS DIVISION 1: NEW ENGLAND

U.S. Registered Community Hospitals
(Nonfederal, short-term general and other special hospitals)

Utilization, Personnel, Revenue and Expenses, Community Health Indicators 1997–2001

	2001	2000	1999	1998	1997
TOTAL FACILITY (Includes Hospital and Nursing Home Units)					
Utilization - Inpatient					
Beds	35,385	34,944	34,915	34,303	35,420
Admissions	1,567,000	1,519,012	1,500,667	1,488,810	1,524,603
Inpatient Days	9,144,828	8,917,327	8,771,404	8,500,264	8,703,966
Average Length of Stay	5.8	5.9	5.8	5.7	5.7
Inpatient Surgeries	444,897	448,066	447,135	448,843	448,806
Births	169,198	170,638	169,142	167,926	171,003
Utilization - Outpatient					
Emergency Outpatient Visits	5,973,441	5,916,202	5,784,739	5,371,671	5,414,695
Other Outpatient Visits	29,179,090	26,862,517	25,245,873	24,883,550	23,077,332
Total Outpatient Visits	35,152,531	32,778,719	31,030,612	30,255,221	28,492,027
Outpatient Surgeries	987,409	956,844	903,825	868,615	805,550
Personnel					
Full Time RNs	34,016	32,203	30,186	29,955	29,726
Full Time LPNs	2,390	2,391	2,078	2,302	2,575
Part Time RNs	33,183	33,845	33,145	32,958	31,959
Part Time LPNs	2,219	2,321	2,272	2,352	2,573
Total Full Time	186,757	173,630	165,298	164,720	166,171
Total Part Time	105,157	107,014	105,196	103,830	104,342
Revenue - Inpatient					
Gross Inpatient Revenue	$23,006,462,654	$21,145,777,686	$19,052,712,630	$17,981,275,871	$17,102,631,114
Revenue - Outpatient					
Gross Outpatient Revenue	$17,354,624,925	$15,014,223,925	$13,647,875,340	$12,012,290,460	$10,695,948,745
Revenue and Expenses - Totals (Includes Inpatient and Outpatient)					
Total Gross Revenue	$40,361,087,579	$36,160,001,611	$32,700,587,970	$29,993,566,331	$27,798,579,859
Deductions from Revenue	19,755,206,105	17,289,206,287	15,008,365,053	12,978,565,939	11,220,128,347
Net Patient Revenue	20,605,881,474	18,870,795,324	17,692,222,917	17,015,000,392	16,578,451,512
Other Operating Revenue	2,061,229,915	1,644,812,612	1,737,545,613	1,802,476,446	1,402,015,028
Other Nonoperating Revenue	256,835,969	706,498,132	665,388,606	654,758,408	716,156,689
Total Net Revenue	22,923,947,358	21,222,106,068	20,095,157,136	19,472,235,246	18,696,623,229
Total Expenses	22,650,945,919	20,923,125,622	19,745,944,243	19,006,482,876	17,839,824,778
HOSPITAL UNIT (Excludes Separate Nursing Home Units)					
Utilization - Inpatient					
Beds	32,730	32,263	32,117	32,505	33,217
Admissions	1,550,961	1,498,475	1,477,023	1,473,480	1,508,816
Inpatient Days	8,190,799	8,007,120	7,885,831	7,942,077	7,973,718
Average Length of Stay	5.3	5.3	5.3	5.4	5.3
Personnel					
Total Full Time	184,640	171,537	163,198	163,025	164,409
Total Part Time	103,487	105,170	103,333	102,503	102,944
Revenue and Expenses - Totals (Includes Inpatient and Outpatient)					
Total Net Revenue	$22,729,636,795	$21,051,443,144	$19,894,763,328	$19,279,686,014	$18,524,638,854
Total Expenses	22,469,904,390	20,769,362,219	19,578,964,509	18,859,372,118	17,710,361,580
COMMUNITY HEALTH INDICATORS PER 1000 POPULATION					
Total Population (in thousands)	14,022	13,923	13,496	13,429	13,378
Inpatient					
Beds	2.5	2.5	2.6	2.6	2.6
Admissions	111.8	109.1	111.2	110.9	114.0
Inpatient Days	652.2	640.5	649.9	633.0	650.6
Inpatient Surgeries	31.7	32.2	33.1	33.4	33.5
Births	12.1	12.3	12.5	12.5	12.8
Outpatient					
Emergency Outpatient Visits	426.0	424.9	428.6	400.0	404.7
Other Outpatient Visits	2,080.9	1,929.4	1,870.6	1,853.0	1,725.0
Total Outpatient Visits	2,506.9	2,354.4	2,299.3	2,253.0	2,129.8
Outpatient Surgeries	70.4	68.7	67.0	64.7	60.2
Expense per Capita (per person)	$1,615.4	$1,502.8	$1,463.1	$1,415.4	$1,333.5

U.S. Census Divisions

TABLE 5

U.S. CENSUS DIVISION 2: MIDDLE ATLANTIC

U.S. Registered Community Hospitals
(Nonfederal, short-term general and other special hospitals)

Overview 1997–2001

	2001	2000	1999	1998	1997
Total U.S. Community Hospitals in Census Division 2, Middle Atlantic	**495**	**502**	**509**	**517**	**527**
Bed Size Category					
6-24	7	8	7	7	7
25-49	22	20	25	23	23
50-99	61	64	59	60	63
100-199	145	152	151	158	150
200-299	111	112	116	110	116
300-399	52	47	52	55	53
400-499	42	46	41	44	49
500 +	55	53	58	60	66
Location					
Hospitals Urban	415	423	428	436	446
Hospitals Rural	80	79	81	81	81
Control					
State and Local Government	29	28	28	28	32
Not for Profit	444	453	461	470	475
Investor owned	22	21	20	19	20
Physician Models					
Independent Practice Association	98	120	126	136	152
Group Practice without Walls	20	26	20	22	25
Open Physician-Hospital Organization	81	104	101	120	135
Closed Physician-Hospital Organization	25	33	44	48	50
Management Service Organization	72	89	96	100	109
Integrated Salary Model	99	112	93	100	109
Equity Model	6	14	13	11	9
Foundation	9	14	17	28	30
Insurance Products					
Health Maintenance Organization	70	97	101	125	118
Preferred Provider Organization	79	98	97	123	135
Indemnity Fee for Service	17	15	15	21	30
Managed Care Contracts					
Health Maintenance Organization	330	351	351	354	389
Preferred Provider Organization	315	332	321	316	333
Affiliations					
Hospitals in a System	236	248	220	224	225
Hospitals in a Network	148	155	146	160	174
Hospitals in a Group Purchasing Organization	350	334	289	287	—

U.S. Census Divisions

TABLE 5

U.S. CENSUS DIVISION 2: MIDDLE ATLANTIC

U.S. Registered Community Hospitals
(Nonfederal, short-term general and other special hospitals)

Utilization, Personnel, Revenue and Expenses, Community Health Indicators 1997–2001

	2001	2000	1999	1998	1997
TOTAL FACILITY (Includes Hospital and Nursing Home Units)					
Utilization - Inpatient					
Beds	134,007	134,044	136,493	139,603	144,785
Admissions	5,303,235	5,285,812	5,230,020	5,199,574	5,223,507
Inpatient Days	35,582,339	35,972,872	36,152,830	36,893,769	37,787,584
Average Length of Stay	6.7	6.8	6.9	7.1	7.2
Inpatient Surgeries	1,530,873	1,570,780	1,573,521	1,615,322	1,582,113
Births	502,368	504,630	506,591	497,211	503,645
Utilization - Outpatient					
Emergency Outpatient Visits	15,262,789	14,855,507	14,638,689	14,081,408	13,832,722
Other Outpatient Visits	80,890,968	79,672,796	76,499,179	75,468,918	68,877,904
Total Outpatient Visits	96,153,757	94,528,303	91,137,868	89,550,326	82,710,626
Outpatient Surgeries	2,688,679	2,673,923	2,560,005	2,597,905	2,384,591
Personnel					
Full Time RNs	125,764	125,727	124,392	123,604	123,249
Full Time LPNs	14,431	14,326	14,634	14,860	15,501
Part Time RNs	55,226	57,785	56,507	56,071	55,335
Part Time LPNs	5,408	5,704	5,939	6,170	6,582
Total Full Time	587,752	580,514	578,915	579,154	581,173
Total Part Time	179,456	182,798	179,758	178,219	184,170
Revenue - Inpatient					
Gross Inpatient Revenue	$102,755,097,357	$88,555,896,320	$79,559,155,616	$75,599,548,059	$71,184,448,051
Revenue - Outpatient					
Gross Outpatient Revenue	$45,742,770,658	$39,791,596,044	$35,350,638,604	$32,012,687,719	$29,395,321,317
Revenue and Expenses - Totals (Includes Inpatient and Outpatient)					
Total Gross Revenue	$148,497,868,015	$128,347,492,364	$114,909,794,220	$107,612,235,778	$100,579,769,368
Deductions from Revenue	87,693,668,174	71,418,197,617	61,003,893,361	54,696,994,230	48,128,749,444
Net Patient Revenue	60,804,199,841	56,929,294,747	53,905,900,859	52,915,241,548	52,451,019,924
Other Operating Revenue	4,858,174,712	4,373,128,371	4,158,957,000	3,768,576,982	3,777,984,669
Other Nonoperating Revenue	879,603,162	1,200,687,387	1,229,111,646	1,553,981,165	1,428,124,864
Total Net Revenue	66,541,977,715	62,503,110,505	59,293,969,505	58,237,799,695	57,657,129,457
Total Expenses	65,738,326,638	61,666,014,763	58,864,243,581	57,242,223,412	55,899,027,634
HOSPITAL UNIT (Excludes Separate Nursing Home Units)					
Utilization - Inpatient					
Beds	122,977	121,947	123,387	126,707	131,176
Admissions	5,251,290	5,228,518	5,165,103	5,140,274	5,172,785
Inpatient Days	31,838,056	31,790,693	31,784,098	32,589,512	33,215,860
Average Length of Stay	6.1	6.1	6.2	6.3	6.4
Personnel					
Total Full Time	570,127	569,721	570,103	570,505	572,224
Total Part Time	175,863	178,618	176,154	174,551	179,981
Revenue and Expenses - Totals (Includes Inpatient and Outpatient)					
Total Net Revenue	$65,632,075,736	$61,678,553,426	$58,381,802,745	$57,275,786,421	$56,751,140,082
Total Expenses	65,050,830,005	61,035,255,854	58,149,232,081	56,519,715,726	55,230,914,621
COMMUNITY HEALTH INDICATORS PER 1000 POPULATION					
Total Population (in thousands)	39,783	39,672	38,334	38,257	38,213
Inpatient					
Beds	3.4	3.4	3.6	3.6	3.8
Admissions	133.3	133.2	136.4	135.9	136.7
Inpatient Days	894.4	906.8	943.1	964.4	988.9
Inpatient Surgeries	38.5	39.6	41.0	42.2	41.4
Births	12.6	12.7	13.2	13.0	13.2
Outpatient					
Emergency Outpatient Visits	383.7	374.5	381.9	368.1	362.0
Other Outpatient Visits	2,033.3	2,008.3	1,995.6	1,972.7	1,802.5
Total Outpatient Visits	2,417.0	2,382.8	2,377.5	2,340.8	2,164.4
Outpatient Surgeries	67.6	67.4	66.8	67.9	62.4
Expense per Capita (per person)	$1,652.4	$1,554.4	$1,535.6	$1,496.3	$1,462.8

TABLE 5

U.S. CENSUS DIVISION 3: SOUTH ATLANTIC

U.S. Registered Community Hospitals
(Nonfederal, short-term general and other special hospitals)

Overview 1997–2001

	2001	2000	1999	1998	1997
Total U.S. Community Hospitals in Census Division 3, South Atlantic	**730**	**739**	**749**	**761**	**767**
Bed Size Category					
6-24	14	17	15	19	15
25-49	101	104	100	98	96
50-99	134	128	131	130	136
100-199	201	212	225	232	227
200-299	121	122	119	125	135
300-399	66	66	76	70	73
400-499	34	35	29	33	31
500 +	59	55	54	54	54
Location					
Hospitals Urban	442	449	456	466	469
Hospitals Rural	288	290	293	295	298
Control					
State and Local Government	142	145	152	154	164
Not for Profit	398	400	404	407	401
Investor owned	190	194	193	200	202
Physician Models					
Independent Practice Association	69	82	90	99	109
Group Practice without Walls	16	23	25	35	48
Open Physician-Hospital Organization	127	136	149	162	148
Closed Physician-Hospital Organization	47	59	68	85	101
Management Service Organization	73	95	114	136	152
Integrated Salary Model	158	162	157	139	134
Equity Model	9	20	23	23	30
Foundation	17	18	27	35	55
Insurance Products					
Health Maintenance Organization	97	122	145	144	146
Preferred Provider Organization	137	158	193	212	237
Indemnity Fee for Service	37	48	47	56	79
Managed Care Contracts					
Health Maintenance Organization	385	407	412	419	440
Preferred Provider Organization	462	476	492	507	527
Affiliations					
Hospitals in a System	361	363	368	336	349
Hospitals in a Network	228	224	235	243	266
Hospitals in a Group Purchasing Organization	460	447	438	393	—

TABLE 5

U.S. CENSUS DIVISION 3: SOUTH ATLANTIC

U.S. Registered Community Hospitals
(Nonfederal, short-term general and other special hospitals)

Utilization, Personnel, Revenue and Expenses, Community Health Indicators 1997–2001

	2001	2000	1999	1998	1997
TOTAL FACILITY (Includes Hospital and Nursing Home Units)					
Utilization - Inpatient					
Beds	152,052	150,851	151,812	153,488	155,237
Admissions	6,453,744	6,262,051	6,069,521	5,921,407	5,818,941
Inpatient Days	36,338,028	35,935,189	35,729,929	35,386,749	35,295,036
Average Length of Stay	5.6	5.7	5.9	6.0	6.1
Inpatient Surgeries	1,975,208	1,890,490	1,838,331	1,839,043	1,798,538
Births	694,845	682,848	644,602	640,494	636,723
Utilization - Outpatient					
Emergency Outpatient Visits	20,100,193	19,803,910	18,439,689	17,836,356	17,331,420
Other Outpatient Visits	58,426,774	56,939,217	52,499,260	49,944,907	47,963,630
Total Outpatient Visits	78,526,967	76,743,127	70,938,949	67,781,263	65,295,050
Outpatient Surgeries	3,193,345	3,038,185	2,975,263	2,848,232	2,675,103
Personnel					
Full Time RNs	149,286	148,599	145,609	144,810	137,132
Full Time LPNs	19,553	19,172	20,456	19,985	21,188
Part Time RNs	66,294	66,561	58,528	55,727	55,403
Part Time LPNs	5,903	6,265	6,674	6,521	6,964
Total Full Time	632,576	616,500	600,721	601,954	591,722
Total Part Time	189,909	197,464	180,821	173,116	175,934
Revenue - Inpatient					
Gross Inpatient Revenue	$94,782,493,433	$86,421,077,582	$77,252,538,734	$72,017,626,254	$67,582,775,006
Revenue - Outpatient					
Gross Outpatient Revenue	$49,302,316,636	$44,278,693,852	$38,501,572,608	$34,478,992,937	$31,337,176,059
Revenue and Expenses - Totals (Includes Inpatient and Outpatient)					
Total Gross Revenue	$144,084,810,069	$130,699,771,434	$115,754,111,342	$106,496,619,191	$98,919,951,065
Deductions from Revenue	77,834,582,485	69,108,825,847	58,573,353,779	51,565,031,185	45,591,148,039
Net Patient Revenue	66,250,227,584	61,590,945,587	57,180,757,563	54,931,588,006	53,328,803,026
Other Operating Revenue	3,560,755,143	3,203,398,523	3,141,920,126	2,740,968,270	2,656,090,845
Other Nonoperating Revenue	1,030,898,593	1,593,464,950	1,555,718,488	1,534,174,491	1,687,942,150
Total Net Revenue	70,841,881,320	66,387,809,060	61,878,396,177	59,206,730,767	57,672,836,021
Total Expenses	66,532,756,720	62,074,155,739	57,070,729,065	54,248,588,217	52,306,033,704
HOSPITAL UNIT (Excludes Separate Nursing Home Units)					
Utilization - Inpatient					
Beds	139,864	137,102	137,364	139,020	141,476
Admissions	6,395,710	6,192,854	5,997,119	5,847,237	5,755,968
Inpatient Days	32,356,811	31,455,354	30,973,296	30,748,971	30,744,954
Average Length of Stay	5.1	5.1	5.2	5.3	5.3
Personnel					
Total Full Time	622,774	605,040	589,107	590,779	578,848
Total Part Time	186,585	193,201	176,916	169,483	171,980
Revenue and Expenses - Totals (Includes Inpatient and Outpatient)					
Total Net Revenue	$70,107,007,948	$64,887,088,976	$61,054,258,380	$58,320,553,086	$56,902,698,161
Total Expenses	65,904,113,552	61,442,541,205	56,365,852,982	53,515,276,584	51,670,789,359
COMMUNITY HEALTH INDICATORS PER 1000 POPULATION					
Total Population (in thousands)	52,763	51,769	49,560	48,927	48,293
Inpatient					
Beds	2.9	2.9	3.1	3.1	3.2
Admissions	122.3	121.0	122.5	121.0	120.5
Inpatient Days	688.7	694.1	720.9	723.3	730.8
Inpatient Surgeries	37.4	36.5	37.1	37.6	37.2
Births	13.2	13.2	13.0	13.1	13.2
Outpatient					
Emergency Outpatient Visits	381.0	382.5	372.1	364.6	358.9
Other Outpatient Visits	1,107.4	1,099.9	1,059.3	1,020.8	993.2
Total Outpatient Visits	1,488.3	1,482.4	1,431.4	1,385.4	1,352.1
Outpatient Surgeries	60.5	58.7	60.0	58.2	55.4
Expense per Capita (per person)	$1,261.0	$1,199.1	$1,151.5	$1,108.8	$1,083.1

TABLE 5

U.S. CENSUS DIVISION 4: EAST NORTH CENTRAL

U.S. Registered Community Hospitals
(Nonfederal, short-term general and other special hospitals)

Overview 1997–2001

	2001	2000	1999	1998	1997
Total U.S. Community Hospitals in Census Division 4, East North Central	**734**	**732**	**744**	**760**	**762**
Bed Size Category					
6-24	22	22	27	25	22
25-49	114	108	107	106	100
50-99	178	171	180	181	185
100-199	193	200	200	205	200
200-299	100	104	103	110	116
300-399	58	56	54	57	62
400-499	30	29	30	34	34
500 +	39	42	43	42	43
Location					
Hospitals Urban	440	443	448	465	463
Hospitals Rural	294	289	296	295	299
Control					
State and Local Government	114	112	119	122	125
Not for Profit	592	591	596	600	602
Investor owned	28	29	29	38	35
Physician Models					
Independent Practice Association	108	111	110	125	140
Group Practice without Walls	47	41	36	37	48
Open Physician-Hospital Organization	195	206	203	214	213
Closed Physician-Hospital Organization	74	82	88	89	79
Management Service Organization	120	136	141	153	154
Integrated Salary Model	229	244	247	233	226
Equity Model	16	18	18	18	20
Foundation	38	41	43	55	60
Insurance Products					
Health Maintenance Organization	154	179	199	212	217
Preferred Provider Organization	165	207	225	238	278
Indemnity Fee for Service	46	62	58	63	87
Managed Care Contracts					
Health Maintenance Organization	515	530	545	557	558
Preferred Provider Organization	565	575	602	604	616
Affiliations					
Hospitals in a System	362	355	361	353	364
Hospitals in a Network	225	218	211	219	231
Hospitals in a Group Purchasing Organization	593	593	550	463	—

TABLE 5

U.S. CENSUS DIVISION 4: EAST NORTH CENTRAL

U.S. Registered Community Hospitals
(Nonfederal, short-term general and other special hospitals)

Utilization, Personnel, Revenue and Expenses, Community Health Indicators 1997–2001

	2001	2000	1999	1998	1997
TOTAL FACILITY (Includes Hospital and Nursing Home Units)					
Utilization - Inpatient					
Beds	130,407	131,722	133,061	137,667	140,357
Admissions	5,418,071	5,299,180	5,188,356	5,184,548	5,177,047
Inpatient Days	29,208,239	29,197,099	29,318,858	29,828,809	30,356,207
Average Length of Stay	5.4	5.5	5.7	5.8	5.9
Inpatient Surgeries	1,532,612	1,536,652	1,471,103	1,507,364	1,565,796
Births	600,441	607,172	593,698	597,087	596,197
Utilization - Outpatient					
Emergency Outpatient Visits	17,712,357	17,307,818	16,699,402	16,553,952	16,115,268
Other Outpatient Visits	87,341,487	84,498,586	78,099,894	75,159,642	72,780,216
Total Outpatient Visits	105,053,844	101,806,404	94,799,296	91,713,594	88,895,484
Outpatient Surgeries	2,952,188	2,876,537	2,818,860	2,772,289	2,763,547
Personnel					
Full Time RNs	118,745	120,794	121,346	121,550	115,881
Full Time LPNs	12,747	12,183	12,823	13,436	13,326
Part Time RNs	88,913	86,191	81,180	82,308	82,120
Part Time LPNs	8,117	7,573	7,764	8,116	8,370
Total Full Time	568,559	560,718	554,898	562,730	549,772
Total Part Time	277,406	267,821	258,605	260,915	264,058
Revenue - Inpatient					
Gross Inpatient Revenue	$77,251,473,672	$69,620,488,497	$63,685,574,779	$61,824,762,835	$59,060,852,695
Revenue - Outpatient					
Gross Outpatient Revenue	$51,950,625,736	$45,806,914,434	$40,204,948,871	$36,725,357,346	$33,622,382,861
Revenue and Expenses - Totals (Includes Inpatient and Outpatient)					
Total Gross Revenue	$129,202,099,408	$115,427,402,931	$103,890,523,650	$98,550,120,181	$92,683,235,556
Deductions from Revenue	65,676,992,538	56,498,399,187	48,691,629,504	44,146,428,562	39,534,972,633
Net Patient Revenue	63,525,106,870	58,929,003,744	55,198,894,146	54,403,691,619	53,148,262,923
Other Operating Revenue	3,607,534,822	3,175,250,858	3,010,491,498	3,056,945,596	3,085,403,252
Other Nonoperating Revenue	917,722,672	2,618,184,368	2,339,165,296	2,184,116,633	1,954,877,424
Total Net Revenue	68,050,364,364	64,722,438,970	60,548,550,940	59,644,753,848	58,188,543,599
Total Expenses	65,691,365,693	60,750,436,230	57,553,715,808	55,835,095,439	53,644,026,600
HOSPITAL UNIT (Excludes Separate Nursing Home Units)					
Utilization - Inpatient					
Beds	119,618	119,146	119,021	124,140	125,955
Admissions	5,346,426	5,218,146	5,091,228	5,093,302	5,065,334
Inpatient Days	25,943,340	25,392,256	25,194,957	25,619,752	25,773,576
Average Length of Stay	4.9	4.9	4.9	5.0	5.1
Personnel					
Total Full Time	561,829	551,564	545,069	552,820	538,509
Total Part Time	273,564	262,824	253,308	255,483	257,716
Revenue and Expenses - Totals (Includes Inpatient and Outpatient)					
Total Net Revenue	$67,427,818,977	$64,122,423,465	$59,695,796,166	$58,792,191,305	$57,255,248,871
Total Expenses	65,195,547,192	60,219,162,173	56,849,086,779	55,104,048,550	52,923,975,256
COMMUNITY HEALTH INDICATORS PER 1000 POPULATION					
Total Population (in thousands)	45,363	45,155	44,442	44,257	44,082
Inpatient					
Beds	2.9	2.9	3.0	3.1	3.2
Admissions	119.4	117.4	116.7	117.1	117.4
Inpatient Days	643.9	646.6	659.7	674.0	688.6
Inpatient Surgeries	33.8	34.0	33.1	34.1	35.5
Births	13.2	13.4	13.4	13.5	13.5
Outpatient					
Emergency Outpatient Visits	390.5	383.3	375.8	374.0	365.6
Other Outpatient Visits	1,925.4	1,871.3	1,757.3	1,698.2	1,651.0
Total Outpatient Visits	2,315.8	2,254.6	2,133.1	2,072.3	2,016.6
Outpatient Surgeries	65.1	63.7	63.4	62.6	62.7
Expense per Capita (per person)	$1,448.1	$1,345.4	$1,295.0	$1,261.6	$1,216.9

TABLE 5

U.S. CENSUS DIVISION 5: EAST SOUTH CENTRAL

U.S. Registered Community Hospitals
(Nonfederal, short-term general and other special hospitals)

Overview 1997–2001

	2001	2000	1999	1998	1997
Total U.S. Community Hospitals in Census Division 5, East South Central	**429**	**429**	**431**	**434**	**437**
Bed Size Category					
6-24	8	8	7	7	7
25-49	81	79	77	71	71
50-99	118	120	131	140	141
100-199	125	126	120	122	119
200-299	42	45	44	42	44
300-399	21	21	24	21	22
400-499	16	12	8	13	12
500 +	18	18	20	18	21
Location					
Hospitals Urban	169	167	168	169	172
Hospitals Rural	260	262	263	265	265
Control					
State and Local Government	125	127	130	134	135
Not for Profit	196	194	197	198	185
Investor owned	108	108	104	102	117
Physician Models					
Independent Practice Association	93	47	54	59	61
Group Practice without Walls	63	16	13	16	18
Open Physician-Hospital Organization	58	56	68	79	81
Closed Physician-Hospital Organization	12	16	20	17	25
Management Service Organization	48	53	61	65	74
Integrated Salary Model	69	62	58	54	57
Equity Model	5	6	7	10	12
Foundation	28	33	29	26	30
Insurance Products					
Health Maintenance Organization	54	60	73	76	91
Preferred Provider Organization	113	103	132	138	170
Indemnity Fee for Service	30	26	32	35	51
Managed Care Contracts					
Health Maintenance Organization	169	150	166	169	212
Preferred Provider Organization	244	183	200	202	304
Affiliations					
Hospitals in a System	203	174	192	189	196
Hospitals in a Network	96	81	86	93	110
Hospitals in a Group Purchasing Organization	219	190	190	166	—

U.S. Census Divisions

TABLE 5

U.S. CENSUS DIVISION 5: EAST SOUTH CENTRAL

U.S. Registered Community Hospitals
(Nonfederal, short-term general and other special hospitals)

Utilization, Personnel, Revenue and Expenses, Community Health Indicators 1997–2001

	2001	2000	1999	1998	1997
TOTAL FACILITY (Includes Hospital and Nursing Home Units)					
Utilization - Inpatient					
Beds	65,898	65,356	65,106	65,925	67,931
Admissions	2,467,417	2,424,100	2,407,150	2,354,428	2,403,693
Inpatient Days	13,998,816	14,074,178	14,113,317	14,054,783	14,585,127
Average Length of Stay	5.7	5.8	5.9	6.0	6.1
Inpatient Surgeries	713,144	721,871	717,980	737,115	732,218
Births	227,383	225,101	226,028	219,666	224,795
Utilization - Outpatient					
Emergency Outpatient Visits	8,156,784	8,104,971	7,978,531	7,536,558	7,401,307
Other Outpatient Visits	21,946,093	22,539,023	20,776,140	19,280,003	18,692,986
Total Outpatient Visits	30,102,877	30,643,994	28,754,671	26,816,561	26,094,293
Outpatient Surgeries	1,213,146	1,188,571	1,137,417	1,092,446	1,029,423
Personnel					
Full Time RNs	53,990	55,378	56,988	56,281	55,900
Full Time LPNs	11,156	10,173	10,980	12,739	12,602
Part Time RNs	20,347	19,888	17,267	16,791	16,509
Part Time LPNs	2,953	2,788	2,706	3,296	3,306
Total Full Time	240,670	234,318	235,391	239,503	238,526
Total Part Time	61,263	63,007	54,327	55,290	54,559
Revenue - Inpatient					
Gross Inpatient Revenue	$33,763,537,509	$30,460,414,643	$28,522,093,205	$26,782,314,962	$25,624,532,917
Revenue - Outpatient					
Gross Outpatient Revenue	$18,799,075,976	$16,791,511,923	$14,755,549,582	$13,281,422,038	$12,370,979,770
Revenue and Expenses - Totals (Includes Inpatient and Outpatient)					
Total Gross Revenue	$52,562,613,485	$47,251,926,566	$43,277,642,787	$40,063,737,000	$37,995,512,687
Deductions from Revenue	29,633,078,052	26,118,962,696	23,230,987,570	20,499,152,910	18,582,677,555
Net Patient Revenue	22,929,535,433	21,132,963,870	20,046,655,217	19,564,584,090	19,412,835,132
Other Operating Revenue	1,079,038,669	1,196,170,102	1,213,648,825	966,961,293	868,503,354
Other Nonoperating Revenue	537,095,911	626,610,283	460,092,660	491,564,566	491,475,527
Total Net Revenue	24,545,670,013	22,955,744,255	21,720,396,702	21,023,109,949	20,772,814,013
Total Expenses	23,153,845,874	21,606,133,823	20,621,277,359	19,556,107,048	18,897,633,039
HOSPITAL UNIT (Excludes Separate Nursing Home Units)					
Utilization - Inpatient					
Beds	60,461	59,945	58,914	59,963	62,005
Admissions	2,440,081	2,396,395	2,374,559	2,327,111	2,377,315
Inpatient Days	12,160,748	12,269,882	12,083,301	12,124,969	12,611,216
Average Length of Stay	5.0	5.1	5.1	5.2	5.3
Personnel					
Total Full Time	236,531	230,035	229,862	234,564	233,842
Total Part Time	60,176	61,799	52,946	54,215	53,331
Revenue and Expenses - Totals (Includes Inpatient and Outpatient)					
Total Net Revenue	$24,261,954,693	$22,629,453,822	$21,349,301,577	$20,725,426,356	$20,493,554,462
Total Expenses	22,927,686,517	21,350,689,942	20,365,677,195	19,324,088,783	18,677,976,725
COMMUNITY HEALTH INDICATORS PER 1000 POPULATION					
Total Population (in thousands)	17,128	17,023	16,583	16,469	16,338
Inpatient					
Beds	3.8	3.8	3.9	4.0	4.2
Admissions	144.1	142.4	145.2	143.0	147.1
Inpatient Days	817.3	826.8	851.1	853.4	892.7
Inpatient Surgeries	41.6	42.4	43.3	44.8	44.8
Births	13.3	13.2	13.6	13.3	13.8
Outpatient					
Emergency Outpatient Visits	476.2	476.1	481.1	457.6	453.0
Other Outpatient Visits	1,281.3	1,324.0	1,252.9	1,170.7	1,144.1
Total Outpatient Visits	1,757.5	1,800.2	1,734.0	1,628.3	1,597.1
Outpatient Surgeries	70.8	69.8	68.6	66.3	63.0
Expense per Capita (per person)	$1,351.8	$1,269.2	$1,243.5	$1,187.4	$1,156.6

TABLE 5

U.S. CENSUS DIVISION 6: WEST NORTH CENTRAL

U.S. Registered Community Hospitals
(Nonfederal, short-term general and other special hospitals)

Overview 1997–2001

	2001	2000	1999	1998	1997
Total U.S. Community Hospitals in Census Division 6, West North Central	**673**	**673**	**672**	**681**	**682**
Bed Size Category					
6-24	85	87	85	88	87
25-49	188	186	183	188	193
50-99	185	182	185	180	176
100-199	112	113	116	121	123
200-299	48	48	44	48	47
300-399	22	25	31	25	26
400-499	14	13	7	9	9
500 +	19	19	21	22	21
Location					
Hospitals Urban	181	176	175	178	180
Hospitals Rural	492	497	497	503	502
Control					
State and Local Government	245	250	248	258	263
Not for Profit	402	403	402	396	391
Investor owned	26	20	22	27	28
Physician Models					
Independent Practice Association	95	95	83	95	109
Group Practice without Walls	22	24	23	32	38
Open Physician-Hospital Organization	97	99	103	113	121
Closed Physician-Hospital Organization	46	50	62	64	58
Management Service Organization	35	37	57	68	79
Integrated Salary Model	230	221	219	204	187
Equity Model	5	7	5	11	15
Foundation	16	17	31	39	44
Insurance Products					
Health Maintenance Organization	90	119	139	140	143
Preferred Provider Organization	130	152	162	176	196
Indemnity Fee for Service	37	41	45	56	64
Managed Care Contracts					
Health Maintenance Organization	338	337	338	339	361
Preferred Provider Organization	501	508	491	483	497
Affiliations					
Hospitals in a System	287	283	280	280	272
Hospitals in a Network	262	262	239	255	250
Hospitals in a Group Purchasing Organization	577	570	527	483	—

TABLE 5

U.S. CENSUS DIVISION 6: WEST NORTH CENTRAL

U.S. Registered Community Hospitals
(Nonfederal, short-term general and other special hospitals)

Utilization, Personnel, Revenue and Expenses, Community Health Indicators 1997–2001

	2001	2000	1999	1998	1997
TOTAL FACILITY (Includes Hospital and Nursing Home Units)					
Utilization - Inpatient					
Beds	75,020	75,842	76,718	76,825	77,086
Admissions	2,481,753	2,411,096	2,346,771	2,305,119	2,290,559
Inpatient Days	16,650,444	16,570,765	16,752,113	16,798,552	16,777,970
Average Length of Stay	6.7	6.9	7.1	7.3	7.3
Inpatient Surgeries	702,686	686,916	685,775	689,445	696,590
Births	261,796	256,291	256,899	256,377	247,114
Utilization - Outpatient					
Emergency Outpatient Visits	6,937,436	6,666,448	6,682,798	5,911,276	5,817,481
Other Outpatient Visits	37,737,290	36,706,774	34,185,839	28,000,033	26,827,201
Total Outpatient Visits	44,674,726	43,373,222	40,868,637	33,911,309	32,644,682
Outpatient Surgeries	1,329,461	1,309,685	1,289,568	1,241,055	1,222,980
Personnel					
Full Time RNs	51,206	51,850	52,237	53,036	49,592
Full Time LPNs	8,162	8,099	8,358	8,990	8,180
Part Time RNs	49,074	46,048	45,113	42,035	44,898
Part Time LPNs	6,465	6,384	6,904	6,630	7,222
Total Full Time	247,196	241,470	240,530	242,835	235,399
Total Part Time	160,957	152,362	145,649	138,554	148,894
Revenue - Inpatient					
Gross Inpatient Revenue	$34,125,326,110	$30,690,964,864	$27,978,962,967	$25,754,385,615	$24,540,540,461
Revenue - Outpatient					
Gross Outpatient Revenue	$21,796,597,517	$18,954,856,055	$16,696,279,258	$14,731,910,689	$13,775,445,692
Revenue and Expenses - Totals (Includes Inpatient and Outpatient)					
Total Gross Revenue	$55,921,923,627	$49,645,820,919	$44,675,242,225	$40,486,296,304	$38,315,986,153
Deductions from Revenue	27,904,622,957	23,918,824,972	20,629,836,841	17,831,563,136	16,003,875,579
Net Patient Revenue	28,017,300,670	25,726,995,947	24,045,405,384	22,654,733,168	22,312,110,574
Other Operating Revenue	1,614,130,546	1,472,106,386	1,441,566,383	1,352,605,326	1,245,827,184
Other Nonoperating Revenue	447,993,850	654,168,860	576,521,233	753,864,537	697,335,694
Total Net Revenue	30,079,425,066	27,853,271,193	26,063,493,000	24,761,203,031	24,255,273,452
Total Expenses	28,645,889,268	26,440,620,590	24,629,816,297	22,971,405,642	22,374,528,707
HOSPITAL UNIT (Excludes Separate Nursing Home Units)					
Utilization - Inpatient					
Beds	60,574	60,766	61,370	60,236	61,123
Admissions	2,428,943	2,348,985	2,275,386	2,205,432	2,212,484
Inpatient Days	12,028,176	11,854,940	11,875,181	11,475,570	11,531,777
Average Length of Stay	5.0	5.0	5.2	5.2	5.2
Personnel					
Total Full Time	239,190	232,906	232,075	233,198	226,415
Total Part Time	153,653	144,687	138,530	130,520	140,698
Revenue and Expenses - Totals (Includes Inpatient and Outpatient)					
Total Net Revenue	$29,384,362,820	$27,176,111,952	$25,386,846,064	$23,955,585,610	$23,538,923,590
Total Expenses	28,042,571,080	25,851,000,851	24,051,512,537	22,296,721,901	21,807,455,342
COMMUNITY HEALTH INDICATORS PER 1000 POPULATION					
Total Population (in thousands)	19,324	19,238	18,800	18,693	18,593
Inpatient					
Beds	3.9	3.9	4.1	4.1	4.1
Admissions	128.4	125.3	124.8	123.3	123.2
Inpatient Days	861.6	861.4	891.1	898.7	902.4
Inpatient Surgeries	36.4	35.7	36.5	36.9	37.5
Births	13.5	13.3	13.7	13.7	13.3
Outpatient					
Emergency Outpatient Visits	359.0	346.5	355.5	316.2	312.9
Other Outpatient Visits	1,952.9	1,908.1	1,818.4	1,497.9	1,442.8
Total Outpatient Visits	2,311.9	2,254.6	2,173.8	1,814.1	1,755.7
Outpatient Surgeries	68.8	68.1	68.6	66.4	65.8
Expense per Capita (per person)	$1,482.4	$1,374.4	$1,310.1	$1,228.9	$1,203.4

U.S. Census Divisions

TABLE 5

U.S. CENSUS DIVISION 7: WEST SOUTH CENTRAL

U.S. Registered Community Hospitals
(Nonfederal, short-term general and other special hospitals)

Overview 1997–2001

	2001	2000	1999	1998	1997
Total U.S. Community Hospitals in Census Division 7, West South Central	**727**	**717**	**722**	**717**	**727**
Bed Size Category					
6-24	80	73	78	71	68
25-49	195	196	187	191	191
50-99	153	151	151	148	150
100-199	155	146	159	160	175
200-299	58	68	63	64	61
300-399	44	41	44	36	40
400-499	15	14	14	19	19
500 +	27	28	26	28	23
Location					
Hospitals Urban	394	384	388	384	391
Hospitals Rural	333	333	334	333	336
Control					
State and Local Government	243	245	252	254	265
Not for Profit	276	271	265	257	252
Investor owned	208	201	205	206	210
Physician Models					
Independent Practice Association	117	124	137	145	146
Group Practice without Walls	25	30	26	32	32
Open Physician-Hospital Organization	151	181	176	189	194
Closed Physician-Hospital Organization	52	50	60	80	96
Management Service Organization	86	119	142	161	190
Integrated Salary Model	101	100	104	113	87
Equity Model	9	18	24	34	21
Foundation	51	60	67	79	82
Insurance Products					
Health Maintenance Organization	104	129	160	169	180
Preferred Provider Organization	131	170	196	219	281
Indemnity Fee for Service	32	43	56	68	71
Managed Care Contracts					
Health Maintenance Organization	452	454	478	462	481
Preferred Provider Organization	550	553	578	547	596
Affiliations					
Hospitals in a System	343	345	339	333	340
Hospitals in a Network	153	171	185	215	240
Hospitals in a Group Purchasing Organization	547	521	417	378	—

U.S. Census Divisions

Table 5

U.S. CENSUS DIVISION 7: WEST SOUTH CENTRAL

U.S. Registered Community Hospitals
(Nonfederal, short-term general and other special hospitals)

Utilization, Personnel, Revenue and Expenses, Community Health Indicators 1997–2001

	2001	2000	1999	1998	1997
TOTAL FACILITY (Includes Hospital and Nursing Home Units)					
Utilization - Inpatient					
Beds	95,071	94,317	94,732	95,291	95,357
Admissions	3,949,513	3,818,189	3,716,015	3,614,369	3,499,916
Inpatient Days	20,782,167	20,064,215	19,957,836	19,575,370	19,313,100
Average Length of Stay	5.3	5.3	5.4	5.4	5.5
Inpatient Surgeries	1,128,483	1,125,604	1,097,488	1,088,948	1,019,868
Births	509,537	503,994	483,514	470,142	458,350
Utilization - Outpatient					
Emergency Outpatient Visits	12,453,535	11,823,842	11,499,044	11,009,388	10,529,194
Other Outpatient Visits	38,124,472	36,704,726	34,854,535	35,091,925	32,264,525
Total Outpatient Visits	50,578,007	48,528,568	46,353,579	46,101,313	42,793,719
Outpatient Surgeries	1,661,253	1,659,492	1,647,551	1,566,478	1,440,784
Personnel					
Full Time RNs	86,746	85,534	85,777	84,100	82,246
Full Time LPNs	20,274	20,174	21,987	21,403	22,010
Part Time RNs	31,071	29,440	27,595	28,301	25,905
Part Time LPNs	6,264	5,767	5,806	5,741	6,426
Total Full Time	382,735	375,496	378,422	376,299	370,669
Total Part Time	100,545	94,690	91,406	96,359	92,541
Revenue - Inpatient					
Gross Inpatient Revenue	$61,419,028,742	$53,960,636,392	$48,750,503,268	$44,816,152,292	$41,326,631,351
Revenue - Outpatient					
Gross Outpatient Revenue	$31,134,758,847	$26,985,710,323	$24,048,411,053	$21,841,270,539	$19,491,181,802
Revenue and Expenses - Totals (Includes Inpatient and Outpatient)					
Total Gross Revenue	$92,553,787,589	$80,946,346,715	$72,758,914,321	$66,657,422,831	$60,817,813,153
Deductions from Revenue	54,100,450,992	46,520,754,796	39,647,718,729	34,734,533,296	30,389,699,912
Net Patient Revenue	38,453,336,597	34,425,591,919	33,111,195,592	31,922,889,535	30,428,113,241
Other Operating Revenue	3,072,362,313	2,917,928,679	2,836,835,943	2,549,861,558	2,348,026,102
Other Nonoperating Revenue	598,918,958	687,359,457	688,647,700	608,344,145	676,895,418
Total Net Revenue	42,124,617,868	38,030,880,055	36,636,679,235	35,081,095,238	33,453,034,761
Total Expenses	39,110,488,373	36,305,621,658	33,769,783,746	32,473,333,390	30,375,897,393
HOSPITAL UNIT (Excludes Separate Nursing Home Units)					
Utilization - Inpatient					
Beds	91,100	89,865	89,550	90,049	89,703
Admissions	3,903,804	3,757,331	3,641,325	3,532,413	3,425,224
Inpatient Days	19,699,547	18,867,455	18,527,824	18,133,098	17,723,877
Average Length of Stay	5.0	5.0	5.1	5.1	5.2
Personnel					
Total Full Time	379,354	371,015	374,262	371,204	364,667
Total Part Time	99,685	93,749	90,326	94,936	89,916
Revenue and Expenses - Totals (Includes Inpatient and Outpatient)					
Total Net Revenue	$41,800,329,627	$37,720,612,218	$36,016,882,393	$34,572,654,887	$32,867,801,813
Total Expenses	38,889,779,063	36,104,024,942	33,477,930,476	32,125,816,230	30,038,541,024
COMMUNITY HEALTH INDICATORS PER 1000 POPULATION					
Total Population (In thousands)	31,943	31,445	30,326	29,953	29,545
Inpatient					
Beds	3.0	3.0	3.1	3.2	3.2
Admissions	123.6	121.4	122.5	120.7	118.5
Inpatient Days	650.6	638.1	658.1	653.5	653.7
Inpatient Surgeries	35.3	35.8	36.2	36.4	34.5
Births	16.0	16.0	15.9	15.7	15.5
Outpatient					
Emergency Outpatient Visits	389.9	376.0	379.2	367.6	356.4
Other Outpatient Visits	1,193.5	1,167.3	1,149.3	1,171.6	1,092.0
Total Outpatient Visits	1,583.4	1,543.3	1,528.5	1,539.1	1,448.4
Outpatient Surgeries	52.0	52.8	54.3	52.3	48.8
Expense per Capita (per person)	$1,224.4	$1,154.6	$1,113.6	$1,084.1	$1,028.1

TABLE 5

U.S. CENSUS DIVISION 8: MOUNTAIN

U.S. Registered Community Hospitals
(Nonfederal, short-term general and other special hospitals)

Overview 1997–2001

	2001	2000	1999	1998	1997
Total U.S. Community Hospitals in Census Division 8, Mountain	**345**	**347**	**346**	**350**	**347**
Bed Size Category					
6-24	35	38	39	40	36
25-49	86	88	82	90	89
50-99	87	87	91	85	88
100-199	69	67	71	69	66
200-299	33	34	32	33	36
300-399	20	18	17	19	19
400-499	9	10	9	10	9
500 +	6	5	5	4	4
Location					
Hospitals Urban	140	136	136	137	135
Hospitals Rural	205	211	210	213	212
Control					
State and Local Government	108	110	116	113	115
Not for Profit	175	176	175	181	178
Investor owned	62	61	55	56	54
Physician Models					
Independent Practice Association	45	60	67	78	81
Group Practice without Walls	11	11	13	14	20
Open Physician-Hospital Organization	36	49	58	66	57
Closed Physician-Hospital Organization	15	22	23	16	28
Management Service Organization	20	26	33	45	53
Integrated Salary Model	87	78	77	71	72
Equity Model	2	1	3	4	4
Foundation	9	13	16	20	32
Insurance Products					
Health Maintenance Organization	56	61	55	71	91
Preferred Provider Organization	55	70	57	79	95
Indemnity Fee for Service	27	31	25	47	54
Managed Care Contracts					
Health Maintenance Organization	143	154	172	165	166
Preferred Provider Organization	176	188	185	178	193
Affiliations					
Hospitals in a System	124	126	124	133	136
Hospitals in a Network	88	85	80	76	85
Hospitals in a Group Purchasing Organization	252	239	215	202	—

U.S. Census Divisions

TABLE 5

U.S. CENSUS DIVISION 8: MOUNTAIN

U.S. Registered Community Hospitals
(Nonfederal, short-term general and other special hospitals)

Utilization, Personnel, Revenue and Expenses, Community Health Indicators 1997–2001

	2001	2000	1999	1998	1997
TOTAL FACILITY (Includes Hospital and Nursing Home Units)					
Utilization - Inpatient					
Beds	42,116	41,536	41,168	40,825	40,941
Admissions	1,825,214	1,773,119	1,708,013	1,646,228	1,604,756
Inpatient Days	9,432,684	9,198,430	9,134,857	8,882,182	8,752,068
Average Length of Stay	5.2	5.2	5.3	5.4	5.5
Inpatient Surgeries	551,364	551,078	554,791	529,048	503,787
Births	277,576	273,536	264,003	253,440	249,484
Utilization - Outpatient					
Emergency Outpatient Visits	5,444,391	5,579,598	5,254,445	4,724,837	4,500,251
Other Outpatient Visits	22,599,897	21,879,555	21,342,609	20,300,196	18,384,385
Total Outpatient Visits	28,044,288	27,459,153	26,597,054	25,025,033	22,884,636
Outpatient Surgeries	813,341	838,426	849,404	784,044	728,932
Personnel					
Full Time RNs	38,561	38,435	37,953	36,847	36,107
Full Time LPNs	4,809	4,412	4,718	4,955	5,088
Part Time RNs	18,430	20,841	18,639	20,723	20,823
Part Time LPNs	1,965	2,185	1,990	2,426	2,417
Total Full Time	170,748	162,370	163,460	155,730	158,226
Total Part Time	60,208	65,617	59,319	64,597	66,211
Revenue - Inpatient					
Gross Inpatient Revenue	$27,813,469,466	$25,420,640,854	$22,802,959,773	$20,124,462,635	$18,599,192,885
Revenue - Outpatient					
Gross Outpatient Revenue	$14,608,268,942	$13,088,918,718	$11,360,904,338	$10,209,844,005	$9,301,418,760
Revenue and Expenses - Totals (Includes Inpatient and Outpatient)					
Total Gross Revenue	$42,421,738,408	$38,509,559,572	$34,163,864,111	$30,334,306,640	$27,900,611,645
Deductions from Revenue	23,195,132,956	20,763,767,673	17,542,214,999	14,865,885,966	13,254,072,518
Net Patient Revenue	19,226,605,452	17,745,791,899	16,621,649,112	15,468,420,674	14,646,539,127
Other Operating Revenue	1,165,866,873	914,977,655	857,114,840	791,106,156	703,240,436
Other Nonoperating Revenue	355,603,623	350,531,542	333,030,721	345,922,560	336,711,894
Total Net Revenue	20,748,075,948	19,011,301,096	17,811,794,673	16,605,449,390	15,686,491,457
Total Expenses	19,222,843,051	17,634,866,621	16,728,824,652	15,200,038,183	14,367,961,824
HOSPITAL UNIT (Excludes Separate Nursing Home Units)					
Utilization - Inpatient					
Beds	37,453	36,716	35,984	35,608	35,601
Admissions	1,804,483	1,750,242	1,659,661	1,613,954	1,570,062
Inpatient Days	7,973,579	7,691,884	7,569,524	7,278,010	7,167,408
Average Length of Stay	4.4	4.4	4.6	4.5	4.6
Personnel					
Total Full Time	167,388	159,111	160,221	152,142	153,929
Total Part Time	58,435	63,895	57,735	62,865	64,403
Revenue and Expenses - Totals (Includes Inpatient and Outpatient)					
Total Net Revenue	$20,511,142,311	$18,801,244,040	$17,573,081,317	$16,327,873,454	$15,383,846,687
Total Expenses	19,017,095,330	17,452,526,303	16,526,820,028	14,988,846,873	14,180,449,695
COMMUNITY HEALTH INDICATORS PER 1000 POPULATION					
Total Population (in thousands)	18,650	18,172	17,127	16,805	16,477
Inpatient					
Beds	2.3	2.3	2.4	2.4	2.5
Admissions	97.9	97.6	99.7	98.0	97.4
Inpatient Days	505.8	506.2	533.3	528.6	531.2
Inpatient Surgeries	29.6	30.3	32.4	31.5	30.6
Births	14.9	15.1	15.4	15.1	15.1
Outpatient					
Emergency Outpatient Visits	291.9	307.0	306.8	281.2	273.1
Other Outpatient Visits	1,211.8	1,204.0	1,246.1	1,208.0	1,115.8
Total Outpatient Visits	1,503.7	1,511.0	1,552.9	1,489.2	1,388.9
Outpatient Surgeries	43.6	46.1	49.6	46.7	44.2
Expense per Capita (per person)	$1,030.7	$970.4	$976.7	$904.5	$872.0

U.S. Census Divisions

TABLE 5

U.S. CENSUS DIVISION 9: PACIFIC

U.S. Registered Community Hospitals
(Nonfederal, short-term general and other special hospitals)

Overview 1997–2001

	2001	2000	1999	1998	1997
Total U.S. Community Hospitals in Census Division 9, Pacific	**570**	**571**	**579**	**588**	**599**
Bed Size Category					
6-24	27	31	36	31	31
25-49	90	91	91	97	94
50-99	110	108	108	111	123
100-199	158	159	162	175	168
200-299	94	97	96	84	95
300-399	49	50	51	58	56
400-499	29	21	21	18	20
500 +	13	14	14	14	12
Location					
Hospitals Urban	432	434	441	451	462
Hospitals Rural	138	137	138	137	137
Control					
State and Local Government	142	138	143	146	150
Not for Profit	329	330	328	330	330
Investor owned	99	103	108	112	119
Physician Models					
Independent Practice Association	142	140	146	172	194
Group Practice without Walls	28	25	24	26	34
Open Physician-Hospital Organization	33	37	39	36	49
Closed Physician-Hospital Organization	25	27	28	30	28
Management Service Organization	55	64	78	91	111
Integrated Salary Model	78	80	80	61	74
Equity Model	2	3	6	5	6
Foundation	29	43	42	48	60
Insurance Products					
Health Maintenance Organization	62	72	100	113	133
Preferred Provider Organization	44	52	72	81	106
Indemnity Fee for Service	16	15	20	30	39
Managed Care Contracts					
Health Maintenance Organization	243	260	285	298	313
Preferred Provider Organization	255	270	290	301	307
Affiliations					
Hospitals in a System	237	224	245	232	242
Hospitals in a Network	80	65	68	66	79
Hospitals in a Group Purchasing Organization	333	295	301	262	—

TABLE 5

U.S. CENSUS DIVISION 9: PACIFIC

U.S. Registered Community Hospitals
(Nonfederal, short-term general and other special hospitals)

Utilization, Personnel, Revenue and Expenses, Community Health Indicators 1997–2001

	2001	2000	1999	1998	1997
TOTAL FACILITY (Includes Hospital and Nursing Home Units)					
Utilization - Inpatient					
Beds	96,010	94,948	95,570	96,061	96,173
Admissions	4,347,642	4,296,908	4,192,529	4,097,190	4,033,938
Inpatient Days	22,968,771	22,490,293	21,953,126	21,509,972	20,932,957
Average Length of Stay	5.3	5.2	5.2	5.2	5.2
Inpatient Surgeries	1,200,316	1,197,879	1,153,469	1,280,577	1,161,365
Births	630,251	665,956	615,818	623,890	654,880
Utilization - Outpatient					
Emergency Outpatient Visits	13,916,852	13,085,734	12,507,125	11,745,959	11,877,554
Other Outpatient Visits	56,276,529	52,457,752	52,358,495	51,292,889	48,451,939
Total Outpatient Visits	70,193,381	65,543,486	64,865,620	63,038,848	60,329,493
Outpatient Surgeries	1,845,904	1,841,711	1,663,599	1,822,550	1,627,380
Personnel					
Full Time RNs	92,781	86,593	84,598	83,182	78,412
Full Time LPNs	11,012	10,753	10,705	11,212	12,047
Part Time RNs	51,294	64,202	59,976	57,708	52,957
Part Time LPNs	4,152	6,024	5,506	5,939	5,629
Total Full Time	411,166	387,216	380,054	371,349	357,203
Total Part Time	150,306	189,923	171,580	171,241	155,883
Revenue - Inpatient					
Gross Inpatient Revenue	$89,170,723,161	$75,477,661,383	$69,198,015,940	$62,749,840,748	$55,603,571,112
Revenue - Outpatient					
Gross Outpatient Revenue	$38,916,573,129	$34,417,684,249	$30,111,292,438	$26,657,715,315	$23,814,436,615
Revenue and Expenses - Totals (Includes Inpatient and Outpatient)					
Total Gross Revenue	$128,087,296,290	$109,895,345,632	$99,309,308,378	$89,407,556,063	$79,418,007,727
Deductions from Revenue	77,374,399,517	62,997,781,765	55,746,141,428	48,651,158,338	41,144,090,067
Net Patient Revenue	50,712,896,773	46,897,563,867	43,563,166,950	40,756,397,725	38,273,917,660
Other Operating Revenue	2,797,221,202	2,794,056,480	2,556,475,389	2,318,011,493	1,976,563,471
Other Nonoperating Revenue	1,328,607,343	1,212,144,701	1,359,542,968	1,195,596,600	1,005,980,393
Total Net Revenue	54,838,725,318	50,903,765,048	47,479,185,307	44,270,005,818	41,256,461,524
Total Expenses	52,988,295,607	49,162,814,581	46,213,076,154	42,300,596,312	40,058,553,714
HOSPITAL UNIT (Excludes Separate Nursing Home Units)					
Utilization - Inpatient					
Beds	88,815	89,168	88,931	89,958	89,249
Admissions	4,286,501	4,248,674	4,133,064	4,032,664	3,959,942
Inpatient Days	20,858,375	20,803,528	20,024,988	19,732,217	18,863,234
Average Length of Stay	4.9	4.9	4.8	4.9	4.8
Personnel					
Total Full Time	406,127	383,153	375,756	366,916	350,807
Total Part Time	148,479	187,897	169,565	168,870	153,263
Revenue and Expenses - Totals (Includes Inpatient and Outpatient)					
Total Net Revenue	$54,279,461,564	$50,442,556,359	$46,970,677,731	$43,805,071,509	$40,742,090,410
Total Expenses	52,589,699,252	48,846,089,081	45,852,689,635	41,975,871,690	39,664,637,791
COMMUNITY HEALTH INDICATORS PER 1000 POPULATION					
Total Population (in thousands)	45,821	45,026	44,023	43,458	42,863
Inpatient					
Beds	2.1	2.1	2.2	2.2	2.2
Admissions	94.9	95.4	95.2	94.3	94.1
Inpatient Days	501.3	499.5	498.7	495.0	488.4
Inpatient Surgeries	26.2	26.6	26.2	29.5	27.1
Births	13.8	14.8	14.0	14.4	15.3
Outpatient					
Emergency Outpatient Visits	303.7	290.6	284.1	270.3	277.1
Other Outpatient Visits	1,228.2	1,165.1	1,189.4	1,180.3	1,130.4
Total Outpatient Visits	1,531.9	1,455.7	1,473.5	1,450.6	1,407.5
Outpatient Surgeries	40.3	40.9	37.8	41.9	38.0
Expense per Capita (per person)	$1,156.4	$1,091.9	$1,049.8	$973.4	$934.6

TABLE 6

ALABAMA

U.S. Registered Community Hospitals
(Nonfederal, short-term general and other special hospitals)

Overview 1997–2001

	2001	2000	1999	1998	1997
Total Community Hospitals	**107**	**108**	**109**	**110**	**111**
Bed Size Category					
6-24	4	4	4	3	4
25-49	18	17	17	13	13
50-99	26	28	29	32	31
100-199	34	34	33	35	35
200-299	11	13	14	13	13
300-399	7	7	6	7	7
400-499	4	3	3	5	2
500 +	3	2	3	2	6
Location					
Hospitals Urban	57	57	57	57	58
Hospitals Rural	50	51	52	53	53
Control					
State and Local Government	40	40	43	44	41
Not for Profit	37	39	40	38	36
Investor owned	30	29	26	28	34
Physician Models					
Independent Practice Association	6	9	13	19	13
Group Practice without Walls	1	4	3	4	3
Open Physician-Hospital Organization	4	7	7	6	8
Closed Physician-Hospital Organization	1	1	2	2	3
Management Service Organization	8	9	15	17	13
Integrated Salary Model	8	11	10	9	15
Equity Model	2	3	1	1	0
Foundation	4	6	2	5	5
Insurance Products					
Health Maintenance Organization	3	14	19	18	21
Preferred Provider Organization	14	20	25	24	26
Indemnity Fee for Service	2	1	4	3	5
Managed Care Contracts					
Health Maintenance Organization	34	40	48	49	53
Preferred Provider Organization	46	56	60	61	66
Affiliations					
Hospitals in a System	42	44	53	55	52
Hospitals in a Network	7	9	9	13	15
Hospitals in a Group Purchasing Organization	52	58	59	52	—

TABLE 6

ALABAMA

U.S. Registered Community Hospitals
(Nonfederal, short-term general and other special hospitals)

Utilization, Personnel, Revenue and Expenses, Community Health Indicators 1997–2001

	2001	2000	1999	1998	1997
TOTAL FACILITY (Includes Hospital and Nursing Home Units)					
Utilization - Inpatient					
Beds	16,627	16,370	16,306	16,998	18,599
Admissions	684,923	680,395	670,059	644,283	684,823
Inpatient Days	3,570,273	3,585,804	3,603,498	3,639,125	3,926,995
Average Length of Stay	5.2	5.3	5.4	5.6	5.7
Inpatient Surgeries	190,655	198,439	196,715	213,314	214,685
Births	55,794	57,501	57,787	55,025	61,663
Utilization - Outpatient					
Emergency Outpatient Visits	1,959,967	2,070,702	1,969,275	1,905,603	1,987,378
Other Outpatient Visits	5,826,096	5,893,511	5,866,213	4,857,719	4,994,889
Total Outpatient Visits	7,786,063	7,964,213	7,835,488	6,763,322	6,982,267
Outpatient Surgeries	293,428	287,725	279,495	276,581	286,116
Personnel					
Full Time RNs	14,825	14,551	14,642	14,317	15,533
Full Time LPNs	2,905	2,693	3,060	4,184	3,384
Part Time RNs	4,799	4,782	4,285	5,078	4,650
Part Time LPNs	695	745	709	1,161	1,033
Total Full Time	62,655	60,209	60,570	60,650	64,312
Total Part Time	13,575	13,408	12,302	15,698	14,104
Revenue - Inpatient					
Gross Inpatient Revenue	$9,398,051,190	$8,966,154,419	$8,625,893,202	$8,129,325,907	$8,337,382,706
Revenue - Outpatient					
Gross Outpatient Revenue	$4,564,975,896	$4,271,722,359	$3,898,882,021	$3,638,475,901	$3,577,549,879
Revenue and Expenses - Totals (Includes Inpatient and Outpatient)					
Total Gross Revenue	$13,963,027,086	$13,237,876,778	$12,524,775,223	$11,767,801,808	$11,914,932,585
Deductions from Revenue	8,380,028,417	8,048,660,850	7,494,355,021	6,852,791,684	6,684,012,334
Net Patient Revenue	5,582,998,669	5,189,215,928	5,030,420,202	4,915,010,124	5,230,920,251
Other Operating Revenue	281,472,509	392,404,366	440,819,124	247,784,982	277,788,474
Other Nonoperating Revenue	112,779,032	138,535,799	137,896,417	176,142,839	159,094,085
Total Net Revenue	5,977,250,210	5,720,156,093	5,609,135,743	5,338,937,945	5,667,802,810
Total Expenses	5,664,284,252	5,461,919,463	5,222,381,900	5,096,414,752	5,103,578,781
HOSPITAL UNIT (Excludes Separate Nursing Home Units)					
Utilization - Inpatient					
Beds	15,704	15,382	15,052	15,704	17,267
Admissions	681,266	676,250	665,857	640,217	680,478
Inpatient Days	3,274,368	3,264,746	3,183,661	3,194,922	3,458,636
Average Length of Stay	4.8	4.8	4.8	5.0	5.1
Personnel					
Total Full Time	62,162	59,546	59,630	59,730	63,169
Total Part Time	13,518	13,272	12,117	15,534	13,880
Revenue and Expenses - Totals (Includes Inpatient and Outpatient)					
Total Net Revenue	$5,942,050,549	$5,695,856,842	$5,567,541,618	$5,288,429,187	$5,620,171,364
Total Expenses	5,626,134,980	5,439,545,167	5,185,831,549	5,050,868,793	5,068,620,503
COMMUNITY HEALTH INDICATORS PER 1000 POPULATION					
Total Population (in thousands)	4,464	4,447	4,370	4,351	4,320
Inpatient					
Beds	3.7	3.7	3.7	3.9	4.3
Admissions	153.4	153.0	153.3	148.1	158.5
Inpatient Days	799.7	806.3	824.6	836.4	909.0
Inpatient Surgeries	42.7	44.6	45.0	49.0	49.7
Births	12.5	12.9	13.2	12.6	14.3
Outpatient					
Emergency Outpatient Visits	439.0	465.6	450.6	438.0	460.0
Other Outpatient Visits	1,305.0	1,325.2	1,342.4	1,116.5	1,156.1
Total Outpatient Visits	1,744.1	1,790.9	1,793.1	1,554.4	1,616.2
Outpatient Surgeries	65.7	64.7	64.0	63.6	66.2
Expense per Capita (per person)	$1,268.8	$1,228.2	$1,195.1	$1,171.3	$1,181.3

TABLE 6

ALASKA

U.S. Registered Community Hospitals
(Nonfederal, short-term general and other special hospitals)

Overview 1997–2001

	2001	2000	1999	1998	1997
Total Community Hospitals	**19**	**18**	**17**	**17**	**17**
Bed Size Category					
6-24	5	4	5	5	5
25-49	6	7	6	6	6
50-99	4	3	3	3	3
100-199	2	2	1	2	1
200-299	1	1	1	0	1
300-399	1	1	1	1	0
400-499	0	0	0	0	0
500 +	0	0	0	0	1
Location					
Hospitals Urban	3	3	2	2	2
Hospitals Rural	16	15	15	15	15
Control					
State and Local Government	8	7	7	8	8
Not for Profit	10	10	9	8	8
Investor owned	1	1	1	1	1
Physician Models					
Independent Practice Association	3	5	2	1	1
Group Practice without Walls	3	4	2	2	2
Open Physician-Hospital Organization	3	4	2	1	1
Closed Physician-Hospital Organization	0	1	0	0	0
Management Service Organization	1	2	2	2	1
Integrated Salary Model	3	3	2	2	1
Equity Model	0	1	0	0	0
Foundation	0	1	0	0	0
Insurance Products					
Health Maintenance Organization	0	0	0	0	0
Preferred Provider Organization	0	1	1	2	2
Indemnity Fee for Service	0	1	1	1	0
Managed Care Contracts					
Health Maintenance Organization	0	0	0	0	0
Preferred Provider Organization	3	7	5	4	4
Affiliations					
Hospitals in a System	4	6	7	5	5
Hospitals in a Network	1	0	0	0	0
Hospitals in a Group Purchasing Organization	9	12	13	10	—

States

TABLE 6

ALASKA

U.S. Registered Community Hospitals
(Nonfederal, short-term general and other special hospitals)

Utilization, Personnel, Revenue and Expenses, Community Health Indicators 1997–2001

	2001	2000	1999	1998	1997
TOTAL FACILITY (Includes Hospital and Nursing Home Units)					
Utilization - Inpatient					
Beds	1,442	1,417	1,250	1,240	1,440
Admissions	49,065	46,887	40,785	41,294	40,493
Inpatient Days	303,092	293,707	246,872	378,357	383,646
Average Length of Stay	6.2	6.3	6.1	9.2	9.5
Inpatient Surgeries	15,888	15,196	12,762	10,914	10,932
Births	7,448	7,728	6,618	6,790	6,942
Utilization - Outpatient					
Emergency Outpatient Visits	205,595	187,226	164,113	160,519	152,725
Other Outpatient Visits	1,182,031	1,083,881	868,170	878,092	785,068
Total Outpatient Visits	1,387,626	1,271,107	1,032,283	1,038,611	937,793
Outpatient Surgeries	37,849	34,678	25,640	20,070	21,794
Personnel					
Full Time RNs	1,504	1,466	1,052	998	977
Full Time LPNs	189	200	86	171	188
Part Time RNs	956	768	832	855	695
Part Time LPNs	97	61	60	97	78
Total Full Time	6,544	5,763	4,154	5,106	4,426
Total Part Time	2,907	2,340	2,216	2,487	2,432
Revenue - Inpatient					
Gross Inpatient Revenue	$875,560,013	$741,246,222	$625,651,216	$616,562,865	$593,765,264
Revenue - Outpatient					
Gross Outpatient Revenue	$579,556,236	$452,257,752	$372,382,270	$373,071,577	$345,416,467
Revenue and Expenses - Totals (Includes Inpatient and Outpatient)					
Total Gross Revenue	$1,455,116,249	$1,193,503,974	$998,033,486	$989,634,442	$939,181,731
Deductions from Revenue	624,227,686	460,734,350	383,654,287	363,552,966	322,475,452
Net Patient Revenue	830,888,563	732,769,624	614,379,199	626,081,476	616,706,279
Other Operating Revenue	72,758,253	34,360,208	29,498,177	29,106,660	28,317,428
Other Nonoperating Revenue	19,704,156	17,142,523	15,285,517	14,512,051	13,947,482
Total Net Revenue	923,350,972	784,272,355	659,162,893	669,700,187	658,971,189
Total Expenses	918,694,601	741,993,877	591,317,689	590,184,996	584,279,297
HOSPITAL UNIT (Excludes Separate Nursing Home Units)					
Utilization - Inpatient					
Beds	1,282	1,199	1,047	1,055	953
Admissions	48,661	46,246	40,167	40,891	39,701
Inpatient Days	252,692	227,379	182,521	319,789	224,165
Average Length of Stay	5.2	4.9	4.5	7.8	5.6
Personnel					
Total Full Time	6,404	5,019	4,021	4,975	4,243
Total Part Time	2,820	2,220	2,093	2,364	2,261
Revenue and Expenses - Totals (Includes Inpatient and Outpatient)					
Total Net Revenue	$902,447,973	$759,807,432	$637,789,467	$651,330,722	$619,309,925
Total Expenses	902,546,954	727,117,622	577,708,366	577,187,974	546,266,493
COMMUNITY HEALTH INDICATORS PER 1000 POPULATION					
Total Population (in thousands)	635	627	620	615	609
Inpatient					
Beds	2.3	2.3	2.0	2.0	2.4
Admissions	77.3	74.8	65.8	67.1	66.5
Inpatient Days	477.4	468.5	398.5	615.0	630.1
Inpatient Surgeries	25.0	24.2	20.6	17.7	18.0
Births	11.7	12.3	10.7	11.0	11.4
Outpatient					
Emergency Outpatient Visits	323.8	298.6	264.9	260.9	250.8
Other Outpatient Visits	1,861.8	1,728.9	1,401.4	1,427.3	1,289.4
Total Outpatient Visits	2,185.6	2,027.5	1,666.3	1,688.2	1,540.3
Outpatient Surgeries	59.6	55.3	41.4	32.6	35.8
Expense per Capita (per person)	$1,447.0	$1,183.5	$954.5	$959.3	$959.7

States

TABLE 6

ARIZONA

U.S. Registered Community Hospitals
(Nonfederal, short-term general and other special hospitals)

Overview 1997–2001

	2001	2000	1999	1998	1997
Total Community Hospitals	**61**	**61**	**61**	**64**	**63**
Bed Size Category					
6-24	1	2	3	3	2
25-49	10	9	8	10	9
50-99	12	13	14	14	16
100-199	16	17	16	15	15
200-299	12	10	12	12	11
300-399	5	5	3	5	5
400-499	2	2	2	3	3
500 +	3	3	3	2	2
Location					
Hospitals Urban	46	46	45	48	48
Hospitals Rural	15	15	16	16	15
Control					
State and Local Government	4	5	6	5	5
Not for Profit	37	37	40	43	41
Investor owned	20	19	15	16	17
Physician Models					
Independent Practice Association	4	8	12	17	22
Group Practice without Walls	4	2	2	3	5
Open Physician-Hospital Organization	3	5	12	15	11
Closed Physician-Hospital Organization	4	6	8	8	16
Management Service Organization	3	5	10	8	14
Integrated Salary Model	10	8	12	8	9
Equity Model	0	0	1	2	4
Foundation	0	0	3	5	11
Insurance Products					
Health Maintenance Organization	6	6	8	13	20
Preferred Provider Organization	3	5	4	11	12
Indemnity Fee for Service	1	2	2	7	9
Managed Care Contracts					
Health Maintenance Organization	28	33	33	35	42
Preferred Provider Organization	30	34	31	33	42
Affiliations					
Hospitals in a System	25	25	30	29	34
Hospitals in a Network	7	5	7	8	8
Hospitals in a Group Purchasing Organization	38	32	28	25	—

TABLE 6

ARIZONA

U.S. Registered Community Hospitals
(Nonfederal, short-term general and other special hospitals)

Utilization, Personnel, Revenue and Expenses, Community Health Indicators 1997–2001

	2001	2000	1999	1998	1997
TOTAL FACILITY (Includes Hospital and Nursing Home Units)					
Utilization - Inpatient					
Beds	10,732	10,864	10,576	10,857	10,624
Admissions	562,824	538,704	511,084	495,155	476,329
Inpatient Days	2,520,301	2,501,003	2,383,512	2,407,367	2,400,418
Average Length of Stay	4.5	4.6	4.7	4.9	5.0
Inpatient Surgeries	159,691	160,251	156,688	150,682	142,639
Births	80,408	77,851	74,255	73,470	71,669
Utilization - Outpatient					
Emergency Outpatient Visits	1,401,509	1,520,393	1,340,258	1,179,377	1,213,179
Other Outpatient Visits	3,670,119	3,779,713	3,602,695	3,404,523	3,226,777
Total Outpatient Visits	5,071,628	5,300,106	4,942,953	4,583,900	4,439,956
Outpatient Surgeries	197,227	212,829	200,933	184,461	158,882
Personnel					
Full Time RNs	10,027	10,777	10,564	9,379	9,671
Full Time LPNs	1,130	1,087	1,074	1,089	1,188
Part Time RNs	4,596	5,489	4,490	5,384	4,560
Part Time LPNs	339	483	342	490	487
Total Full Time	43,534	44,168	45,637	39,692	40,443
Total Part Time	13,146	16,142	12,958	16,233	14,267
Revenue - Inpatient					
Gross Inpatient Revenue	$9,022,219,011	$9,060,359,014	$7,422,253,864	$6,671,768,461	$6,257,590,592
Revenue - Outpatient					
Gross Outpatient Revenue	$3,772,046,879	$3,805,828,209	$2,988,190,051	$2,751,942,554	$2,535,871,461
Revenue and Expenses - Totals (Includes Inpatient and Outpatient)					
Total Gross Revenue	$12,794,265,890	$12,866,187,223	$10,410,443,915	$9,423,711,015	$8,793,462,053
Deductions from Revenue	7,796,688,881	7,953,167,237	6,128,351,767	5,261,902,297	4,970,141,242
Net Patient Revenue	4,997,577,009	4,913,019,986	4,282,092,148	4,161,808,718	3,823,320,811
Other Operating Revenue	208,436,718	181,210,600	216,768,538	218,272,428	137,297,537
Other Nonoperating Revenue	50,890,354	82,678,089	92,131,062	86,281,497	76,691,223
Total Net Revenue	5,256,904,081	5,176,908,675	4,590,991,748	4,466,362,643	4,037,309,571
Total Expenses	4,986,268,299	4,797,810,319	4,496,686,959	4,146,260,978	3,848,207,981
HOSPITAL UNIT (Excludes Separate Nursing Home Units)					
Utilization - Inpatient					
Beds	10,325	10,205	9,687	9,879	9,620
Admissions	556,648	529,994	480,299	481,335	459,622
Inpatient Days	2,377,612	2,296,954	2,130,184	2,131,761	2,107,233
Average Length of Stay	4.3	4.3	4.4	4.4	4.6
Personnel					
Total Full Time	42,966	43,521	44,926	39,061	39,360
Total Part Time	13,025	15,952	12,773	16,056	14,056
Revenue and Expenses - Totals (Includes Inpatient and Outpatient)					
Total Net Revenue	$5,225,561,891	$5,127,715,363	$4,525,282,814	$4,392,952,619	$3,927,149,144
Total Expenses	4,951,790,513	4,752,834,132	4,438,540,156	4,083,472,789	3,803,767,955
COMMUNITY HEALTH INDICATORS PER 1000 POPULATION					
Total Population (in thousands)	5,307	5,131	4,778	4,667	4,552
Inpatient					
Beds	2.0	2.1	2.2	2.3	2.3
Admissions	106.0	105.0	107.0	106.1	104.6
Inpatient Days	474.9	487.5	498.8	515.8	527.3
Inpatient Surgeries	30.1	31.2	32.8	32.3	31.3
Births	15.2	15.2	15.5	15.7	15.7
Outpatient					
Emergency Outpatient Visits	264.1	296.3	280.5	252.7	266.5
Other Outpatient Visits	691.5	736.7	754.0	729.4	708.8
Total Outpatient Visits	955.6	1,033.0	1,034.5	982.1	975.3
Outpatient Surgeries	37.2	41.5	42.1	39.5	34.9
Expense per Capita (per person)	$939.5	$935.1	$941.1	$888.4	$845.3

States

TABLE 6

ARKANSAS

U.S. Registered Community Hospitals
(Nonfederal, short-term general and other special hospitals)

Overview 1997–2001

	2001	2000	1999	1998	1997
Total Community Hospitals	**83**	**83**	**83**	**82**	**82**
Bed Size Category					
6-24	8	5	4	3	3
25-49	17	18	17	18	18
50-99	26	28	29	26	25
100-199	19	18	19	22	22
200-299	6	8	7	7	7
300-399	5	3	4	3	4
400-499	0	0	0	0	1
500 +	2	3	3	3	2
Location					
Hospitals Urban	28	28	28	27	27
Hospitals Rural	55	55	55	55	55
Control					
State and Local Government	15	15	16	15	17
Not for Profit	49	49	48	48	46
Investor owned	19	19	19	19	19
Physician Models					
Independent Practice Association	12	11	7	10	10
Group Practice without Walls	4	4	4	1	2
Open Physician-Hospital Organization	24	30	24	22	26
Closed Physician-Hospital Organization	6	7	9	12	18
Management Service Organization	12	10	15	16	15
Integrated Salary Model	11	10	7	9	7
Equity Model	0	1	0	0	2
Foundation	11	13	14	15	15
Insurance Products					
Health Maintenance Organization	17	18	14	15	21
Preferred Provider Organization	22	24	19	22	40
Indemnity Fee for Service	3	7	6	7	10
Managed Care Contracts					
Health Maintenance Organization	47	48	36	32	45
Preferred Provider Organization	69	68	54	49	67
Affiliations					
Hospitals in a System	38	39	32	30	37
Hospitals in a Network	24	25	18	20	25
Hospitals in a Group Purchasing Organization	74	70	51	40	—

TABLE 6

ARKANSAS

U.S. Registered Community Hospitals
(Nonfederal, short-term general and other special hospitals)

Utilization, Personnel, Revenue and Expenses, Community Health Indicators 1997–2001

	2001	2000	1999	1998	1997
TOTAL FACILITY (Includes Hospital and Nursing Home Units)					
Utilization - Inpatient					
Beds	9,535	9,784	10,051	9,876	10,111
Admissions	371,080	368,287	375,297	358,068	346,426
Inpatient Days	2,034,589	2,092,183	2,195,965	2,108,469	2,126,384
Average Length of Stay	5.5	5.7	5.9	5.9	6.1
Inpatient Surgeries	109,244	111,178	104,278	98,224	111,399
Births	36,863	37,723	36,561	34,702	34,386
Utilization - Outpatient					
Emergency Outpatient Visits	1,152,995	1,170,079	1,073,440	931,213	996,491
Other Outpatient Visits	3,340,779	3,237,000	2,882,432	3,236,970	3,180,179
Total Outpatient Visits	4,493,774	4,407,079	3,955,872	4,168,183	4,176,670
Outpatient Surgeries	151,651	154,713	154,726	147,547	143,322
Personnel					
Full Time RNs	8,359	8,817	9,235	8,418	8,288
Full Time LPNs	2,742	2,956	3,088	2,682	2,853
Part Time RNs	3,461	3,192	3,186	2,668	2,868
Part Time LPNs	976	879	888	645	878
Total Full Time	35,358	36,051	38,857	37,029	35,650
Total Part Time	11,629	11,110	10,349	10,143	10,959
Revenue - Inpatient					
Gross Inpatient Revenue	$4,758,131,946	$4,388,134,177	$3,950,394,296	$3,586,801,167	$3,292,550,631
Revenue - Outpatient					
Gross Outpatient Revenue	$2,687,321,039	$2,451,987,458	$2,145,741,679	$1,995,030,902	$1,723,174,525
Revenue and Expenses - Totals (Includes Inpatient and Outpatient)					
Total Gross Revenue	$7,445,452,985	$6,840,121,635	$6,096,135,975	$5,581,832,069	$5,015,725,156
Deductions from Revenue	4,144,999,443	3,722,444,602	3,162,771,954	2,722,206,991	2,302,373,072
Net Patient Revenue	3,300,453,542	3,117,677,033	2,933,364,021	2,859,625,078	2,713,352,084
Other Operating Revenue	103,461,117	95,650,547	95,687,603	103,252,406	74,227,059
Other Nonoperating Revenue	42,618,122	48,896,908	42,627,476	49,083,754	47,620,583
Total Net Revenue	3,446,532,781	3,262,224,488	3,071,679,100	3,011,961,238	2,835,199,726
Total Expenses	3,249,943,830	3,176,562,841	2,972,492,256	2,802,389,937	2,583,850,005
HOSPITAL UNIT (Excludes Separate Nursing Home Units)					
Utilization - Inpatient					
Beds	9,041	9,018	9,372	9,188	9,231
Admissions	368,569	364,432	371,400	353,300	339,848
Inpatient Days	1,875,344	1,855,365	1,967,250	1,881,151	1,826,791
Average Length of Stay	5.1	5.1	5.3	5.3	5.4
Personnel					
Total Full Time	35,066	35,476	38,481	36,506	34,817
Total Part Time	11,549	10,979	10,282	10,023	10,740
Revenue and Expenses - Totals (Includes Inpatient and Outpatient)					
Total Net Revenue	$3,427,559,010	$3,241,028,997	$3,048,845,221	$2,983,447,352	$2,805,490,868
Total Expenses	3,238,102,085	3,158,262,454	2,951,957,813	2,780,940,022	2,560,001,108
COMMUNITY HEALTH INDICATORS PER 1000 POPULATION					
Total Population (in thousands)	2,692	2,673	2,551	2,538	2,524
Inpatient					
Beds	3.5	3.7	3.9	3.9	4.0
Admissions	137.8	137.8	147.1	141.1	137.3
Inpatient Days	755.8	782.6	860.7	830.7	842.5
Inpatient Surgeries	40.6	41.6	40.9	38.7	44.1
Births	13.7	14.1	14.3	13.7	13.6
Outpatient					
Emergency Outpatient Visits	428.3	437.7	420.7	366.9	394.8
Other Outpatient Visits	1,241.0	1,210.8	1,129.8	1,275.3	1,260.0
Total Outpatient Visits	1,669.3	1,648.5	1,550.5	1,642.2	1,654.8
Outpatient Surgeries	56.3	57.9	60.6	58.1	56.8
Expense per Capita (per person)	$1,207.2	$1,188.2	$1,165.1	$1,104.1	$1,023.7

States

TABLE 6

CALIFORNIA

U.S. Registered Community Hospitals
(Nonfederal, short-term general and other special hospitals)

Overview 1997–2001

	2001	2000	1999	1998	1997
Total Community Hospitals	**384**	**389**	**395**	**405**	**414**
Bed Size Category					
6-24	10	14	16	14	14
25-49	39	38	38	43	41
50-99	67	72	74	77	82
100-199	121	123	121	130	130
200-299	74	73	76	68	76
300-399	38	40	40	45	45
400-499	24	17	18	16	17
500 +	11	12	12	12	9
Location					
Hospitals Urban	344	348	354	364	373
Hospitals Rural	40	41	41	41	41
Control					
State and Local Government	75	71	73	76	81
Not for Profit	220	224	222	226	224
Investor owned	89	94	100	103	109
Physician Models					
Independent Practice Association	100	98	109	135	142
Group Practice without Walls	17	19	18	20	26
Open Physician-Hospital Organization	10	13	11	14	17
Closed Physician-Hospital Organization	17	20	18	21	18
Management Service Organization	39	48	60	74	93
Integrated Salary Model	27	30	35	26	31
Equity Model	1	0	3	3	6
Foundation	24	37	37	44	51
Insurance Products					
Health Maintenance Organization	40	50	64	78	89
Preferred Provider Organization	21	26	36	49	68
Indemnity Fee for Service	10	8	11	20	26
Managed Care Contracts					
Health Maintenance Organization	153	172	187	211	206
Preferred Provider Organization	155	170	185	210	200
Affiliations					
Hospitals in a System	158	153	170	169	167
Hospitals in a Network	37	31	32	33	41
Hospitals in a Group Purchasing Organization	199	172	173	152	—

TABLE 6

CALIFORNIA

U.S. Registered Community Hospitals
(Nonfederal, short-term general and other special hospitals)

Utilization, Personnel, Revenue and Expenses, Community Health Indicators 1997–2001

	2001	2000	1999	1998	1997
TOTAL FACILITY (Includes Hospital and Nursing Home Units)					
Utilization - Inpatient					
Beds	73,291	72,707	73,672	74,482	74,119
Admissions	3,332,839	3,315,316	3,244,086	3,170,435	3,110,316
Inpatient Days	17,835,799	17,481,600	17,150,813	16,658,170	16,117,513
Average Length of Stay	5.4	5.3	5.3	5.3	5.2
Inpatient Surgeries	882,138	884,506	843,269	989,428	856,631
Births	493,383	528,444	480,910	488,930	518,468
Utilization - Outpatient					
Emergency Outpatient Visits	10,262,726	9,704,390	9,294,157	8,717,395	9,006,700
Other Outpatient Visits	38,284,808	35,240,037	35,484,904	36,312,939	34,631,906
Total Outpatient Visits	48,547,534	44,944,427	44,779,061	45,030,334	43,638,606
Outpatient Surgeries	1,270,674	1,331,626	1,181,547	1,348,773	1,176,306
Personnel					
Full Time RNs	69,584	63,988	65,955	63,560	59,125
Full Time LPNs	8,885	8,535	8,855	9,032	9,837
Part Time RNs	32,774	45,077	40,309	40,093	35,020
Part Time LPNs	3,008	4,430	3,840	4,395	4,169
Total Full Time	304,856	288,372	291,859	281,708	267,082
Total Part Time	97,102	133,503	115,347	118,499	105,022
Revenue - Inpatient					
Gross Inpatient Revenue	$75,039,514,757	$62,888,212,691	$57,872,210,168	$52,606,987,346	$46,084,240,849
Revenue - Outpatient					
Gross Outpatient Revenue	$29,444,438,788	$26,342,290,083	$22,979,554,909	$20,697,199,456	$18,256,476,724
Revenue and Expenses - Totals (Includes Inpatient and Outpatient)					
Total Gross Revenue	$104,483,953,545	$89,230,502,774	$80,851,765,077	$73,304,186,802	$64,340,717,573
Deductions from Revenue	66,687,816,045	54,071,554,980	48,233,268,070	42,424,919,273	35,696,369,324
Net Patient Revenue	37,796,137,500	35,158,947,794	32,618,497,007	30,879,267,529	28,644,348,249
Other Operating Revenue	1,977,991,741	2,111,614,257	1,920,808,322	1,758,564,441	1,507,260,090
Other Nonoperating Revenue	1,133,993,257	931,691,027	1,113,488,295	930,586,609	777,659,776
Total Net Revenue	40,908,122,498	38,202,253,078	35,652,793,624	33,568,418,579	30,929,268,115
Total Expenses	39,559,376,603	37,075,150,430	34,970,489,094	32,167,200,150	30,199,407,775
HOSPITAL UNIT (Excludes Separate Nursing Home Units)					
Utilization - Inpatient					
Beds	67,949	69,021	69,254	70,008	69,315
Admissions	3,282,183	3,276,996	3,197,409	3,115,912	3,045,967
Inpatient Days	16,282,337	16,393,006	15,871,206	15,371,332	14,697,286
Average Length of Stay	5.0	5.0	5.0	4.9	4.8
Personnel					
Total Full Time	301,146	285,607	289,021	278,659	262,952
Total Part Time	95,942	132,111	114,039	116,817	103,188
Revenue and Expenses - Totals (Includes Inpatient and Outpatient)					
Total Net Revenue	$40,457,487,441	$37,843,321,779	$35,260,844,072	$33,192,772,385	$30,545,198,840
Total Expenses	39,259,239,984	36,841,630,156	34,701,831,498	31,918,474,511	29,909,912,379
COMMUNITY HEALTH INDICATORS PER 1000 POPULATION					
Total Population (in thousands)	34,501	33,872	33,145	32,683	32,218
Inpatient					
Beds	2.1	2.1	2.2	2.3	2.3
Admissions	96.6	97.9	97.9	97.0	96.5
Inpatient Days	517.0	516.1	517.4	509.7	500.3
Inpatient Surgeries	25.6	26.1	25.4	30.3	26.6
Births	14.3	15.6	14.5	15.0	16.1
Outpatient					
Emergency Outpatient Visits	297.5	286.5	280.4	266.7	279.6
Other Outpatient Visits	1,109.7	1,040.4	1,070.6	1,111.1	1,074.9
Total Outpatient Visits	1,407.1	1,326.9	1,351.0	1,377.8	1,354.5
Outpatient Surgeries	36.8	39.3	35.6	41.3	36.5
Expense per Capita (per person)	$1,146.6	$1,094.6	$1,055.1	$984.2	$937.4

TABLE 6

COLORADO

U.S. Registered Community Hospitals
(Nonfederal, short-term general and other special hospitals)

Overview 1997–2001

	2001	2000	1999	1998	1997
Total Community Hospitals	**66**	**69**	**67**	**69**	**67**
Bed Size Category					
6-24	7	9	8	9	8
25-49	16	17	16	19	17
50-99	16	16	16	13	14
100-199	8	8	9	10	10
200-299	7	8	6	6	6
300-399	8	6	8	8	9
400-499	3	5	4	4	3
500 +	1	0	0	0	0
Location					
Hospitals Urban	31	32	32	33	32
Hospitals Rural	35	37	35	36	35
Control					
State and Local Government	26	28	27	27	26
Not for Profit	32	32	32	32	32
Investor owned	8	9	8	10	9
Physician Models					
Independent Practice Association	8	7	9	15	13
Group Practice without Walls	1	2	3	4	5
Open Physician-Hospital Organization	8	14	16	14	13
Closed Physician-Hospital Organization	3	8	4	3	5
Management Service Organization	6	7	7	16	14
Integrated Salary Model	18	16	17	17	12
Equity Model	0	1	1	1	0
Foundation	4	5	4	4	6
Insurance Products					
Health Maintenance Organization	8	11	11	12	14
Preferred Provider Organization	8	13	13	15	17
Indemnity Fee for Service	2	4	4	12	9
Managed Care Contracts					
Health Maintenance Organization	38	45	51	48	47
Preferred Provider Organization	39	46	48	43	43
Affiliations					
Hospitals in a System	22	26	19	22	23
Hospitals in a Network	20	21	17	22	26
Hospitals in a Group Purchasing Organization	46	50	46	38	—

States

TABLE 6 — COLORADO

U.S. Registered Community Hospitals
(Nonfederal, short-term general and other special hospitals)

Utilization, Personnel, Revenue and Expenses, Community Health Indicators 1997–2001

	2001	2000	1999	1998	1997
TOTAL FACILITY (Includes Hospital and Nursing Home Units)					
Utilization - Inpatient					
Beds	9,442	9,391	9,349	9,179	9,122
Admissions	413,605	397,026	383,283	373,257	366,494
Inpatient Days	2,111,549	1,986,526	1,947,693	1,875,297	1,829,756
Average Length of Stay	5.1	5.0	5.1	5.0	5.0
Inpatient Surgeries	124,570	125,630	121,742	132,188	111,126
Births	61,708	61,859	54,800	54,806	54,298
Utilization - Outpatient					
Emergency Outpatient Visits	1,380,740	1,377,130	1,324,504	1,176,404	951,705
Other Outpatient Visits	5,531,785	5,335,591	5,115,007	4,869,311	5,236,416
Total Outpatient Visits	6,912,525	6,712,721	6,439,511	6,045,715	6,188,121
Outpatient Surgeries	201,029	219,396	207,411	192,979	192,801
Personnel					
Full Time RNs	10,136	9,656	9,417	9,609	8,385
Full Time LPNs	824	694	820	957	881
Part Time RNs	4,179	4,346	4,221	4,656	5,735
Part Time LPNs	280	283	317	390	457
Total Full Time	43,027	39,556	39,830	40,766	39,885
Total Part Time	12,781	13,204	12,649	14,345	17,589
Revenue - Inpatient					
Gross Inpatient Revenue	$7,227,257,609	$5,902,881,921	$5,465,908,323	$4,873,956,748	$4,341,256,545
Revenue - Outpatient					
Gross Outpatient Revenue	$4,189,489,714	$3,614,340,221	$3,052,304,763	$2,621,444,182	$2,404,195,914
Revenue and Expenses - Totals (Includes Inpatient and Outpatient)					
Total Gross Revenue	$11,416,747,323	$9,517,222,142	$8,518,213,086	$7,495,400,930	$6,745,452,459
Deductions from Revenue	6,439,372,017	4,994,563,358	4,429,949,594	3,602,908,633	3,041,810,547
Net Patient Revenue	4,977,375,306	4,522,658,784	4,088,263,492	3,892,492,297	3,703,641,912
Other Operating Revenue	479,100,659	321,544,924	244,779,945	191,236,964	213,583,407
Other Nonoperating Revenue	141,537,462	106,349,090	99,153,654	79,577,825	130,353,598
Total Net Revenue	5,590,013,427	4,950,552,798	4,432,197,091	4,163,307,086	4,047,578,917
Total Expenses	4,948,616,302	4,453,861,107	4,188,116,091	3,797,350,129	3,637,019,617
HOSPITAL UNIT (Excludes Separate Nursing Home Units)					
Utilization - Inpatient					
Beds	8,661	8,715	8,695	8,532	8,572
Admissions	410,743	394,223	379,249	369,151	362,333
Inpatient Days	1,867,438	1,767,350	1,749,055	1,672,531	1,653,358
Average Length of Stay	4.5	4.5	4.6	4.5	4.6
Personnel					
Total Full Time	42,445	39,050	39,350	40,100	39,402
Total Part Time	12,595	12,997	12,420	14,113	17,316
Revenue and Expenses - Totals (Includes Inpatient and Outpatient)					
Total Net Revenue	$5,547,464,684	$4,922,342,002	$4,401,477,273	$4,130,522,694	$4,014,005,028
Total Expenses	4,910,277,563	4,425,039,103	4,161,145,943	3,772,942,264	3,613,519,840
COMMUNITY HEALTH INDICATORS PER 1000 POPULATION					
Total Population (in thousands)	4,418	4,301	4,056	3,969	3,891
Inpatient					
Beds	2.1	2.2	2.3	2.3	2.3
Admissions	93.6	92.3	94.5	94.0	94.2
Inpatient Days	478.0	461.8	480.2	472.5	470.2
Inpatient Surgeries	28.2	29.2	30.0	33.3	28.6
Births	14.0	14.4	13.5	13.8	14.0
Outpatient					
Emergency Outpatient Visits	312.5	320.2	326.5	296.4	244.6
Other Outpatient Visits	1,252.2	1,240.5	1,261.1	1,226.8	1,345.7
Total Outpatient Visits	1,564.7	1,560.6	1,587.6	1,523.2	1,590.2
Outpatient Surgeries	45.5	51.0	51.1	48.6	49.5
Expense per Capita (per person)	$1,120.2	$1,035.5	$1,032.5	$956.8	$934.7

TABLE 6

CONNECTICUT

U.S. Registered Community Hospitals
(Nonfederal, short-term general and other special hospitals)

Overview 1997–2001

	2001	2000	1999	1998	1997
Total Community Hospitals	**35**	**35**	**35**	**33**	**34**
Bed Size Category					
6-24	0	0	0	0	0
25-49	1	1	0	0	0
50-99	10	10	10	10	10
100-199	9	11	11	11	12
200-299	6	4	7	7	7
300-399	4	4	2	1	1
400-499	1	1	1	1	1
500 +	4	4	4	3	3
Location					
Hospitals Urban	29	29	29	27	28
Hospitals Rural	6	6	6	6	6
Control					
State and Local Government	1	1	2	2	2
Not for Profit	34	33	33	31	31
Investor owned	0	1	0	0	1
Physician Models					
Independent Practice Association	12	12	15	16	16
Group Practice without Walls	2	3	5	3	4
Open Physician-Hospital Organization	13	14	17	14	11
Closed Physician-Hospital Organization	2	2	4	3	4
Management Service Organization	7	8	10	14	11
Integrated Salary Model	5	5	8	8	5
Equity Model	0	0	0	1	2
Foundation	2	2	1	1	2
Insurance Products					
Health Maintenance Organization	9	12	15	18	9
Preferred Provider Organization	7	7	7	11	9
Indemnity Fee for Service	0	0	0	0	1
Managed Care Contracts					
Health Maintenance Organization	28	32	32	31	29
Preferred Provider Organization	27	30	29	28	29
Affiliations					
Hospitals in a System	16	17	18	17	16
Hospitals in a Network	11	15	12	10	9
Hospitals in a Group Purchasing Organization	29	32	31	24	—

TABLE 6

CONNECTICUT

U.S. Registered Community Hospitals
(Nonfederal, short-term general and other special hospitals)

Utilization, Personnel, Revenue and Expenses, Community Health Indicators 1997–2001

	2001	2000	1999	1998	1997
TOTAL FACILITY (Includes Hospital and Nursing Home Units)					
Utilization - Inpatient					
Beds	8,041	7,719	7,872	6,949	7,238
Admissions	360,007	348,780	337,821	330,091	338,108
Inpatient Days	2,184,918	2,114,362	2,070,480	1,758,052	1,815,702
Average Length of Stay	6.1	6.1	6.1	5.3	5.4
Inpatient Surgeries	102,924	101,548	105,211	105,163	104,797
Births	42,694	42,839	43,063	42,915	43,296
Utilization - Outpatient					
Emergency Outpatient Visits	1,328,651	1,323,999	1,344,816	1,164,247	1,164,834
Other Outpatient Visits	5,160,775	5,409,523	5,473,361	5,334,173	6,060,431
Total Outpatient Visits	6,489,426	6,733,522	6,818,177	6,498,420	7,225,265
Outpatient Surgeries	192,473	192,522	185,381	179,562	183,645
Personnel					
Full Time RNs	6,817	6,784	6,597	6,664	6,212
Full Time LPNs	323	360	331	345	379
Part Time RNs	6,866	5,413	5,727	5,378	6,178
Part Time LPNs	397	321	363	415	477
Total Full Time	35,996	34,079	33,264	33,281	33,435
Total Part Time	22,275	19,311	19,557	18,364	21,485
Revenue - Inpatient					
Gross Inpatient Revenue	$5,235,105,389	$4,793,838,712	$4,607,260,826	$4,282,299,864	$4,221,900,534
Revenue - Outpatient					
Gross Outpatient Revenue	$3,092,163,110	$2,787,895,246	$2,554,529,729	$2,215,490,372	$2,032,728,915
Revenue and Expenses - Totals (Includes Inpatient and Outpatient)					
Total Gross Revenue	$8,327,268,499	$7,581,733,958	$7,161,790,555	$6,497,790,236	$6,254,629,449
Deductions from Revenue	3,787,142,271	3,417,644,028	3,082,461,893	2,620,865,505	2,448,420,386
Net Patient Revenue	4,540,126,228	4,164,089,930	4,079,328,662	3,876,924,731	3,806,209,063
Other Operating Revenue	187,046,158	180,038,222	235,827,532	221,385,804	146,383,079
Other Nonoperating Revenue	89,196,050	139,597,475	130,391,249	131,068,417	116,142,663
Total Net Revenue	4,816,368,436	4,483,725,627	4,445,547,443	4,229,378,952	4,068,734,805
Total Expenses	4,718,315,413	4,396,429,072	4,339,548,425	4,060,531,565	3,859,139,320
HOSPITAL UNIT (Excludes Separate Nursing Home Units)					
Utilization - Inpatient					
Beds	7,262	6,854	7,007	6,845	7,009
Admissions	358,242	347,414	336,878	329,790	337,868
Inpatient Days	1,863,319	1,795,186	1,781,174	1,721,983	1,733,956
Average Length of Stay	5.2	5.2	5.3	5.2	5.1
Personnel					
Total Full Time	35,093	33,092	32,782	33,200	33,253
Total Part Time	21,647	18,570	19,062	18,306	21,292
Revenue and Expenses - Totals (Includes Inpatient and Outpatient)					
Total Net Revenue	$4,750,389,473	$4,425,572,619	$4,401,579,596	$4,214,483,042	$4,047,871,486
Total Expenses	4,644,731,988	4,334,999,636	4,295,663,582	4,051,497,724	3,842,649,773
COMMUNITY HEALTH INDICATORS PER 1000 POPULATION					
Total Population (in thousands)	3,425	3,406	3,282	3,273	3,269
Inpatient					
Beds	2.3	2.3	2.1	2.1	2.2
Admissions	105.1	102.4	102.9	100.9	103.4
Inpatient Days	637.9	620.9	630.9	537.2	555.5
Inpatient Surgeries	30.1	29.8	32.1	32.1	32.1
Births	12.5	12.6	13.1	13.1	13.2
Outpatient					
Emergency Outpatient Visits	387.9	388.8	409.8	355.8	356.4
Other Outpatient Visits	1,506.8	1,588.4	1,667.7	1,630.0	1,854.2
Total Outpatient Visits	1,894.7	1,977.2	2,077.4	1,985.7	2,210.6
Outpatient Surgeries	56.2	56.5	56.5	54.9	56.2
Expense per Capita (per person)	$1,377.6	$1,291.0	$1,322.2	$1,240.8	$1,180.7

States

TABLE 6

DELAWARE

U.S. Registered Community Hospitals
(Nonfederal, short-term general and other special hospitals)

Overview 1997–2001

	2001	2000	1999	1998	1997
Total Community Hospitals	**5**	**5**	**6**	**6**	**6**
Bed Size Category					
6-24	0	0	0	0	0
25-49	0	0	0	0	0
50-99	0	0	0	0	0
100-199	1	0	1	1	1
200-299	2	3	3	3	3
300-399	1	1	1	1	1
400-499	0	0	0	0	0
500 +	1	1	1	1	1
Location					
Hospitals Urban	3	3	4	4	4
Hospitals Rural	2	2	2	2	2
Control					
State and Local Government	0	0	0	0	0
Not for Profit	5	5	6	6	6
Investor owned	0	0	0	0	0
Physician Models					
Independent Practice Association	0	1	1	1	1
Group Practice without Walls	0	0	0	0	0
Open Physician-Hospital Organization	1	1	2	2	3
Closed Physician-Hospital Organization	0	1	1	1	1
Management Service Organization	0	0	0	0	0
Integrated Salary Model	2	3	2	2	4
Equity Model	0	0	0	0	0
Foundation	0	0	1	1	0
Insurance Products					
Health Maintenance Organization	1	1	1	2	1
Preferred Provider Organization	0	0	0	0	1
Indemnity Fee for Service	0	0	0	0	1
Managed Care Contracts					
Health Maintenance Organization	4	3	6	6	6
Preferred Provider Organization	4	3	6	6	6
Affiliations					
Hospitals in a System	3	2	4	4	4
Hospitals in a Network	0	0	0	0	3
Hospitals in a Group Purchasing Organization	5	4	6	4	—

States

Table 6

DELAWARE

U.S. Registered Community Hospitals
(Nonfederal, short-term general and other special hospitals)

Utilization, Personnel, Revenue and Expenses, Community Health Indicators 1997–2001

	2001	2000	1999	1998	1997
TOTAL FACILITY (Includes Hospital and Nursing Home Units)					
Utilization - Inpatient					
Beds	1,853	1,839	2,000	1,977	1,888
Admissions	83,047	83,318	87,200	84,319	80,602
Inpatient Days	502,238	505,422	492,551	508,870	488,879
Average Length of Stay	6.0	6.1	5.6	6.0	6.1
Inpatient Surgeries	24,321	25,878	27,295	27,420	23,621
Births	11,286	11,375	10,896	10,775	10,299
Utilization - Outpatient					
Emergency Outpatient Visits	268,517	286,231	285,276	267,369	255,986
Other Outpatient Visits	1,216,401	1,175,657	1,062,037	1,028,481	970,477
Total Outpatient Visits	1,484,918	1,461,888	1,347,313	1,295,850	1,226,463
Outpatient Surgeries	57,342	52,972	66,234	61,375	61,109
Personnel					
Full Time RNs	2,058	2,179	2,455	2,042	2,504
Full Time LPNs	171	174	173	163	226
Part Time RNs	1,522	1,433	1,347	1,061	541
Part Time LPNs	77	74	84	79	57
Total Full Time	9,465	9,412	8,772	8,775	9,663
Total Part Time	3,936	3,798	3,933	3,234	1,500
Revenue - Inpatient					
Gross Inpatient Revenue	$934,270,274	$899,982,681	$931,058,817	$866,020,507	$840,967,806
Revenue - Outpatient					
Gross Outpatient Revenue	$543,554,090	$465,864,889	$474,399,061	$454,760,376	$403,668,599
Revenue and Expenses - Totals (Includes Inpatient and Outpatient)					
Total Gross Revenue	$1,477,824,364	$1,365,847,570	$1,405,457,878	$1,320,780,883	$1,244,636,405
Deductions from Revenue	535,555,319	484,935,362	489,660,170	412,465,075	380,365,779
Net Patient Revenue	942,269,045	880,912,208	915,797,708	908,315,808	864,270,626
Other Operating Revenue	64,471,002	120,518,768	102,355,170	88,643,163	78,916,675
Other Nonoperating Revenue	-6,015,492	39,475,261	43,155,449	39,565,691	41,377,659
Total Net Revenue	1,000,724,555	1,040,906,237	1,061,308,327	1,036,524,662	984,564,960
Total Expenses	1,049,014,326	1,020,468,822	990,513,404	962,105,695	906,632,552
HOSPITAL UNIT (Excludes Separate Nursing Home Units)					
Utilization - Inpatient					
Beds	1,561	1,561	1,786	1,699	1,709
Admissions	81,719	82,238	85,787	83,107	79,908
Inpatient Days	395,736	405,399	421,774	416,541	427,073
Average Length of Stay	4.8	4.9	4.9	5.0	5.3
Personnel					
Total Full Time	9,181	9,194	8,625	8,516	9,474
Total Part Time	3,806	3,736	3,846	3,139	1,429
Revenue and Expenses - Totals (Includes Inpatient and Outpatient)					
Total Net Revenue	$978,200,536	$1,003,754,485	$1,042,456,545	$1,019,156,844	$974,529,878
Total Expenses	1,023,947,668	1,004,383,808	968,889,580	945,393,771	896,656,999
COMMUNITY HEALTH INDICATORS PER 1000 POPULATION					
Total Population (in thousands)	796	784	754	744	735
Inpatient					
Beds	2.3	2.3	2.7	2.7	2.6
Admissions	104.3	106.3	115.7	113.3	109.7
Inpatient Days	630.8	645.0	653.7	683.9	665.1
Inpatient Surgeries	30.5	33.0	36.2	36.9	32.1
Births	14.2	14.5	14.5	14.5	14.0
Outpatient					
Emergency Outpatient Visits	337.3	365.3	378.6	359.3	348.3
Other Outpatient Visits	1,527.8	1,500.3	1,409.4	1,382.2	1,320.3
Total Outpatient Visits	1,865.1	1,865.6	1,788.0	1,741.6	1,668.6
Outpatient Surgeries	72.0	67.6	87.9	82.5	83.1
Expense per Capita (per person)	$1,317.6	$1,302.3	$1,314.5	$1,293.0	$1,233.5

TABLE 6

DISTRICT OF COLUMBIA

U.S. Registered Community Hospitals
(Nonfederal, short-term general and other special hospitals)

Overview 1997–2001

	2001	2000	1999	1998	1997
Total Community Hospitals	**10**	**11**	**12**	**12**	**12**
Bed Size Category					
6-24	0	0	0	0	0
25-49	0	0	0	0	0
50-99	0	1	1	1	1
100-199	3	3	3	3	3
200-299	2	3	4	4	4
300-399	3	2	2	2	2
400-499	0	0	0	0	0
500 +	2	2	2	2	2
Location					
Hospitals Urban	10	11	12	12	12
Hospitals Rural	0	0	0	0	0
Control					
State and Local Government	0	0	1	1	1
Not for Profit	7	8	8	9	10
Investor owned	3	3	3	2	1
Physician Models					
Independent Practice Association	0	0	2	2	2
Group Practice without Walls	1	1	0	1	0
Open Physician-Hospital Organization	1	2	1	1	3
Closed Physician-Hospital Organization	2	2	3	2	2
Management Service Organization	1	2	3	3	1
Integrated Salary Model	5	4	5	6	6
Equity Model	0	0	0	0	0
Foundation	0	0	0	0	2
Insurance Products					
Health Maintenance Organization	4	4	5	5	3
Preferred Provider Organization	1	2	0	1	3
Indemnity Fee for Service	0	1	0	0	1
Managed Care Contracts					
Health Maintenance Organization	8	7	9	11	10
Preferred Provider Organization	7	7	6	9	10
Affiliations					
Hospitals in a System	6	4	5	5	5
Hospitals in a Network	2	2	1	1	2
Hospitals in a Group Purchasing Organization	7	7	8	9	—

DISTRICT OF COLUMBIA

U.S. Registered Community Hospitals
(Nonfederal, short-term general and other special hospitals)

Utilization, Personnel, Revenue and Expenses, Community Health Indicators 1997–2001

	2001	2000	1999	1998	1997
TOTAL FACILITY (Includes Hospital and Nursing Home Units)					
Utilization - Inpatient					
Beds	3,372	3,339	3,541	3,552	3,620
Admissions	131,906	129,056	138,408	140,293	129,062
Inpatient Days	903,469	901,167	984,094	977,258	939,547
Average Length of Stay	6.8	7.0	7.1	7.0	7.3
Inpatient Surgeries	42,789	58,333	61,982	47,272	45,890
Births	12,583	11,439	11,824	15,211	14,072
Utilization - Outpatient					
Emergency Outpatient Visits	337,851	284,075	330,143	354,334	311,911
Other Outpatient Visits	1,081,197	1,047,332	1,053,206	1,101,426	919,760
Total Outpatient Visits	1,419,048	1,331,407	1,383,349	1,455,760	1,231,671
Outpatient Surgeries	55,491	74,848	95,860	62,753	62,808
Personnel					
Full Time RNs	3,731	4,041	4,249	3,940	3,452
Full Time LPNs	261	286	324	237	383
Part Time RNs	1,695	1,908	1,328	1,852	1,501
Part Time LPNs	64	93	99	66	68
Total Full Time	18,187	18,519	17,209	17,756	17,666
Total Part Time	4,877	5,266	4,514	4,937	3,650
Revenue - Inpatient					
Gross Inpatient Revenue	$3,109,126,002	$2,730,685,206	$2,761,995,772	$2,704,578,426	$2,428,335,299
Revenue - Outpatient					
Gross Outpatient Revenue	$1,192,439,734	$963,364,001	$972,983,386	$853,089,506	$809,239,402
Revenue and Expenses - Totals (Includes Inpatient and Outpatient)					
Total Gross Revenue	$4,301,565,736	$3,694,049,207	$3,734,979,158	$3,557,667,932	$3,237,574,701
Deductions from Revenue	2,344,359,123	1,987,583,335	2,036,092,141	1,956,975,216	1,592,347,618
Net Patient Revenue	1,957,206,613	1,706,465,872	1,698,887,017	1,600,692,716	1,645,227,083
Other Operating Revenue	151,214,377	111,158,200	144,298,148	181,047,807	158,006,259
Other Nonoperating Revenue	42,742,302	53,069,156	97,579,393	82,508,594	85,093,865
Total Net Revenue	2,151,160,292	1,870,693,220	1,940,704,550	1,004,249,117	1,000,327,207
Total Expenses	2,157,226,423	1,845,801,885	1,971,499,970	1,819,975,151	1,812,028,792
HOSPITAL UNIT (Excludes Separate Nursing Home Units)					
Utilization - Inpatient					
Beds	3,080	3,056	3,256	3,199	3,258
Admissions	130,307	127,615	136,998	139,094	128,095
Inpatient Days	804,586	803,418	880,583	858,824	824,061
Average Length of Stay	6.2	6.3	6.4	6.2	6.4
Personnel					
Total Full Time	17,000	18,235	16,977	17,403	17,360
Total Part Time	4,755	5,163	4,409	4,747	3,535
Revenue and Expenses - Totals (Includes Inpatient and Outpatient)					
Total Net Revenue	$2,119,026,870	$1,846,118,330	$1,910,666,848	$1,828,063,922	$1,853,499,085
Total Expenses	2,130,816,375	1,824,373,545	1,946,444,149	1,804,493,901	1,789,783,819
COMMUNITY HEALTH INDICATORS PER 1000 POPULATION					
Total Population (in thousands)	572	572	519	521	529
Inpatient					
Beds	5.9	5.8	6.8	6.8	6.8
Admissions	230.7	225.6	266.7	269.1	244.1
Inpatient Days	1,580.0	1,575.3	1,896.1	1,874.2	1,776.9
Inpatient Surgeries	74.8	102.0	119.4	90.7	86.8
Births	22.0	20.0	22.8	29.2	26.6
Outpatient					
Emergency Outpatient Visits	590.8	496.6	636.1	679.5	589.9
Other Outpatient Visits	1,890.8	1,830.8	2,029.3	2,112.3	1,739.5
Total Outpatient Visits	2,481.6	2,327.4	2,665.4	2,791.9	2,329.4
Outpatient Surgeries	97.0	130.8	184.7	120.3	118.8
Expense per Capita (per person)	$3,772.5	$3,226.6	$3,798.7	$3,490.4	$3,427.0

TABLE 6

FLORIDA

U.S. Registered Community Hospitals
(Nonfederal, short-term general and other special hospitals)

Overview 1997–2001

	2001	2000	1999	1998	1997
Total Community Hospitals	**202**	**202**	**203**	**204**	**206**
Bed Size Category					
6-24	2	2	3	5	4
25-49	21	22	20	15	17
50-99	30	27	32	29	30
100-199	51	53	52	57	53
200-299	37	38	37	41	45
300-399	24	24	24	23	21
400-499	14	14	13	13	15
500 +	23	22	22	21	21
Location					
Hospitals Urban	170	171	172	173	175
Hospitals Rural	32	31	31	31	31
Control					
State and Local Government	20	19	24	21	24
Not for Profit	87	88	86	90	87
Investor owned	95	95	93	93	95
Physician Models					
Independent Practice Association	22	22	21	27	31
Group Practice without Walls	6	7	7	10	10
Open Physician-Hospital Organization	20	24	23	29	40
Closed Physician-Hospital Organization	7	13	18	22	23
Management Service Organization	16	27	30	37	43
Integrated Salary Model	30	29	31	30	28
Equity Model	1	2	3	1	3
Foundation	1	2	4	4	7
Insurance Products					
Health Maintenance Organization	20	25	30	30	37
Preferred Provider Organization	19	22	34	38	45
Indemnity Fee for Service	8	10	3	7	9
Managed Care Contracts					
Health Maintenance Organization	90	94	97	103	119
Preferred Provider Organization	97	96	96	106	124
Affiliations					
Hospitals in a System	88	88	91	84	101
Hospitals in a Network	31	31	38	29	44
Hospitals in a Group Purchasing Organization	98	93	89	73	—

TABLE 6

FLORIDA

U.S. Registered Community Hospitals
(Nonfederal, short-term general and other special hospitals)

Utilization, Personnel, Revenue and Expenses, Community Health Indicators 1997–2001

	2001	2000	1999	1998	1997
TOTAL FACILITY (Includes Hospital and Nursing Home Units)					
Utilization - Inpatient					
Beds	51,762	51,170	49,434	49,231	49,762
Admissions	2,207,147	2,119,052	2,020,073	1,947,024	1,882,928
Inpatient Days	11,521,025	11,345,469	11,135,544	10,839,718	10,659,344
Average Length of Stay	5.2	5.4	5.5	5.6	5.7
Inpatient Surgeries	660,330	614,345	570,283	597,151	547,981
Births	204,753	193,344	180,857	180,131	183,852
Utilization - Outpatient					
Emergency Outpatient Visits	5,879,596	6,041,546	5,488,609	5,285,638	5,041,372
Other Outpatient Visits	14,891,198	15,752,042	14,210,881	14,160,604	13,631,515
Total Outpatient Visits	20,770,794	21,793,588	19,699,490	19,446,242	18,672,887
Outpatient Surgeries	857,272	816,677	803,554	825,987	738,491
Personnel					
Full Time RNs	48,277	47,635	45,140	44,510	41,234
Full Time LPNs	6,224	6,258	6,898	6,345	6,455
Part Time RNs	14,235	17,432	15,741	14,439	14,334
Part Time LPNs	1,550	1,799	1,894	1,614	2,124
Total Full Time	198,925	193,653	186,175	186,555	180,678
Total Part Time	40,983	52,267	48,474	43,501	43,555
Revenue - Inpatient					
Gross Inpatient Revenue	$38,526,016,053	$36,166,618,934	$30,772,909,076	$28,063,792,535	$26,272,191,774
Revenue - Outpatient					
Gross Outpatient Revenue	$17,579,375,385	$16,339,412,601	$14,207,698,162	$12,690,404,737	$11,732,584,498
Revenue and Expenses - Totals (Includes Inpatient and Outpatient)					
Total Gross Revenue	$56,105,391,438	$52,506,031,535	$44,980,607,238	$40,754,197,272	$38,004,776,272
Deductions from Revenue	35,545,733,610	33,270,201,252	27,234,827,859	23,887,698,462	21,512,040,371
Net Patient Revenue	20,559,657,828	19,235,830,283	17,745,779,379	16,866,498,810	16,492,735,901
Other Operating Revenue	1,232,856,710	1,060,248,158	993,711,653	915,677,497	861,581,186
Other Nonoperating Revenue	287,972,889	516,162,789	438,224,356	404,349,404	414,907,897
Total Net Revenue	22,080,487,427	20,812,241,230	19,177,715,388	18,186,525,711	17,769,224,984
Total Expenses	20,475,866,330	19,289,627,098	17,522,447,345	16,741,873,851	16,131,930,686
HOSPITAL UNIT (Excludes Separate Nursing Home Units)					
Utilization - Inpatient					
Beds	49,865	48,979	47,342	46,735	47,108
Admissions	2,193,104	2,098,216	1,999,574	1,923,396	1,862,937
Inpatient Days	10,918,750	10,688,767	10,464,347	10,058,943	9,830,054
Average Length of Stay	5.0	5.1	5.2	5.2	5.3
Personnel					
Total Full Time	197,587	191,191	183,992	184,283	178,054
Total Part Time	40,716	51,396	47,889	42,974	43,100
Revenue and Expenses - Totals (Includes Inpatient and Outpatient)					
Total Net Revenue	$21,928,434,635	$20,649,613,293	$18,999,058,161	$17,971,784,870	$17,563,050,900
Total Expenses	20,345,809,450	19,160,212,008	17,374,197,783	16,582,856,855	15,984,189,115
COMMUNITY HEALTH INDICATORS PER 1000 POPULATION					
Total Population (in thousands)	16,397	15,982	15,111	14,908	14,683
Inpatient					
Beds	3.2	3.2	3.3	3.3	3.4
Admissions	134.6	132.6	133.7	130.6	128.2
Inpatient Days	702.7	709.9	736.9	727.1	725.9
Inpatient Surgeries	40.3	38.4	37.7	40.1	37.3
Births	12.5	12.1	12.0	12.1	12.5
Outpatient					
Emergency Outpatient Visits	358.6	378.0	363.2	354.5	343.3
Other Outpatient Visits	908.2	985.6	940.4	949.9	928.4
Total Outpatient Visits	1,266.8	1,363.6	1,303.6	1,304.4	1,271.7
Outpatient Surgeries	52.3	51.1	53.2	55.4	50.3
Expense per Capita (per person)	$1,248.8	$1,206.9	$1,159.6	$1,123.0	$1,098.7

TABLE 6

GEORGIA

U.S. Registered Community Hospitals
(Nonfederal, short-term general and other special hospitals)

Overview 1997–2001

	2001	2000	1999	1998	1997
Total Community Hospitals	**147**	**151**	**154**	**156**	**158**
Bed Size Category					
6-24	4	5	4	5	2
25-49	34	36	36	36	33
50-99	28	28	23	24	31
100-199	42	43	51	49	49
200-299	13	14	14	16	14
300-399	10	11	14	13	18
400-499	9	9	9	10	7
500 +	7	5	3	3	4
Location					
Hospitals Urban	64	67	68	68	70
Hospitals Rural	83	84	86	88	88
Control					
State and Local Government	53	56	55	60	65
Not for Profit	62	62	63	58	54
Investor owned	32	33	36	38	39
Physician Models					
Independent Practice Association	16	18	16	15	10
Group Practice without Walls	2	4	2	3	5
Open Physician-Hospital Organization	22	21	21	21	18
Closed Physician-Hospital Organization	24	25	16	19	22
Management Service Organization	17	17	15	16	20
Integrated Salary Model	18	26	14	10	12
Equity Model	2	2	1	2	3
Foundation	4	4	3	2	12
Insurance Products					
Health Maintenance Organization	14	16	20	18	26
Preferred Provider Organization	41	36	43	42	53
Indemnity Fee for Service	10	9	8	11	13
Managed Care Contracts					
Health Maintenance Organization	58	65	60	56	59
Preferred Provider Organization	98	103	111	102	101
Affiliations					
Hospitals in a System	73	75	76	60	58
Hospitals in a Network	69	61	58	54	56
Hospitals in a Group Purchasing Organization	109	103	98	79	—

States

TABLE 6

GEORGIA

U.S. Registered Community Hospitals
(Nonfederal, short-term general and other special hospitals)

Utilization, Personnel, Revenue and Expenses, Community Health Indicators 1997–2001

	2001	2000	1999	1998	1997
TOTAL FACILITY (Includes Hospital and Nursing Home Units)					
Utilization - Inpatient					
Beds	24,113	23,875	24,784	25,236	25,735
Admissions	903,663	862,797	824,376	821,895	856,076
Inpatient Days	5,484,805	5,479,389	5,625,261	5,471,839	5,529,715
Average Length of Stay	6.1	6.4	6.8	6.7	6.5
Inpatient Surgeries	284,283	257,624	257,164	270,264	268,798
Births	130,673	129,084	113,784	113,640	115,005
Utilization - Outpatient					
Emergency Outpatient Visits	3,149,115	3,128,275	2,854,136	2,731,084	2,705,906
Other Outpatient Visits	8,865,939	8,113,649	7,984,774	7,574,974	7,499,550
Total Outpatient Visits	12,015,054	11,241,924	10,838,910	10,306,058	10,205,456
Outpatient Surgeries	497,614	459,852	429,526	417,725	402,741
Personnel					
Full Time RNs	21,881	22,259	20,681	21,335	21,394
Full Time LPNs	3,888	3,466	3,854	3,793	3,931
Part Time RNs	12,896	11,977	8,977	8,896	9,448
Part Time LPNs	1,224	1,147	1,147	1,447	1,256
Total Full Time	95,397	92,094	90,711	92,013	89,378
Total Part Time	34,238	32,304	27,457	26,545	27,504
Revenue - Inpatient					
Gross Inpatient Revenue	$12,699,629,255	$11,757,965,146	$10,148,108,959	$9,941,881,557	$9,204,473,808
Revenue - Outpatient					
Gross Outpatient Revenue	$7,748,463,309	$7,353,248,681	$5,911,411,142	$5,326,318,708	$4,649,637,696
Revenue and Expenses - Totals (Includes Inpatient and Outpatient)					
Total Gross Revenue	$20,448,092,564	$19,111,213,827	$16,059,520,101	$15,268,200,265	$13,854,111,504
Deductions from Revenue	10,910,867,874	9,922,910,066	7,822,591,409	7,054,393,279	6,032,026,948
Net Patient Revenue	9,537,224,690	9,188,303,761	8,236,928,692	8,213,806,986	7,822,084,556
Other Operating Revenue	582,210,731	496,378,760	632,168,142	437,251,429	501,485,177
Other Nonoperating Revenue	247,374,354	242,231,703	227,205,059	252,900,681	229,398,604
Total Net Revenue	10,366,809,775	9,926,914,224	9,096,301,893	8,903,959,096	8,552,968,337
Total Expenses	9,839,984,105	9,217,250,307	8,225,718,150	7,934,635,819	7,676,386,463
HOSPITAL UNIT (Excludes Separate Nursing Home Units)					
Utilization - Inpatient					
Beds	20,813	20,138	20,540	21,826	22,529
Admissions	898,539	856,482	816,709	815,273	849,808
Inpatient Days	4,396,989	4,184,817	4,200,321	4,378,494	4,459,945
Average Length of Stay	4.9	4.9	5.1	5.4	5.2
Personnel					
Total Full Time	93,155	89,656	88,053	89,896	86,089
Total Part Time	33,810	31,527	20,714	25,932	20,733
Revenue and Expenses - Totals (Includes Inpatient and Outpatient)					
Total Net Revenue	$10,228,892,959	$9,802,309,486	$8,956,729,154	$8,778,169,228	$8,435,648,421
Total Expenses	9,716,646,918	9,104,562,407	8,091,415,980	7,806,605,169	7,580,016,737
COMMUNITY HEALTH INDICATORS PER 1000 POPULATION					
Total Population (in thousands)	8,384	8,186	7,788	7,637	7,486
Inpatient					
Beds	2.9	2.9	3.2	3.3	3.4
Admissions	107.8	105.4	105.8	107.6	114.4
Inpatient Days	654.2	669.3	722.3	716.5	738.7
Inpatient Surgeries	33.9	31.5	33.0	35.4	35.9
Births	15.6	15.8	14.6	14.9	15.4
Outpatient					
Emergency Outpatient Visits	375.6	382.1	366.5	357.6	361.5
Other Outpatient Visits	1,057.5	991.1	1,025.2	991.9	1,001.8
Total Outpatient Visits	1,433.1	1,373.2	1,391.7	1,349.6	1,363.3
Outpatient Surgeries	59.4	56.2	55.2	54.7	53.8
Expense per Capita (per person)	$1,173.7	$1,125.9	$1,056.2	$1,039.0	$1,025.4

TABLE 6

HAWAII

U.S. Registered Community Hospitals
(Nonfederal, short-term general and other special hospitals)

Overview 1997–2001

	2001	2000	1999	1998	1997
Total Community Hospitals	**23**	**21**	**22**	**20**	**19**
Bed Size Category					
6-24	2	2	2	2	2
25-49	4	3	4	3	2
50-99	4	3	3	2	2
100-199	8	8	10	10	9
200-299	4	4	2	2	3
300-399	0	0	0	0	0
400-499	1	1	1	1	1
500 +	0	0	0	0	0
Location					
Hospitals Urban	13	12	12	12	11
Hospitals Rural	10	9	10	8	8
Control					
State and Local Government	8	7	8	6	6
Not for Profit	14	13	13	13	12
Investor owned	1	1	1	1	1
Physician Models					
Independent Practice Association	4	6	5	4	5
Group Practice without Walls	0	0	1	1	1
Open Physician-Hospital Organization	3	4	5	5	3
Closed Physician-Hospital Organization	0	0	0	0	0
Management Service Organization	0	0	1	1	1
Integrated Salary Model	2	2	2	2	2
Equity Model	0	0	1	1	0
Foundation	1	1	1	1	3
Insurance Products					
Health Maintenance Organization	3	3	6	7	5
Preferred Provider Organization	2	2	5	5	3
Indemnity Fee for Service	1	1	1	2	1
Managed Care Contracts					
Health Maintenance Organization	11	11	14	11	10
Preferred Provider Organization	9	7	10	9	6
Affiliations					
Hospitals in a System	13	13	15	10	10
Hospitals in a Network	2	3	2	1	2
Hospitals in a Group Purchasing Organization	16	14	14	7	—

TABLE 6

HAWAII

U.S. Registered Community Hospitals
(Nonfederal, short-term general and other special hospitals)

Utilization, Personnel, Revenue and Expenses, Community Health Indicators 1997–2001

	2001	2000	1999	1998	1997
TOTAL FACILITY (Includes Hospital and Nursing Home Units)					
Utilization - Inpatient					
Beds	3,235	3,057	2,913	2,791	2,783
Admissions	108,252	99,937	99,191	97,717	96,743
Inpatient Days	879,258	847,352	769,824	776,392	829,757
Average Length of Stay	8.1	8.5	7.8	7.9	8.6
Inpatient Surgeries	31,003	28,912	30,001	31,497	30,141
Births	10,007	9,903	10,148	11,054	14,409
Utilization - Outpatient					
Emergency Outpatient Visits	287,017	253,452	239,560	306,804	295,946
Other Outpatient Visits	2,880,570	2,212,552	2,197,092	2,153,289	2,143,391
Total Outpatient Visits	3,167,587	2,466,004	2,436,652	2,460,093	2,439,337
Outpatient Surgeries	52,624	46,250	45,328	49,842	45,259
Personnel					
Full Time RNs	2,727	3,002	2,738	2,778	2,792
Full Time LPNs	420	395	423	459	473
Part Time RNs	1,409	968	1,053	1,198	1,106
Part Time LPNs	138	93	81	107	114
Total Full Time	12,621	11,854	11,697	13,116	12,274
Total Part Time	3,953	3,051	2,978	3,521	3,195
Revenue - Inpatient					
Gross Inpatient Revenue	$1,932,544,979	$1,803,657,551	$1,649,885,281	$1,555,005,916	$1,541,452,700
Revenue - Outpatient					
Gross Outpatient Revenue	$1,063,359,978	$826,991,000	$730,624,505	$668,609,149	$633,526,244
Revenue and Expenses - Totals (Includes Inpatient and Outpatient)					
Total Gross Revenue	$2,995,904,957	$2,630,648,551	$2,380,509,786	$2,223,615,065	$2,174,978,944
Deductions from Revenue	1,574,104,007	1,382,408,955	1,199,936,747	1,076,694,668	1,040,942,379
Net Patient Revenue	1,421,800,950	1,248,239,596	1,180,573,039	1,146,920,397	1,134,036,565
Other Operating Revenue	82,464,076	70,164,871	74,945,697	58,805,480	82,141,707
Other Nonoperating Revenue	30,318,193	33,274,738	28,166,307	29,810,902	38,141,387
Total Net Revenue	1,534,583,219	1,351,679,205	1,283,685,043	1,235,536,770	1,254,319,659
Total Expenses	1,587,146,492	1,360,759,208	1,273,162,963	1,207,907,910	1,207,258,257
HOSPITAL UNIT (Excludes Separate Nursing Home Units)					
Utilization - Inpatient					
Beds	2,704	2,511	2,386	2,459	2,341
Admissions	106,717	97,822	96,915	95,879	94,798
Inpatient Days	704,963	676,735	594,519	664,731	677,632
Average Length of Stay	6.6	6.9	6.1	6.9	7.1
Personnel					
Total Full Time	12,228	11,517	11,200	12,720	11,791
Total Part Time	3,889	2,992	2,885	3,429	3,092
Revenue and Expenses - Totals (Includes Inpatient and Outpatient)					
Total Net Revenue	$1,513,078,577	$1,331,297,637	$1,255,628,493	$1,215,412,826	$1,228,109,953
Total Expenses	1,567,775,123	1,342,654,703	1,246,855,789	1,189,371,784	1,187,926,995
COMMUNITY HEALTH INDICATORS PER 1000 POPULATION					
Total Population (in thousands)	1,224	1,212	1,185	1,190	1,189
Inpatient					
Beds	2.6	2.5	2.5	2.3	2.3
Admissions	88.4	82.5	83.7	82.1	81.3
Inpatient Days	718.1	699.4	649.4	652.2	697.7
Inpatient Surgeries	25.3	23.9	25.3	26.5	25.3
Births	8.2	8.2	8.6	9.3	12.1
Outpatient					
Emergency Outpatient Visits	234.4	209.2	202.1	257.7	248.8
Other Outpatient Visits	2,352.6	1,826.2	1,853.3	1,808.8	1,802.2
Total Outpatient Visits	2,587.1	2,035.4	2,055.4	2,066.5	2,051.0
Outpatient Surgeries	43.0	38.2	38.2	41.9	38.1
Expense per Capita (per person)	$1,296.3	$1,123.2	$1,073.9	$1,014.6	$1,015.1

TABLE 6

IDAHO

U.S. Registered Community Hospitals
(Nonfederal, short-term general and other special hospitals)

Overview 1997–2001

	2001	2000	1999	1998	1997
Total Community Hospitals	**40**	**42**	**42**	**42**	**42**
Bed Size Category					
6-24	9	8	8	8	7
25-49	8	11	10	13	13
50-99	12	12	13	10	11
100-199	6	6	6	6	6
200-299	3	3	4	4	4
300-399	2	2	1	1	1
400-499	0	0	0	0	0
500 +	0	0	0	0	0
Location					
Hospitals Urban	7	7	7	7	7
Hospitals Rural	33	35	35	35	35
Control					
State and Local Government	27	28	28	26	26
Not for Profit	11	11	11	13	13
Investor owned	2	3	3	3	3
Physician Models					
Independent Practice Association	6	5	7	5	8
Group Practice without Walls	1	0	2	1	0
Open Physician-Hospital Organization	6	8	10	12	12
Closed Physician-Hospital Organization	5	4	2	2	0
Management Service Organization	1	1	2	1	1
Integrated Salary Model	7	5	5	7	7
Equity Model	1	0	1	0	0
Foundation	0	0	3	2	2
Insurance Products					
Health Maintenance Organization	7	6	5	6	9
Preferred Provider Organization	8	9	6	6	8
Indemnity Fee for Service	4	5	5	4	7
Managed Care Contracts					
Health Maintenance Organization	12	11	13	17	12
Preferred Provider Organization	22	19	19	22	22
Affiliations					
Hospitals in a System	6	7	8	7	8
Hospitals in a Network	17	13	14	11	8
Hospitals in a Group Purchasing Organization	28	29	27	26	—

TABLE 6

IDAHO

U.S. Registered Community Hospitals
(Nonfederal, short-term general and other special hospitals)

Utilization, Personnel, Revenue and Expenses, Community Health Indicators 1997–2001

	2001	2000	1999	1998	1997
TOTAL FACILITY (Includes Hospital and Nursing Home Units)					
Utilization - Inpatient					
Beds	3,439	3,485	3,499	3,414	3,467
Admissions	122,510	123,187	119,928	115,248	108,440
Inpatient Days	682,010	669,186	694,361	697,744	679,075
Average Length of Stay	5.6	5.4	5.8	6.1	6.3
Inpatient Surgeries	41,062	38,270	38,624	35,403	38,423
Births	19,672	17,738	17,990	17,258	17,426
Utilization - Outpatient					
Emergency Outpatient Visits	411,533	409,030	414,388	380,805	361,189
Other Outpatient Visits	2,228,545	1,748,372	1,767,925	1,795,095	1,762,802
Total Outpatient Visits	2,640,078	2,157,402	2,182,313	2,175,900	2,123,991
Outpatient Surgeries	57,886	53,171	60,607	66,258	56,902
Personnel					
Full Time RNs	2,411	2,370	2,556	2,337	2,432
Full Time LPNs	489	502	525	502	525
Part Time RNs	1,918	1,759	1,676	1,736	1,596
Part Time LPNs	275	310	324	330	289
Total Full Time	11,650	11,074	11,354	10,698	10,727
Total Part Time	6,681	5,678	5,373	6,036	5,469
Revenue - Inpatient					
Gross Inpatient Revenue	$1,311,305,096	$1,243,357,709	$1,132,120,798	$1,028,373,427	$888,962,434
Revenue - Outpatient					
Gross Outpatient Revenue	$841,069,903	$785,301,536	$682,496,769	$625,389,911	$549,001,983
Revenue and Expenses - Totals (Includes Inpatient and Outpatient)					
Total Gross Revenue	$2,152,374,999	$2,028,659,245	$1,814,617,567	$1,653,763,338	$1,437,964,417
Deductions from Revenue	817,619,918	826,933,247	675,699,809	581,633,458	441,055,211
Net Patient Revenue	1,334,755,081	1,201,725,998	1,138,917,758	1,072,129,880	996,909,206
Other Operating Revenue	43,219,742	42,583,119	55,873,470	35,587,970	28,216,566
Other Nonoperating Revenue	38,074,932	28,837,697	31,708,471	33,445,442	32,498,388
Total Net Revenue	1,416,049,755	1,273,146,814	1,226,499,699	1,141,163,292	1,057,624,160
Total Expenses	1,313,949,886	1,167,101,520	1,116,899,654	1,005,344,536	910,642,288
HOSPITAL UNIT (Excludes Separate Nursing Home Units)					
Utilization - Inpatient					
Beds	2,828	2,874	2,816	2,785	2,766
Admissions	119,945	120,655	115,670	111,251	105,247
Inpatient Days	504,028	497,049	503,844	512,257	458,658
Average Length of Stay	4.2	4.1	4.4	4.6	4.4
Personnel					
Total Full Time	11,265	10,801	10,039	10,163	9,933
Total Part Time	6,431	5,396	5,097	5,743	5,109
Revenue and Expenses - Totals (Includes Inpatient and Outpatient)					
Total Net Revenue	$1,390,073,406	$1,249,236,753	$1,191,632,434	$1,104,782,133	$1,020,503,487
Total Expenses	1,292,299,636	1,151,521,698	1,093,475,829	978,344,737	891,759,561
COMMUNITY HEALTH INDICATORS PER 1000 POPULATION					
Total Population (in thousands)	1,321	1,294	1,252	1,231	1,211
Inpatient					
Beds	2.6	2.7	2.8	2.8	2.9
Admissions	92.7	95.2	95.8	93.6	89.6
Inpatient Days	516.3	517.2	554.7	566.8	560.9
Inpatient Surgeries	31.1	29.6	30.9	28.8	31.7
Births	14.9	13.7	14.4	14.0	14.4
Outpatient					
Emergency Outpatient Visits	311.5	316.1	331.1	309.4	298.3
Other Outpatient Visits	1,687.0	1,351.2	1,412.4	1,458.3	1,456.1
Total Outpatient Visits	1,998.5	1,667.3	1,743.5	1,767.7	1,754.4
Outpatient Surgeries	43.8	41.1	48.4	53.8	47.0
Expense per Capita (per person)	$994.7	$902.0	$892.3	$816.7	$752.2

TABLE 6

ILLINOIS

U.S. Registered Community Hospitals
(Nonfederal, short-term general and other special hospitals)

Overview 1997–2001

	2001	2000	1999	1998	1997
Total Community Hospitals	**192**	**196**	**198**	**203**	**202**
Bed Size Category					
6-24	3	4	3	2	1
25-49	18	18	20	18	20
50-99	36	34	37	42	40
100-199	67	68	66	69	63
200-299	29	33	34	32	35
300-399	21	21	19	18	20
400-499	7	7	6	9	9
500 +	11	11	13	13	14
Location					
Hospitals Urban	120	124	125	131	129
Hospitals Rural	72	72	73	72	73
Control					
State and Local Government	28	28	30	31	34
Not for Profit	156	159	161	158	156
Investor owned	8	9	7	14	12
Physician Models					
Independent Practice Association	36	42	42	49	52
Group Practice without Walls	8	9	7	9	15
Open Physician-Hospital Organization	53	51	51	53	56
Closed Physician-Hospital Organization	14	19	26	29	29
Management Service Organization	37	42	48	50	47
Integrated Salary Model	50	65	65	60	63
Equity Model	2	2	4	3	5
Foundation	9	11	10	15	21
Insurance Products					
Health Maintenance Organization	27	35	48	57	47
Preferred Provider Organization	29	35	44	53	65
Indemnity Fee for Service	10	15	11	12	24
Managed Care Contracts					
Health Maintenance Organization	122	140	143	144	148
Preferred Provider Organization	141	153	161	157	167
Affiliations					
Hospitals in a System	98	102	103	104	104
Hospitals in a Network	32	32	38	41	45
Hospitals in a Group Purchasing Organization	150	158	153	143	—

States

TABLE 6

ILLINOIS

U.S. Registered Community Hospitals
(Nonfederal, short-term general and other special hospitals)

Utilization, Personnel, Revenue and Expenses, Community Health Indicators 1997–2001

	2001	2000	1999	1998	1997
TOTAL FACILITY (Includes Hospital and Nursing Home Units)					
Utilization - Inpatient					
Beds	36,834	37,310	37,658	39,218	40,254
Admissions	1,559,357	1,530,800	1,508,816	1,466,273	1,442,514
Inpatient Days	8,215,380	8,189,818	8,267,158	8,640,319	8,542,006
Average Length of Stay	5.3	5.4	5.5	5.9	5.9
Inpatient Surgeries	414,121	404,231	387,355	391,333	399,971
Births	173,967	179,057	176,435	175,567	170,914
Utilization - Outpatient					
Emergency Outpatient Visits	4,582,408	4,497,815	4,420,908	4,325,178	4,207,882
Other Outpatient Visits	20,687,505	20,601,748	19,495,093	18,449,726	17,799,270
Total Outpatient Visits	25,269,913	25,099,563	23,916,001	22,774,904	22,007,152
Outpatient Surgeries	710,346	691,824	654,078	634,897	634,378
Personnel					
Full Time RNs	33,093	33,905	34,481	33,335	30,665
Full Time LPNs	2,781	2,789	3,042	3,280	3,173
Part Time RNs	23,596	21,807	21,044	21,929	21,634
Part Time LPNs	1,116	1,239	1,186	1,332	1,342
Total Full Time	160,545	161,303	157,818	155,054	149,634
Total Part Time	71,502	69,069	65,200	71,091	71,394
Revenue - Inpatient					
Gross Inpatient Revenue	$24,926,910,293	$22,597,529,237	$20,652,014,700	$19,762,078,685	$18,210,731,941
Revenue - Outpatient					
Gross Outpatient Revenue	$14,044,549,597	$12,699,517,400	$11,241,559,394	$10,261,730,664	$9,117,294,079
Revenue and Expenses - Totals (Includes Inpatient and Outpatient)					
Total Gross Revenue	$38,971,459,890	$35,297,046,637	$31,893,574,094	$30,023,809,349	$27,328,026,020
Deductions from Revenue	21,796,610,516	19,210,165,443	17,010,439,012	15,152,657,271	13,020,508,048
Net Patient Revenue	17,174,849,374	16,086,881,194	14,883,135,082	14,871,152,078	14,307,517,972
Other Operating Revenue	1,057,250,792	984,694,243	846,212,294	960,315,367	1,135,032,573
Other Nonoperating Revenue	384,325,832	937,308,890	975,103,585	804,130,431	621,121,427
Total Net Revenue	18,616,425,998	18,008,884,327	16,704,450,961	16,635,597,876	16,063,671,972
Total Expenses	18,304,829,361	17,215,623,885	16,050,659,864	15,467,918,335	14,744,229,289
HOSPITAL UNIT (Excludes Separate Nursing Home Units)					
Utilization - Inpatient					
Beds	33,998	33,695	33,806	34,791	35,499
Admissions	1,526,030	1,495,873	1,469,587	1,425,365	1,388,863
Inpatient Days	7,417,273	7,180,518	7,202,654	7,335,025	7,033,489
Average Length of Stay	4.9	4.8	4.9	5.1	5.1
Personnel					
Total Full Time	158,634	158,538	154,891	151,705	145,424
Total Part Time	70,507	67,735	63,943	69,441	69,412
Revenue and Expenses - Totals (Includes Inpatient and Outpatient)					
Total Net Revenue	$18,410,732,829	$17,824,208,519	$16,449,642,798	$16,317,362,510	$15,722,176,986
Total Expenses	18,152,199,024	17,076,598,221	15,858,782,696	15,180,165,418	14,445,004,962
COMMUNITY HEALTH INDICATORS PER 1000 POPULATION					
Total Population (in thousands)	12,482	12,419	12,128	12,070	12,012
Inpatient					
Beds	3.0	3.0	3.1	3.2	3.4
Admissions	124.9	123.3	124.4	121.5	120.1
Inpatient Days	658.2	659.4	681.6	715.9	711.2
Inpatient Surgeries	33.2	32.5	31.9	32.4	33.3
Births	13.9	14.4	14.5	14.5	14.2
Outpatient					
Emergency Outpatient Visits	367.1	362.2	364.5	358.3	350.3
Other Outpatient Visits	1,657.3	1,658.9	1,607.4	1,528.6	1,481.9
Total Outpatient Visits	2,024.5	2,021.0	1,971.9	1,886.9	1,832.2
Outpatient Surgeries	56.9	55.7	53.9	52.6	52.8
Expense per Capita (per person)	$1,466.5	$1,386.2	$1,323.4	$1,281.5	$1,227.5

TABLE 6

INDIANA

U.S. Registered Community Hospitals
(Nonfederal, short-term general and other special hospitals)

Overview 1997–2001

	2001	2000	1999	1998	1997
Total Community Hospitals	**110**	**109**	**111**	**111**	**112**
Bed Size Category					
6-24	5	4	5	3	2
25-49	21	22	23	22	19
50-99	30	29	30	29	33
100-199	24	24	23	27	26
200-299	13	13	13	13	16
300-399	5	5	5	5	5
400-499	4	3	4	5	4
500 +	8	9	8	7	7
Location					
Hospitals Urban	64	64	65	65	65
Hospitals Rural	46	45	46	46	47
Control					
State and Local Government	41	41	45	45	45
Not for Profit	57	56	54	55	57
Investor owned	12	12	12	11	10
Physician Models					
Independent Practice Association	15	15	10	13	10
Group Practice without Walls	4	1	0	2	7
Open Physician-Hospital Organization	26	32	31	35	38
Closed Physician-Hospital Organization	14	16	14	14	11
Management Service Organization	17	20	19	24	28
Integrated Salary Model	31	32	36	31	30
Equity Model	1	1	1	2	2
Foundation	2	1	4	5	7
Insurance Products					
Health Maintenance Organization	20	32	34	32	37
Preferred Provider Organization	28	42	42	41	45
Indemnity Fee for Service	8	11	11	11	14
Managed Care Contracts					
Health Maintenance Organization	60	73	72	73	74
Preferred Provider Organization	71	82	86	89	89
Affiliations					
Hospitals in a System	34	41	36	35	39
Hospitals in a Network	36	40	32	37	39
Hospitals in a Group Purchasing Organization	78	87	84	86	—

TABLE 6

INDIANA

U.S. Registered Community Hospitals
(Nonfederal, short-term general and other special hospitals)

Utilization, Personnel, Revenue and Expenses, Community Health Indicators 1997–2001

	2001	2000	1999	1998	1997
TOTAL FACILITY (Includes Hospital and Nursing Home Units)					
Utilization - Inpatient					
Beds	19,036	19,160	19,225	19,401	19,406
Admissions	718,369	699,511	683,264	704,396	695,279
Inpatient Days	3,944,457	3,943,695	3,998,799	4,076,111	4,077,184
Average Length of Stay	5.5	5.6	5.9	5.8	5.9
Inpatient Surgeries	195,206	216,204	189,678	196,317	202,058
Births	80,485	81,052	75,076	76,706	76,880
Utilization - Outpatient					
Emergency Outpatient Visits	2,385,242	2,187,447	2,120,329	2,154,402	2,148,386
Other Outpatient Visits	12,008,043	11,946,547	10,993,509	10,580,210	10,250,954
Total Outpatient Visits	14,393,285	14,133,994	13,113,838	12,734,612	12,399,340
Outpatient Surgeries	386,704	388,192	408,893	393,135	393,378
Personnel					
Full Time RNs	15,997	17,308	17,831	17,156	16,656
Full Time LPNs	2,486	2,430	2,373	2,222	2,207
Part Time RNs	10,944	11,696	10,222	11,039	10,764
Part Time LPNs	1,344	1,403	1,207	1,286	1,328
Total Full Time	77,258	76,219	75,902	76,533	73,507
Total Part Time	35,540	35,901	32,134	33,137	34,086
Revenue - Inpatient					
Gross Inpatient Revenue	$9,449,404,551	$8,288,484,221	$7,574,440,688	$7,344,203,384	$7,125,602,842
Revenue - Outpatient					
Gross Outpatient Revenue	$6,380,741,910	$5,799,391,724	$5,058,777,890	$4,638,804,328	$4,198,110,613
Revenue and Expenses - Totals (Includes Inpatient and Outpatient)					
Total Gross Revenue	$15,830,146,461	$14,087,875,945	$12,633,218,578	$11,983,007,712	$11,323,713,455
Deductions from Revenue	7,243,961,000	6,058,831,246	5,130,679,610	4,768,195,948	4,345,392,045
Net Patient Revenue	8,586,185,461	8,029,044,699	7,502,538,968	7,214,811,764	6,978,321,410
Other Operating Revenue	501,261,342	496,781,927	439,652,541	416,591,590	343,260,841
Other Nonoperating Revenue	145,445,011	282,308,259	262,145,842	235,353,311	240,604,074
Total Net Revenue	9,232,891,814	8,808,134,885	8,204,337,351	7,866,756,665	7,562,186,325
Total Expenses	8,446,387,337	7,865,789,801	7,490,717,665	7,192,794,077	6,845,781,906
HOSPITAL UNIT (Excludes Separate Nursing Home Units)					
Utilization - Inpatient					
Beds	17,157	16,957	16,801	17,110	17,200
Admissions	705,746	684,461	664,977	687,644	671,438
Inpatient Days	3,404,916	3,337,863	3,341,593	3,393,449	3,424,139
Average Length of Stay	4.8	4.9	5.0	4.9	5.1
Personnel					
Total Full Time	75,807	74,693	74,041	74,493	71,280
Total Part Time	34,952	35,169	31,265	32,362	33,061
Revenue and Expenses - Totals (Includes Inpatient and Outpatient)					
Total Net Revenue	$9,142,546,269	$8,721,330,380	$8,064,204,896	$7,720,270,403	$7,365,509,598
Total Expenses	8,353,731,881	7,780,952,771	7,368,487,400	7,062,481,912	6,735,464,282
COMMUNITY HEALTH INDICATORS PER 1000 POPULATION					
Total Population (in thousands)	6,115	6,080	5,943	5,908	5,872
Inpatient					
Beds	3.1	3.2	3.2	3.3	3.3
Admissions	117.5	115.0	115.0	119.2	118.4
Inpatient Days	645.1	648.6	672.9	690.0	694.3
Inpatient Surgeries	31.9	35.6	31.9	33.2	34.4
Births	13.2	13.3	12.6	13.0	13.1
Outpatient					
Emergency Outpatient Visits	390.1	359.7	356.8	364.7	365.8
Other Outpatient Visits	1,963.8	1,964.7	1,849.9	1,790.9	1,745.6
Total Outpatient Visits	2,353.9	2,324.5	2,206.6	2,155.6	2,111.5
Outpatient Surgeries	63.2	63.8	68.8	66.5	67.0
Expense per Capita (per person)	$1,381.3	$1,293.6	$1,260.4	$1,217.5	$1,165.8

TABLE 6

IOWA

U.S. Registered Community Hospitals
(Nonfederal, short-term general and other special hospitals)

Overview 1997–2001

	2001	2000	1999	1998	1997
Total Community Hospitals	**116**	**115**	**115**	**116**	**115**
Bed Size Category					
6-24	12	11	11	12	11
25-49	42	41	40	39	40
50-99	31	29	31	31	28
100-199	15	17	18	18	22
200-299	7	8	6	7	5
300-399	5	5	5	4	5
400-499	2	2	2	3	1
500 +	2	2	2	2	3
Location					
Hospitals Urban	21	21	21	21	21
Hospitals Rural	95	94	94	95	94
Control					
State and Local Government	59	58	59	61	60
Not for Profit	56	57	56	54	53
Investor owned	1	0	0	1	2
Physician Models					
Independent Practice Association	14	15	17	14	17
Group Practice without Walls	4	3	3	4	5
Open Physician-Hospital Organization	21	21	20	20	21
Closed Physician-Hospital Organization	17	19	20	21	17
Management Service Organization	14	13	15	14	18
Integrated Salary Model	44	41	39	35	29
Equity Model	1	1	0	4	3
Foundation	4	6	7	9	8
Insurance Products					
Health Maintenance Organization	17	18	21	20	22
Preferred Provider Organization	34	40	40	39	47
Indemnity Fee for Service	7	6	6	7	12
Managed Care Contracts					
Health Maintenance Organization	69	69	70	64	67
Preferred Provider Organization	98	100	104	97	93
Affiliations					
Hospitals in a System	52	50	49	46	40
Hospitals in a Network	55	52	46	38	33
Hospitals in a Group Purchasing Organization	109	108	104	100	—

TABLE 6

IOWA

U.S. Registered Community Hospitals
(Nonfederal, short-term general and other special hospitals)

Utilization, Personnel, Revenue and Expenses, Community Health Indicators 1997–2001

	2001	2000	1999	1998	1997
TOTAL FACILITY (Includes Hospital and Nursing Home Units)					
Utilization - Inpatient					
Beds	11,538	11,811	11,838	12,219	12,248
Admissions	370,885	359,682	359,142	374,245	366,703
Inpatient Days	2,491,172	2,493,185	2,498,984	2,528,052	2,508,509
Average Length of Stay	6.7	6.9	7.0	6.8	6.8
Inpatient Surgeries	107,252	105,897	105,951	110,705	106,210
Births	37,628	37,692	37,162	37,496	36,609
Utilization - Outpatient					
Emergency Outpatient Visits	1,063,304	1,050,606	1,051,682	982,497	999,586
Other Outpatient Visits	8,336,049	8,106,385	7,511,574	6,768,865	6,452,387
Total Outpatient Visits	9,399,353	9,156,991	8,563,256	7,751,362	7,451,973
Outpatient Surgeries	289,647	289,715	280,264	266,352	246,790
Personnel					
Full Time RNs	8,519	8,855	8,581	9,049	8,315
Full Time LPNs	904	897	826	940	862
Part Time RNs	7,027	6,698	6,988	6,848	6,842
Part Time LPNs	818	757	781	887	831
Total Full Time	40,716	40,602	39,836	39,655	37,815
Total Part Time	25,215	23,512	23,967	23,606	23,321
Revenue - Inpatient					
Gross Inpatient Revenue	$3,868,944,808	$3,523,992,700	$3,291,048,997	$3,155,651,791	$3,015,799,276
Revenue - Outpatient					
Gross Outpatient Revenue	$2,990,618,965	$2,693,739,475	$2,389,853,804	$2,158,066,967	$1,970,879,302
Revenue and Expenses - Totals (Includes Inpatient and Outpatient)					
Total Gross Revenue	$6,859,563,773	$6,217,732,175	$5,680,902,801	$5,313,718,758	$4,986,678,578
Deductions from Revenue	2,824,125,097	2,466,317,174	2,114,838,477	1,958,777,267	1,747,510,227
Net Patient Revenue	4,035,438,676	3,751,415,001	3,566,064,324	3,354,941,491	3,239,168,351
Other Operating Revenue	319,656,799	308,982,657	265,943,571	257,812,692	257,601,031
Other Nonoperating Revenue	93,484,169	83,255,612	90,128,303	101,543,557	81,765,984
Total Net Revenue	4,448,579,644	4,143,653,270	3,922,136,198	3,714,297,740	3,578,535,366
Total Expenses	4,202,394,287	3,932,103,219	3,669,806,143	3,452,505,145	3,314,717,535
HOSPITAL UNIT (Excludes Separate Nursing Home Units)					
Utilization - Inpatient					
Beds	9,251	9,481	9,440	9,677	9,898
Admissions	359,577	347,688	345,654	340,869	351,618
Inpatient Days	1,748,201	1,739,816	1,733,617	1,705,889	1,736,239
Average Length of Stay	4.9	5.0	5.0	5.0	4.9
Personnel					
Total Full Time	39,690	39,540	38,830	38,421	36,594
Total Part Time	24,220	22,599	23,099	22,445	22,151
Revenue and Expenses - Totals (Includes Inpatient and Outpatient)					
Total Net Revenue	$4,348,039,384	$4,048,875,825	$3,830,086,493	$3,580,062,378	$3,474,023,931
Total Expenses	4,123,430,546	3,857,836,935	3,590,355,032	3,333,491,525	3,233,534,087
COMMUNITY HEALTH INDICATORS PER 1000 POPULATION					
Total Population (in thousands)	2,923	2,926	2,869	2,861	2,854
Inpatient					
Beds	3.9	4.0	4.1	4.3	4.3
Admissions	126.9	122.9	125.2	130.8	128.5
Inpatient Days	852.2	852.0	870.9	883.6	878.8
Inpatient Surgeries	36.7	36.2	36.9	38.7	37.2
Births	12.9	12.9	13.0	13.1	12.8
Outpatient					
Emergency Outpatient Visits	363.7	359.0	366.5	343.4	350.2
Other Outpatient Visits	2,851.7	2,770.2	2,617.8	2,365.9	2,260.5
Total Outpatient Visits	3,215.5	3,129.2	2,984.3	2,709.3	2,610.7
Outpatient Surgeries	99.1	99.0	97.7	93.1	86.5
Expense per Capita (per person)	$1,437.6	$1,343.7	$1,278.9	$1,206.7	$1,161.3

TABLE 6

KANSAS

U.S. Registered Community Hospitals
(Nonfederal, short-term general and other special hospitals)

Overview 1997–2001

	2001	2000	1999	1998	1997
Total Community Hospitals	**133**	**129**	**131**	**129**	**130**
Bed Size Category					
6-24	15	18	17	16	17
25-49	44	39	41	47	48
50-99	46	46	44	36	37
100-199	18	16	17	19	17
200-299	5	5	7	6	6
300-399	2	3	3	2	2
400-499	2	1	0	1	1
500 +	1	1	2	2	2
Location					
Hospitals Urban	28	25	26	24	25
Hospitals Rural	105	104	105	105	105
Control					
State and Local Government	62	63	63	65	65
Not for Profit	62	60	61	57	56
Investor owned	9	6	7	7	9
Physician Models					
Independent Practice Association	19	15	12	15	17
Group Practice without Walls	9	7	7	7	6
Open Physician-Hospital Organization	19	19	21	22	23
Closed Physician-Hospital Organization	3	4	3	3	3
Management Service Organization	5	6	12	15	12
Integrated Salary Model	45	42	43	38	31
Equity Model	0	0	0	1	1
Foundation	2	5	10	9	5
Insurance Products					
Health Maintenance Organization	9	15	16	18	19
Preferred Provider Organization	21	23	27	28	28
Indemnity Fee for Service	6	7	6	9	12
Managed Care Contracts					
Health Maintenance Organization	48	41	45	43	48
Preferred Provider Organization	108	106	103	100	104
Affiliations					
Hospitals in a System	56	54	55	52	56
Hospitals in a Network	76	79	76	74	76
Hospitals in a Group Purchasing Organization	124	119	115	110	—

TABLE 6

KANSAS

U.S. Registered Community Hospitals
(Nonfederal, short-term general and other special hospitals)

Utilization, Personnel, Revenue and Expenses, Community Health Indicators 1997–2001

	2001	2000	1999	1998	1997
TOTAL FACILITY (Includes Hospital and Nursing Home Units)					
Utilization - Inpatient					
Beds	11,211	10,821	11,615	10,923	10,829
Admissions	322,067	310,256	326,352	299,701	298,451
Inpatient Days	2,175,989	2,081,932	2,232,737	2,148,493	2,095,243
Average Length of Stay	6.8	6.7	6.8	7.2	7.0
Inpatient Surgeries	86,949	84,051	91,259	81,732	89,222
Births	37,847	37,599	38,971	36,168	34,902
Utilization - Outpatient					
Emergency Outpatient Visits	907,083	889,390	921,066	809,296	787,809
Other Outpatient Visits	4,486,945	4,365,883	4,103,314	3,894,843	3,930,904
Total Outpatient Visits	5,394,028	5,255,273	5,024,380	4,704,139	4,718,713
Outpatient Surgeries	161,789	162,669	176,375	159,197	163,458
Personnel					
Full Time RNs	6,906	7,158	7,601	7,196	7,409
Full Time LPNs	1,079	1,038	1,075	1,025	1,038
Part Time RNs	4,041	4,072	4,415	3,826	4,098
Part Time LPNs	549	523	590	520	562
Total Full Time	32,609	31,548	33,931	34,496	32,861
Total Part Time	14,668	13,944	12,984	11,555	12,928
Revenue - Inpatient					
Gross Inpatient Revenue	$4,299,715,760	$3,829,510,816	$3,772,245,204	$3,394,554,236	$3,242,966,681
Revenue - Outpatient					
Gross Outpatient Revenue	$2,632,758,324	$2,374,823,658	$2,198,345,422	$1,926,917,284	$1,844,127,624
Revenue and Expenses - Totals (Includes Inpatient and Outpatient)					
Total Gross Revenue	$6,932,474,084	$6,204,334,474	$5,970,590,626	$5,321,471,520	$5,087,094,305
Deductions from Revenue	3,693,649,527	3,189,390,696	2,949,255,620	2,551,924,564	2,309,581,670
Net Patient Revenue	3,238,824,557	3,014,943,778	3,021,335,006	2,769,546,956	2,777,512,635
Other Operating Revenue	162,388,962	147,629,759	144,033,337	128,359,530	120,567,863
Other Nonoperating Revenue	42,943,502	71,565,700	65,565,230	80,111,039	58,397,270
Total Net Revenue	3,444,157,021	3,234,139,237	3,230,933,573	2,978,017,525	2,956,477,768
Total Expenses	3,285,567,037	3,065,466,141	3,036,739,861	2,712,003,392	2,723,941,300
HOSPITAL UNIT (Excludes Separate Nursing Home Units)					
Utilization - Inpatient					
Beds	9,171	8,658	9,380	8,730	8,890
Admissions	314,556	301,101	316,200	288,353	282,539
Inpatient Days	1,576,671	1,489,124	1,615,520	1,506,584	1,512,993
Average Length of Stay	5.0	4.9	5.1	5.2	5.4
Personnel					
Total Full Time	31,407	30,303	32,649	33,205	31,627
Total Part Time	13,885	13,199	12,225	10,801	12,162
Revenue and Expenses - Totals (Includes Inpatient and Outpatient)					
Total Net Revenue	$3,372,688,086	$3,169,162,014	$3,160,271,291	$2,901,003,496	$2,887,145,416
Total Expenses	3,229,152,871	3,011,711,334	2,981,430,308	2,652,210,976	2,675,695,076
COMMUNITY HEALTH INDICATORS PER 1000 POPULATION					
Total Population (in thousands)	2,695	2,688	2,654	2,639	2,616
Inpatient					
Beds	4.2	4.0	4.4	4.1	4.1
Admissions	119.5	115.4	123.0	113.6	114.1
Inpatient Days	807.5	774.4	841.3	814.2	800.8
Inpatient Surgeries	32.3	31.3	34.4	31.0	34.1
Births	14.0	14.0	14.7	13.7	13.3
Outpatient					
Emergency Outpatient Visits	336.6	330.8	347.0	306.7	301.1
Other Outpatient Visits	1,665.1	1,624.0	1,546.1	1,476.1	1,502.4
Total Outpatient Visits	2,001.8	1,954.8	1,893.1	1,782.8	1,803.6
Outpatient Surgeries	60.0	60.5	66.5	60.3	62.5
Expense per Capita (per person)	$1,219.3	$1,140.2	$1,144.2	$1,027.8	$1,041.1

TABLE 6

KENTUCKY

U.S. Registered Community Hospitals
(Nonfederal, short-term general and other special hospitals)

Overview 1997–2001

	2001	2000	1999	1998	1997
Total Community Hospitals	**103**	**105**	**105**	**106**	**105**
Bed Size Category					
6-24	1	3	2	1	1
25-49	20	19	22	19	19
50-99	33	30	29	37	38
100-199	22	27	27	26	22
200-299	14	14	12	9	11
300-399	6	6	9	7	6
400-499	5	4	2	5	7
500 +	2	2	2	2	1
Location					
Hospitals Urban	32	33	33	34	33
Hospitals Rural	71	72	72	72	72
Control					
State and Local Government	14	15	14	13	14
Not for Profit	71	72	73	73	69
Investor owned	18	18	18	20	22
Physician Models					
Independent Practice Association	7	6	8	7	14
Group Practice without Walls	2	3	1	3	5
Open Physician-Hospital Organization	11	12	15	18	17
Closed Physician-Hospital Organization	1	1	6	3	4
Management Service Organization	3	12	14	13	15
Integrated Salary Model	29	24	21	21	13
Equity Model	0	0	1	3	3
Foundation	10	11	10	6	7
Insurance Products					
Health Maintenance Organization	22	17	20	22	25
Preferred Provider Organization	17	8	18	27	33
Indemnity Fee for Service	2	0	3	6	12
Managed Care Contracts					
Health Maintenance Organization	53	48	52	57	51
Preferred Provider Organization	68	54	69	68	69
Affiliations					
Hospitals in a System	52	45	51	47	44
Hospitals in a Network	13	13	15	22	25
Hospitals in a Group Purchasing Organization	76	63	62	57	—

TABLE 6 KENTUCKY

U.S. Registered Community Hospitals
(Nonfederal, short-term general and other special hospitals)

Utilization, Personnel, Revenue and Expenses, Community Health Indicators 1997–2001

	2001	2000	1999	1998	1997
TOTAL FACILITY (Includes Hospital and Nursing Home Units)					
Utilization - Inpatient					
Beds	15,001	14,827	14,956	15,240	15,351
Admissions	594,899	581,620	569,792	551,325	542,640
Inpatient Days	3,315,218	3,333,314	3,296,591	3,173,476	3,187,922
Average Length of Stay	5.6	5.7	5.8	5.8	5.9
Inpatient Surgeries	167,283	170,029	164,304	179,309	165,189
Births	52,818	53,547	51,637	51,107	50,348
Utilization - Outpatient					
Emergency Outpatient Visits	1,985,284	1,953,727	1,990,266	1,761,831	1,645,843
Other Outpatient Visits	6,692,104	6,742,993	5,991,574	5,630,880	5,158,502
Total Outpatient Visits	8,677,388	8,696,720	7,981,840	7,392,711	6,804,345
Outpatient Surgeries	359,153	349,830	333,683	313,438	271,997
Personnel					
Full Time RNs	12,892	13,138	13,532	13,576	12,932
Full Time LPNs	2,427	2,206	2,362	2,496	2,419
Part Time RNs	5,229	5,041	5,217	4,582	4,711
Part Time LPNs	540	544	648	683	642
Total Full Time	57,175	55,775	54,147	55,425	52,391
Total Part Time	17,162	17,452	16,457	14,345	15,324
Revenue - Inpatient					
Gross Inpatient Revenue	$7,787,598,143	$6,926,847,867	$6,349,440,581	$5,934,530,227	$5,389,064,850
Revenue - Outpatient					
Gross Outpatient Revenue	$4,733,719,223	$4,237,568,311	$3,654,809,995	$3,246,317,231	$2,868,511,231
Revenue and Expenses - Totals (Includes Inpatient and Outpatient)					
Total Gross Revenue	$12,521,317,366	$11,164,416,178	$10,004,250,576	$9,180,847,458	$8,257,576,081
Deductions from Revenue	6,819,797,436	5,892,730,890	5,113,919,722	4,401,939,860	3,753,249,649
Net Patient Revenue	5,701,519,930	5,271,685,288	4,890,330,854	4,778,907,598	4,504,326,432
Other Operating Revenue	264,715,481	250,730,317	237,393,468	218,060,479	192,217,386
Other Nonoperating Revenue	61,362,641	91,895,438	108,001,346	132,156,395	105,985,221
Total Net Revenue	6,027,598,052	5,614,311,043	5,235,725,668	5,129,124,472	4,802,529,039
Total Expenses	5,731,885,674	5,262,215,893	4,962,196,037	4,790,309,964	4,407,574,434
HOSPITAL UNIT (Excludes Separate Nursing Home Units)					
Utilization - Inpatient					
Beds	13,587	13,295	13,125	13,511	14,055
Admissions	584,628	570,135	555,394	539,916	533,355
Inpatient Days	2,863,991	2,844,864	2,716,093	2,667,045	2,786,334
Average Length of Stay	4.9	5.0	4.9	4.9	5.2
Personnel					
Total Full Time	55,916	54,545	52,598	54,031	51,331
Total Part Time	16,843	17,049	15,919	13,917	14,945
Revenue and Expenses - Totals (Includes Inpatient and Outpatient)					
Total Net Revenue	$5,922,961,820	$5,467,691,050	$5,083,079,627	$5,015,843,495	$4,717,397,316
Total Expenses	5,659,683,174	5,142,390,665	4,876,938,853	4,713,425,656	4,344,747,735
COMMUNITY HEALTH INDICATORS PER 1000 POPULATION					
Total Population (in thousands)	4,066	4,042	3,961	3,934	3,908
Inpatient					
Beds	3.7	3.7	3.8	3.9	3.9
Admissions	146.3	143.9	143.9	140.1	138.9
Inpatient Days	815.4	824.7	832.3	806.6	815.8
Inpatient Surgeries	41.1	42.1	41.5	45.6	42.3
Births	13.0	13.2	13.0	13.0	12.9
Outpatient					
Emergency Outpatient Visits	488.3	483.4	502.5	447.8	421.2
Other Outpatient Visits	1,646.0	1,668.3	1,512.7	1,431.2	1,320.0
Total Outpatient Visits	2,134.4	2,151.7	2,015.2	1,879.0	1,741.2
Outpatient Surgeries	88.3	86.6	84.2	79.7	69.6
Expense per Capita (per person)	$1,409.9	$1,302.0	$1,252.8	$1,217.6	$1,127.9

Table 6

LOUISIANA

U.S. Registered Community Hospitals
(Nonfederal, short-term general and other special hospitals)

Overview 1997–2001

	2001	2000	1999	1998	1997
Total Community Hospitals	**125**	**123**	**122**	**126**	**127**
Bed Size Category					
6-24	9	6	5	5	4
25-49	29	29	29	29	29
50-99	30	33	31	32	30
100-199	30	27	32	34	37
200-299	11	11	8	10	10
300-399	6	8	11	8	9
400-499	4	4	4	3	3
500 +	6	5	2	5	5
Location					
Hospitals Urban	76	75	74	78	78
Hospitals Rural	49	48	48	48	49
Control					
State and Local Government	55	55	55	57	57
Not for Profit	33	31	30	30	29
Investor owned	37	37	37	39	41
Physician Models					
Independent Practice Association	17	15	11	12	20
Group Practice without Walls	2	3	1	4	3
Open Physician-Hospital Organization	17	25	20	19	28
Closed Physician-Hospital Organization	15	14	13	23	22
Management Service Organization	10	15	18	23	28
Integrated Salary Model	16	19	14	18	15
Equity Model	0	0	1	2	5
Foundation	2	2	1	2	3
Insurance Products					
Health Maintenance Organization	9	12	18	25	29
Preferred Provider Organization	15	19	27	37	49
Indemnity Fee for Service	2	3	5	7	9
Managed Care Contracts					
Health Maintenance Organization	54	55	57	66	60
Preferred Provider Organization	69	70	72	80	80
Affiliations					
Hospitals in a System	39	41	37	44	48
Hospitals in a Network	18	22	17	29	31
Hospitals in a Group Purchasing Organization	71	62	60	58	—

States

LOUISIANA

U.S. Registered Community Hospitals
(Nonfederal, short-term general and other special hospitals)

Utilization, Personnel, Revenue and Expenses, Community Health Indicators 1997–2001

	2001	2000	1999	1998	1997
TOTAL FACILITY (Includes Hospital and Nursing Home Units)					
Utilization - Inpatient					
Beds	17,975	17,544	16,782	17,820	18,605
Admissions	682,586	654,323	626,801	637,892	650,104
Inpatient Days	3,736,536	3,569,621	3,472,409	3,564,901	3,682,678
Average Length of Stay	5.5	5.5	5.5	5.6	5.7
Inpatient Surgeries	172,824	179,651	174,051	173,281	170,682
Births	63,248	64,904	63,553	63,976	62,528
Utilization - Outpatient					
Emergency Outpatient Visits	2,267,490	2,143,846	2,182,109	2,254,789	2,198,306
Other Outpatient Visits	7,792,891	7,882,211	7,331,885	7,952,356	6,396,365
Total Outpatient Visits	10,060,381	10,026,057	9,513,994	10,207,145	8,594,671
Outpatient Surgeries	285,927	278,438	272,852	267,370	253,198
Personnel					
Full Time RNs	14,845	15,634	15,460	15,939	15,674
Full Time LPNs	3,202	3,711	3,849	3,787	3,988
Part Time RNs	5,472	5,630	4,586	4,881	4,014
Part Time LPNs	1,046	1,073	1,018	912	988
Total Full Time	68,540	70,010	68,263	73,149	71,692
Total Part Time	18,200	18,093	16,056	17,568	15,951
Revenue - Inpatient					
Gross Inpatient Revenue	$9,096,048,174	$8,243,500,319	$7,543,819,679	$7,549,027,025	$7,316,534,192
Revenue - Outpatient					
Gross Outpatient Revenue	$4,760,161,472	$4,251,539,053	$3,934,910,084	$3,827,901,719	$3,439,171,448
Revenue and Expenses - Totals (Includes Inpatient and Outpatient)					
Total Gross Revenue	$13,856,209,646	$12,495,039,372	$11,478,729,763	$11,376,928,744	$10,755,705,640
Deductions from Revenue	7,622,952,381	6,598,655,986	5,462,495,406	5,494,978,293	5,129,882,169
Net Patient Revenue	6,233,257,265	5,896,383,386	6,016,234,357	5,881,950,451	5,625,823,471
Other Operating Revenue	267,094,438	242,589,117	431,151,639	255,734,431	283,360,339
Other Nonoperating Revenue	118,755,497	132,937,013	123,928,310	107,524,057	118,308,925
Total Net Revenue	6,619,107,200	6,271,000,516	6,571,314,306	6,245,208,030	6,027,492,735
Total Expenses	6,231,829,149	5,944,697,229	5,552,067,184	5,874,665,596	5,384,026,729
HOSPITAL UNIT (Excludes Separate Nursing Home Units)					
Utilization - Inpatient					
Beds	16,772	16,724	16,031	17,118	17,568
Admissions	676,446	645,795	617,298	627,610	641,360
Inpatient Days	3,433,204	3,333,668	3,256,709	3,361,008	3,376,509
Average Length of Stay	5.1	5.2	5.3	5.4	5.3
Personnel					
Total Full Time	67,052	68,743	67,579	72,324	70,307
Total Part Time	17,972	17,855	15,884	17,368	15,523
Revenue and Expenses - Totals (Includes Inpatient and Outpatient)					
Total Net Revenue	$6,575,698,935	$6,196,038,147	$6,306,351,941	$6,173,466,062	$5,879,812,346
Total Expenses	6,196,893,942	5,901,358,320	5,509,175,610	5,814,898,961	5,329,049,016
COMMUNITY HEALTH INDICATORS PER 1000 POPULATION					
Total Population (in thousands)	4,465	4,469	4,372	4,363	4,351
Inpatient					
Beds	4.0	3.9	3.8	4.1	4.3
Admissions	152.9	146.4	143.4	146.2	149.4
Inpatient Days	836.8	798.8	794.2	817.1	846.3
Inpatient Surgeries	38.7	40.2	39.8	39.7	39.2
Births	14.2	14.5	14.5	14.7	14.4
Outpatient					
Emergency Outpatient Visits	507.8	479.7	499.1	516.8	505.2
Other Outpatient Visits	1,745.2	1,763.8	1,677.0	1,822.8	1,470.0
Total Outpatient Visits	2,252.9	2,243.5	2,176.1	2,339.6	1,975.2
Outpatient Surgeries	64.0	62.3	62.4	61.3	58.2
Expense per Capita (per person)	$1,395.6	$1,330.2	$1,269.9	$1,346.5	$1,237.3

TABLE 6

MAINE

U.S. Registered Community Hospitals
(Nonfederal, short-term general and other special hospitals)

Overview 1997–2001

	2001	2000	1999	1998	1997
Total Community Hospitals	**37**	**37**	**37**	**38**	**38**
Bed Size Category					
6-24	0	1	2	1	3
25-49	14	13	12	14	13
50-99	11	12	12	13	12
100-199	9	8	8	7	7
200-299	0	0	0	0	0
300-399	2	2	2	2	2
400-499	0	0	0	0	0
500 +	1	1	1	1	1
Location					
Hospitals Urban	8	8	8	9	9
Hospitals Rural	29	29	29	29	29
Control					
State and Local Government	3	3	3	3	3
Not for Profit	33	33	33	34	34
Investor owned	1	1	1	1	1
Physician Models					
Independent Practice Association	4	3	3	2	2
Group Practice without Walls	1	1	2	4	4
Open Physician-Hospital Organization	16	12	13	13	10
Closed Physician-Hospital Organization	0	2	2	2	3
Management Service Organization	4	4	5	5	7
Integrated Salary Model	13	14	16	13	14
Equity Model	2	2	2	2	3
Foundation	2	0	0	0	0
Insurance Products					
Health Maintenance Organization	2	3	6	7	7
Preferred Provider Organization	3	4	7	9	11
Indemnity Fee for Service	2	2	2	3	4
Managed Care Contracts					
Health Maintenance Organization	28	28	27	28	28
Preferred Provider Organization	24	25	22	27	26
Affiliations					
Hospitals in a System	20	16	18	16	16
Hospitals in a Network	16	15	13	13	14
Hospitals in a Group Purchasing Organization	31	31	30	30	—

States

TABLE 6

MAINE

U.S. Registered Community Hospitals
(Nonfederal, short-term general and other special hospitals)

Utilization, Personnel, Revenue and Expenses, Community Health Indicators 1997–2001

	2001	2000	1999	1998	1997
TOTAL FACILITY (Includes Hospital and Nursing Home Units)					
Utilization - Inpatient					
Beds	3,844	3,700	3,691	3,768	3,691
Admissions	148,612	147,236	146,378	144,363	143,351
Inpatient Days	898,059	867,352	872,635	843,811	857,274
Average Length of Stay	6.0	5.9	6.0	5.8	6.0
Inpatient Surgeries	45,682	45,114	44,045	41,907	43,196
Births	13,320	13,294	13,284	13,252	13,283
Utilization - Outpatient					
Emergency Outpatient Visits	700,510	673,853	579,803	636,973	603,070
Other Outpatient Visits	2,812,088	2,573,641	2,197,596	2,037,267	2,058,575
Total Outpatient Visits	3,512,598	3,247,494	2,777,399	2,674,240	2,661,645
Outpatient Surgeries	114,146	108,086	96,653	91,545	74,672
Personnel					
Full Time RNs	3,573	3,628	3,517	3,514	3,500
Full Time LPNs	270	302	352	364	408
Part Time RNs	3,005	2,964	2,725	2,652	2,838
Part Time LPNs	183	212	199	215	340
Total Full Time	16,599	16,403	15,485	16,028	14,864
Total Part Time	9,641	9,180	7,239	8,293	8,923
Revenue - Inpatient					
Gross Inpatient Revenue	$1,812,197,212	$1,698,718,945	$1,520,624,429	$1,421,620,856	$1,362,740,940
Revenue - Outpatient					
Gross Outpatient Revenue	$1,304,548,466	$1,154,754,197	$999,290,257	$858,420,867	$758,777,729
Revenue and Expenses - Totals (Includes Inpatient and Outpatient)					
Total Gross Revenue	$3,116,745,678	$2,853,473,142	$2,519,914,686	$2,280,041,723	$2,121,518,669
Deductions from Revenue	1,217,966,635	1,115,439,062	915,152,948	726,791,652	648,177,224
Net Patient Revenue	1,898,779,043	1,738,034,080	1,604,761,738	1,553,250,071	1,473,341,445
Other Operating Revenue	65,237,618	57,843,349	55,504,484	59,938,444	60,812,728
Other Nonoperating Revenue	44,611,020	65,070,578	60,959,561	56,650,639	56,956,623
Total Net Revenue	2,008,627,681	1,860,948,007	1,721,225,783	1,669,839,154	1,591,110,796
Total Expenses	1,895,302,775	1,728,203,811	1,590,697,508	1,529,313,309	1,439,968,708
HOSPITAL UNIT (Excludes Separate Nursing Home Units)					
Utilization - Inpatient					
Beds	3,266	3,308	3,146	3,287	3,217
Admissions	146,398	145,274	144,095	142,153	141,387
Inpatient Days	715,018	744,933	702,828	698,519	701,875
Average Length of Stay	4.9	5.1	4.9	4.9	5.0
Personnel					
Total Full Time	16,166	16,052	15,042	15,485	14,464
Total Part Time	9,376	8,910	6,920	7,946	8,577
Revenue and Expenses - Totals (Includes Inpatient and Outpatient)					
Total Net Revenue	$1,978,598,927	$1,840,086,132	$1,689,929,697	$1,646,474,939	$1,565,864,525
Total Expenses	1,864,078,445	1,710,294,770	1,569,334,589	1,512,040,904	1,420,044,749
COMMUNITY HEALTH INDICATORS PER 1000 POPULATION					
Total Population (in thousands)	1,287	1,275	1,253	1,248	1,245
Inpatient					
Beds	3.0	2.9	2.9	3.0	3.0
Admissions	115.5	115.5	116.8	115.7	115.1
Inpatient Days	698.0	680.3	696.4	676.4	688.5
Inpatient Surgeries	35.5	35.4	35.2	33.6	34.7
Births	10.4	10.4	10.6	10.6	10.7
Outpatient					
Emergency Outpatient Visits	544.4	528.5	462.7	510.6	484.3
Other Outpatient Visits	2,185.6	2,018.7	1,753.8	1,633.0	1,653.2
Total Outpatient Visits	2,730.0	2,547.2	2,216.5	2,143.6	2,137.5
Outpatient Surgeries	88.7	84.8	77.1	73.4	60.0
Expense per Capita (per person)	$1,473.0	$1,355.5	$1,269.5	$1,225.8	$1,156.4

TABLE 6

MARYLAND

U.S. Registered Community Hospitals
(Nonfederal, short-term general and other special hospitals)

Overview 1997–2001

	2001	2000	1999	1998	1997
Total Community Hospitals	49	49	49	51	51
Bed Size Category					
6-24	0	0	0	0	0
25-49	3	3	3	3	3
50-99	6	5	4	6	6
100-199	15	18	19	19	18
200-299	12	11	9	7	10
300-399	8	6	9	9	7
400-499	2	3	1	3	3
500 +	3	3	4	4	4
Location					
Hospitals Urban	40	40	40	42	42
Hospitals Rural	9	9	9	9	9
Control					
State and Local Government	0	0	0	0	0
Not for Profit	47	47	47	49	49
Investor owned	2	2	2	2	2
Physician Models					
Independent Practice Association	6	7	11	15	16
Group Practice without Walls	1	1	2	3	2
Open Physician-Hospital Organization	7	9	11	14	9
Closed Physician-Hospital Organization	5	4	7	9	13
Management Service Organization	3	5	15	18	26
Integrated Salary Model	23	19	20	19	18
Equity Model	3	4	5	4	7
Foundation	2	2	4	7	7
Insurance Products					
Health Maintenance Organization	16	14	10	11	8
Preferred Provider Organization	8	10	10	14	13
Indemnity Fee for Service	3	3	4	3	4
Managed Care Contracts					
Health Maintenance Organization	38	37	33	32	43
Preferred Provider Organization	34	32	29	34	41
Affiliations					
Hospitals in a System	37	36	32	28	31
Hospitals in a Network	8	6	5	8	16
Hospitals in a Group Purchasing Organization	43	41	34	37	—

Table 6

MARYLAND

U.S. Registered Community Hospitals
(Nonfederal, short-term general and other special hospitals)

Utilization, Personnel, Revenue and Expenses, Community Health Indicators 1997–2001

	2001	2000	1999	1998	1997
TOTAL FACILITY (Includes Hospital and Nursing Home Units)					
Utilization - Inpatient					
Beds	11,234	11,192	11,629	12,670	12,680
Admissions	608,165	586,809	576,551	564,913	570,234
Inpatient Days	2,981,003	2,993,513	3,023,508	3,144,315	3,129,218
Average Length of Stay	4.9	5.1	5.2	5.6	5.5
Inpatient Surgeries	183,287	178,327	175,733	190,587	194,173
Births	63,843	64,030	62,251	62,307	63,216
Utilization - Outpatient					
Emergency Outpatient Visits	1,854,562	1,765,739	1,667,655	1,505,744	1,611,360
Other Outpatient Visits	4,411,827	4,251,883	4,275,428	3,514,579	3,807,263
Total Outpatient Visits	6,266,389	6,017,622	5,943,083	5,020,323	5,418,623
Outpatient Surgeries	330,571	335,445	320,799	299,859	315,331
Personnel					
Full Time RNs	11,196	11,629	12,145	12,201	11,324
Full Time LPNs	593	629	702	795	898
Part Time RNs	8,804	8,458	7,152	7,756	8,073
Part Time LPNs	338	365	515	354	446
Total Full Time	54,035	52,045	51,194	50,745	53,164
Total Part Time	25,913	25,896	23,098	24,357	29,771
Revenue - Inpatient					
Gross Inpatient Revenue	$5,524,686,729	$4,869,935,847	$4,872,474,817	$4,945,479,136	$4,632,198,518
Revenue - Outpatient					
Gross Outpatient Revenue	$2,614,614,189	$2,239,872,994	$2,014,087,252	$1,976,311,835	$1,759,834,838
Revenue and Expenses - Totals (Includes Inpatient and Outpatient)					
Total Gross Revenue	$8,139,300,918	$7,109,808,841	$6,886,562,069	$6,921,790,971	$6,392,033,356
Deductions from Revenue	1,898,515,253	1,433,510,257	1,603,233,392	1,690,984,916	1,171,336,368
Net Patient Revenue	6,240,785,665	5,676,298,584	5,283,328,677	5,230,806,055	5,220,696,988
Other Operating Revenue	266,638,563	255,723,354	217,607,190	228,596,574	215,778,382
Other Nonoperating Revenue	43,785,690	91,201,507	82,290,784	103,389,417	96,638,703
Total Net Revenue	6,551,209,918	6,023,223,445	5,583,226,651	5,562,792,046	5,533,114,073
Total Expenses	6,345,348,924	5,872,418,845	5,457,297,063	5,305,756,896	5,251,525,530
HOSPITAL UNIT (Excludes Separate Nursing Home Units)					
Utilization - Inpatient					
Beds	10,575	10,297	10,699	11,350	11,589
Admissions	598,350	574,952	564,358	553,916	562,604
Inpatient Days	2,773,678	2,708,689	2,753,302	2,768,381	2,824,000
Average Length of Stay	4.6	4.7	4.9	5.0	5.0
Personnel					
Total Full Time	53,463	51,409	50,461	49,810	52,321
Total Part Time	25,579	25,392	22,627	23,861	29,239
Revenue and Expenses - Totals (Includes Inpatient and Outpatient)					
Total Net Revenue	$6,462,828,420	$5,938,396,900	$5,486,858,411	$5,441,766,935	$5,470,218,810
Total Expenses	6,281,919,803	5,796,277,170	5,372,382,741	5,198,032,054	5,195,988,028
COMMUNITY HEALTH INDICATORS PER 1000 POPULATION					
Total Population (in thousands)	5,375	5,296	5,172	5,130	5,093
Inpatient					
Beds	2.1	2.1	2.2	2.5	2.5
Admissions	113.1	110.8	111.5	110.1	112.0
Inpatient Days	554.6	565.2	584.6	612.9	614.4
Inpatient Surgeries	34.1	33.7	34.0	37.2	38.1
Births	11.9	12.1	12.0	12.1	12.4
Outpatient					
Emergency Outpatient Visits	345.0	333.4	322.5	293.5	316.4
Other Outpatient Visits	820.8	802.8	826.7	685.1	747.6
Total Outpatient Visits	1,165.8	1,136.2	1,149.2	978.6	1,064.0
Outpatient Surgeries	61.5	63.3	62.0	58.5	61.9
Expense per Capita (per person)	$1,180.5	$1,108.7	$1,055.2	$1,034.2	$1,031.1

States

TABLE 6

MASSACHUSETTS

U.S. Registered Community Hospitals
(Nonfederal, short-term general and other special hospitals)

Overview 1997–2001

	2001	2000	1999	1998	1997
Total Community Hospitals	**80**	**80**	**79**	**82**	**84**
Bed Size Category					
6-24	2	2	3	3	4
25-49	13	13	12	12	11
50-99	6	6	6	9	7
100-199	28	27	29	27	28
200-299	16	16	12	17	18
300-399	8	9	10	6	9
400-499	1	1	1	1	1
500 +	6	6	6	7	6
Location					
Hospitals Urban	69	69	68	71	75
Hospitals Rural	11	11	11	11	9
Control					
State and Local Government	4	4	4	4	6
Not for Profit	70	70	69	72	72
Investor owned	6	6	6	6	6
Physician Models					
Independent Practice Association	31	31	37	31	36
Group Practice without Walls	10	9	9	10	10
Open Physician-Hospital Organization	18	19	21	22	29
Closed Physician-Hospital Organization	10	10	10	11	9
Management Service Organization	17	17	24	19	13
Integrated Salary Model	28	28	24	25	31
Equity Model	1	1	2	2	3
Foundation	5	6	10	10	13
Insurance Products					
Health Maintenance Organization	8	9	8	13	19
Preferred Provider Organization	4	5	6	12	16
Indemnity Fee for Service	1	1	2	4	8
Managed Care Contracts					
Health Maintenance Organization	60	56	62	62	70
Preferred Provider Organization	57	53	57	57	65
Affiliations					
Hospitals in a System	43	40	50	42	49
Hospitals in a Network	22	21	22	18	23
Hospitals in a Group Purchasing Organization	55	50	53	51	—

TABLE 6

MASSACHUSETTS

U.S. Registered Community Hospitals
(Nonfederal, short-term general and other special hospitals)

Utilization, Personnel, Revenue and Expenses, Community Health Indicators 1997–2001

	2001	2000	1999	1998	1997
TOTAL FACILITY (Includes Hospital and Nursing Home Units)					
Utilization - Inpatient					
Beds	16,504	16,586	16,309	16,493	17,431
Admissions	766,708	740,286	739,375	738,018	764,322
Inpatient Days	4,382,048	4,289,840	4,210,454	4,186,012	4,283,021
Average Length of Stay	5.7	5.8	5.7	5.7	5.6
Inpatient Surgeries	212,539	217,649	214,009	219,487	215,878
Births	79,908	81,640	79,484	78,257	80,598
Utilization - Outpatient					
Emergency Outpatient Visits	2,717,815	2,715,812	2,726,113	2,473,668	2,559,125
Other Outpatient Visits	16,060,322	13,994,541	12,982,756	12,952,045	11,065,537
Total Outpatient Visits	18,778,137	16,710,353	15,708,869	15,425,713	13,624,662
Outpatient Surgeries	467,917	458,544	440,958	423,601	385,558
Personnel					
Full Time RNs	18,018	16,359	14,936	14,465	14,374
Full Time LPNs	1,236	1,207	854	1,052	1,141
Part Time RNs	16,968	18,591	17,782	18,695	16,758
Part Time LPNs	1,067	1,171	1,111	1,109	1,126
Total Full Time	101,474	93,354	87,466	86,242	87,993
Total Part Time	52,916	56,902	56,698	57,013	55,208
Revenue - Inpatient					
Gross Inpatient Revenue	$12,173,968,661	$11,247,798,711	$9,839,772,237	$9,196,917,700	$8,657,400,754
Revenue - Outpatient					
Gross Outpatient Revenue	$9,610,590,844	$8,231,186,269	$7,625,652,302	$6,711,695,879	$5,950,486,217
Revenue and Expenses - Totals (Includes Inpatient and Outpatient)					
Total Gross Revenue	$21,784,559,505	$19,478,984,980	$17,465,424,539	$15,908,613,579	$14,607,886,971
Deductions from Revenue	11,457,845,346	10,026,437,014	8,646,920,813	7,346,543,961	6,262,106,585
Net Patient Revenue	10,326,714,159	9,452,547,966	8,818,503,726	8,562,069,618	8,345,780,386
Other Operating Revenue	1,636,890,502	1,232,552,918	1,299,771,155	1,364,112,758	1,071,184,180
Other Nonoperating Revenue	124,637,693	365,783,979	341,554,169	369,873,327	375,913,482
Total Net Revenue	12,088,242,354	11,050,884,863	10,459,829,050	10,290,055,703	9,792,878,048
Total Expenses	12,055,797,429	11,148,180,478	10,518,160,942	10,315,437,574	9,539,109,117
HOSPITAL UNIT (Excludes Separate Nursing Home Units)					
Utilization - Inpatient					
Beds	15,814	15,662	15,515	15,907	16,539
Admissions	757,011	725,509	720,669	726,626	751,742
Inpatient Days	4,140,284	3,993,613	3,980,792	4,023,095	3,999,786
Average Length of Stay	5.5	5.5	5.5	5.5	5.3
Personnel					
Total Full Time	101,143	92,938	86,618	85,515	87,298
Total Part Time	52,480	56,327	55,971	56,441	54,648
Revenue and Expenses - Totals (Includes Inpatient and Outpatient)					
Total Net Revenue	$12,032,855,996	$10,993,289,677	$10,367,408,392	$10,176,513,120	$9,695,593,011
Total Expenses	12,015,811,316	11,098,723,636	10,444,538,511	10,225,709,796	9,467,991,953
COMMUNITY HEALTH INDICATORS PER 1000 POPULATION					
Total Population (in thousands)	6,379	6,349	6,175	6,144	6,115
Inpatient					
Beds	2.6	2.6	2.6	2.7	2.9
Admissions	120.2	116.6	119.7	120.1	125.0
Inpatient Days	686.9	675.7	681.8	681.3	700.4
Inpatient Surgeries	33.3	34.3	34.7	35.7	35.3
Births	12.5	12.9	12.9	12.7	13.2
Outpatient					
Emergency Outpatient Visits	426.0	427.7	441.5	402.6	418.5
Other Outpatient Visits	2,517.6	2,204.2	2,102.4	2,107.9	1,809.4
Total Outpatient Visits	2,943.6	2,631.9	2,543.9	2,510.5	2,227.9
Outpatient Surgeries	73.3	72.2	71.4	68.9	63.0
Expense per Capita (per person)	$1,889.8	$1,755.9	$1,703.3	$1,678.8	$1,559.8

TABLE 6

MICHIGAN

U.S. Registered Community Hospitals
(Nonfederal, short-term general and other special hospitals)

Overview 1997–2001

	2001	2000	1999	1998	1997
Total Community Hospitals	**145**	**146**	**145**	**151**	**154**
Bed Size Category					
6-24	7	7	10	11	11
25-49	23	20	17	22	17
50-99	50	51	51	47	51
100-199	17	18	19	20	20
200-299	17	21	18	18	21
300-399	16	13	14	16	19
400-499	7	7	7	8	7
500 +	8	9	9	9	8
Location					
Hospitals Urban	86	88	87	92	95
Hospitals Rural	59	58	58	59	59
Control					
State and Local Government	20	19	19	21	21
Not for Profit	122	124	122	128	130
Investor owned	3	3	4	2	3
Physician Models					
Independent Practice Association	22	23	25	32	37
Group Practice without Walls	13	13	7	10	12
Open Physician-Hospital Organization	58	55	44	46	48
Closed Physician-Hospital Organization	14	20	23	21	18
Management Service Organization	27	26	23	29	28
Integrated Salary Model	59	68	56	59	57
Equity Model	1	1	3	2	2
Foundation	4	5	6	8	9
Insurance Products					
Health Maintenance Organization	45	52	47	50	57
Preferred Provider Organization	52	66	60	67	82
Indemnity Fee for Service	11	18	14	17	24
Managed Care Contracts					
Health Maintenance Organization	117	114	106	106	108
Preferred Provider Organization	125	123	122	121	127
Affiliations					
Hospitals in a System	77	79	77	74	89
Hospitals in a Network	50	56	46	45	54
Hospitals in a Group Purchasing Organization	124	125	119	110	—

States

MICHIGAN

U.S. Registered Community Hospitals
(Nonfederal, short-term general and other special hospitals)

Utilization, Personnel, Revenue and Expenses, Community Health Indicators 1997–2001

	2001	2000	1999	1998	1997
TOTAL FACILITY (Includes Hospital and Nursing Home Units)					
Utilization - Inpatient					
Beds	25,630	26,074	26,144	27,168	27,923
Admissions	1,122,004	1,106,045	1,084,277	1,104,883	1,111,527
Inpatient Days	6,108,896	6,176,230	6,295,931	6,380,260	6,591,143
Average Length of Stay	5.4	5.6	5.8	5.8	5.9
Inpatient Surgeries	321,558	334,190	323,881	329,527	339,255
Births	126,846	131,092	128,720	127,816	128,280
Utilization - Outpatient					
Emergency Outpatient Visits	3,753,945	3,703,509	3,528,497	3,462,575	3,422,070
Other Outpatient Visits	22,230,144	21,157,782	18,843,667	18,309,759	17,769,222
Total Outpatient Visits	25,984,089	24,861,291	22,372,164	21,772,334	21,191,292
Outpatient Surgeries	702,275	650,872	661,422	644,153	638,220
Personnel					
Full Time RNs	25,106	25,678	24,608	25,232	24,754
Full Time LPNs	2,768	2,631	2,657	2,996	2,818
Part Time RNs	17,888	16,721	17,554	17,752	16,746
Part Time LPNs	2,420	1,764	2,068	2,160	2,214
Total Full Time	120,138	122,715	119,054	127,456	124,145
Total Part Time	60,068	54,816	58,407	59,512	58,902
Revenue - Inpatient					
Gross Inpatient Revenue	$15,269,814,888	$14,753,771,125	$13,703,264,931	$13,735,570,282	$13,229,424,941
Revenue - Outpatient					
Gross Outpatient Revenue	$12,008,967,077	$10,951,098,666	$9,612,610,858	$9,165,570,745	$8,449,790,072
Revenue and Expenses - Totals (Includes Inpatient and Outpatient)					
Total Gross Revenue	$27,278,781,965	$25,704,869,791	$23,315,875,789	$22,901,141,027	$21,679,215,013
Deductions from Revenue	13,827,622,183	12,700,091,926	10,906,847,788	10,215,663,891	9,366,767,420
Net Patient Revenue	13,451,159,782	13,004,777,865	12,409,028,001	12,685,477,136	12,312,447,593
Other Operating Revenue	634,303,135	647,130,579	581,407,288	588,209,470	510,759,600
Other Nonoperating Revenue	122,735,458	687,142,951	515,479,497	471,734,694	402,277,716
Total Net Revenue	14,208,198,375	14,339,051,395	13,505,914,786	13,745,421,300	13,225,404,909
Total Expenses	13,891,061,790	13,456,111,469	12,897,935,106	12,920,233,262	12,374,846,831
HOSPITAL UNIT (Excludes Separate Nursing Home Units)					
Utilization - Inpatient					
Beds	23,868	24,012	23,841	24,993	25,751
Admissions	1,117,366	1,100,448	1,077,852	1,099,675	1,106,483
Inpatient Days	5,539,802	5,510,749	5,582,723	5,647,658	5,866,018
Average Length of Stay	5.0	5.0	5.2	5.1	5.3
Personnel					
Total Full Time	118,969	121,360	117,733	126,146	122,700
Total Part Time	59,286	54,005	57,651	58,775	58,065
Revenue and Expenses - Totals (Includes Inpatient and Outpatient)					
Total Net Revenue	$14,113,345,021	$14,241,432,247	$13,399,295,963	$13,646,478,835	$13,130,156,196
Total Expenses	13,820,531,836	13,364,180,983	12,804,079,036	12,830,389,161	12,295,926,785
COMMUNITY HEALTH INDICATORS PER 1000 POPULATION					
Total Population (in thousands)	9,991	9,938	9,864	9,820	9,785
Inpatient					
Beds	2.6	2.6	2.7	2.8	2.9
Admissions	112.3	111.3	109.9	112.5	113.6
Inpatient Days	611.5	621.4	638.3	649.7	673.6
Inpatient Surgeries	32.2	33.6	32.8	33.6	34.7
Births	12.7	13.2	13.0	13.0	13.1
Outpatient					
Emergency Outpatient Visits	375.7	372.6	357.7	352.6	349.7
Other Outpatient Visits	2,225.1	2,128.9	1,910.4	1,864.5	1,815.9
Total Outpatient Visits	2,600.8	2,501.5	2,268.1	2,217.1	2,165.6
Outpatient Surgeries	70.3	65.5	67.1	65.6	65.2
Expense per Capita (per person)	$1,390.4	$1,353.9	$1,307.6	$1,315.7	$1,264.6

TABLE 6

MINNESOTA

U.S. Registered Community Hospitals
(Nonfederal, short-term general and other special hospitals)

Overview 1997–2001

	2001	2000	1999	1998	1997
Total Community Hospitals	**133**	**135**	**134**	**136**	**137**
Bed Size Category					
6-24	16	16	16	17	17
25-49	23	25	25	26	26
50-99	39	38	40	39	37
100-199	38	39	37	37	39
200-299	6	6	5	6	7
300-399	3	3	6	6	6
400-499	4	4	1	1	1
500 +	4	4	4	4	4
Location					
Hospitals Urban	45	45	44	45	47
Hospitals Rural	88	90	90	91	90
Control					
State and Local Government	43	44	42	48	53
Not for Profit	90	91	92	88	84
Investor owned	0	0	0	0	0
Physician Models					
Independent Practice Association	24	21	15	18	21
Group Practice without Walls	2	1	1	4	6
Open Physician-Hospital Organization	9	8	7	12	14
Closed Physician-Hospital Organization	5	4	10	7	5
Management Service Organization	3	3	3	7	7
Integrated Salary Model	37	28	31	31	29
Equity Model	2	2	1	1	2
Foundation	3	1	5	8	12
Insurance Products					
Health Maintenance Organization	19	19	26	24	22
Preferred Provider Organization	18	22	20	25	29
Indemnity Fee for Service	3	5	9	11	15
Managed Care Contracts					
Health Maintenance Organization	70	62	60	64	70
Preferred Provider Organization	78	68	66	63	65
Affiliations					
Hospitals in a System	54	45	49	48	44
Hospitals in a Network	21	17	14	27	28
Hospitals in a Group Purchasing Organization	104	94	75	42	—

TABLE 6

MINNESOTA

U.S. Registered Community Hospitals
(Nonfederal, short-term general and other special hospitals)

Utilization, Personnel, Revenue and Expenses, Community Health Indicators 1997–2001

	2001	2000	1999	1998	1997
TOTAL FACILITY (Includes Hospital and Nursing Home Units)					
Utilization - Inpatient					
Beds	16,508	16,705	16,458	16,486	17,076
Admissions	586,016	570,672	534,692	515,813	526,742
Inpatient Days	4,102,576	4,089,075	4,046,050	4,110,360	4,254,912
Average Length of Stay	7.0	7.2	7.6	8.0	8.1
Inpatient Surgeries	173,787	162,709	158,632	157,630	167,887
Births	67,706	61,900	65,535	65,944	59,958
Utilization - Outpatient					
Emergency Outpatient Visits	1,506,825	1,454,970	1,364,802	1,143,117	1,195,116
Other Outpatient Visits	7,059,035	5,880,642	5,085,822	4,372,094	4,573,855
Total Outpatient Visits	8,565,860	7,335,612	6,450,624	5,515,211	5,768,971
Outpatient Surgeries	269,459	265,564	267,683	243,258	253,073
Personnel					
Full Time RNs	7,296	7,235	8,404	9,198	6,753
Full Time LPNs	1,463	1,420	1,857	1,922	1,427
Part Time RNs	18,377	16,856	14,906	12,433	16,240
Part Time LPNs	2,612	2,614	2,845	2,356	3,036
Total Full Time	42,981	40,907	44,027	43,315	39,947
Total Part Time	56,308	52,536	47,798	41,291	53,320
Revenue - Inpatient					
Gross Inpatient Revenue	$8,594,174,827	$7,576,893,093	$6,735,210,305	$5,967,869,859	$5,868,932,670
Revenue - Outpatient					
Gross Outpatient Revenue	$5,096,222,863	$4,321,208,532	$3,755,772,176	$3,119,336,088	$2,963,588,396
Revenue and Expenses - Totals (Includes Inpatient and Outpatient)					
Total Gross Revenue	$13,690,397,690	$11,898,101,625	$10,490,982,481	$9,087,205,947	$8,832,521,066
Deductions from Revenue	6,733,859,329	5,560,355,139	4,745,177,001	3,891,787,468	3,588,802,638
Net Patient Revenue	6,956,538,361	6,337,746,486	5,745,805,480	5,195,418,479	5,243,718,428
Other Operating Revenue	371,921,708	325,155,610	312,210,657	299,354,500	280,663,453
Other Nonoperating Revenue	77,288,116	160,470,734	137,362,929	148,114,241	141,305,312
Total Net Revenue	7,405,748,185	6,823,372,830	6,195,379,066	5,642,887,220	5,665,687,193
Total Expenses	7,067,072,024	6,411,848,478	5,807,149,050	5,265,388,159	5,270,452,689
HOSPITAL UNIT (Excludes Separate Nursing Home Units)					
Utilization - Inpatient					
Beds	12,558	12,669	12,737	11,874	12,423
Admissions	581,569	565,919	528,535	508,463	520,956
Inpatient Days	2,715,146	2,714,883	2,789,190	2,540,143	2,636,102
Average Length of Stay	4.7	4.8	5.3	5.0	5.1
Personnel					
Total Full Time	40,988	38,802	42,095	41,327	37,809
Total Part Time	53,557	49,441	45,255	38,314	50,080
Revenue and Expenses - Totals (Includes Inpatient and Outpatient)					
Total Net Revenue	$7,227,917,429	$6,659,630,244	$6,039,668,626	$5,453,930,915	$5,487,450,520
Total Expenses	6,891,386,470	6,245,744,327	5,647,638,456	5,088,046,865	5,118,463,978
COMMUNITY HEALTH INDICATORS PER 1000 POPULATION					
Total Population (in thousands)	4,972	4,919	4,776	4,726	4,688
Inpatient					
Beds	3.3	3.4	3.4	3.5	3.6
Admissions	117.9	116.0	112.0	109.1	112.4
Inpatient Days	825.1	831.2	847.3	869.7	907.7
Inpatient Surgeries	35.0	33.1	33.2	33.4	35.8
Births	13.6	12.6	13.7	14.0	12.8
Outpatient					
Emergency Outpatient Visits	303.0	295.8	285.8	241.9	254.9
Other Outpatient Visits	1,419.7	1,195.4	1,065.0	925.0	975.7
Total Outpatient Visits	1,722.7	1,491.1	1,350.8	1,166.9	1,230.7
Outpatient Surgeries	54.2	54.0	56.1	51.5	54.0
Expense per Capita (per person)	$1,421.3	$1,303.4	$1,216.0	$1,114.0	$1,124.3

TABLE 6

MISSISSIPPI

U.S. Registered Community Hospitals
(Nonfederal, short-term general and other special hospitals)

Overview 1997–2001

	2001	2000	1999	1998	1997
Total Community Hospitals	96	95	96	96	97
Bed Size Category					
6-24	2	1	1	1	1
25-49	17	18	18	16	17
50-99	29	29	34	36	34
100-199	33	31	27	28	31
200-299	6	8	7	7	6
300-399	2	1	4	3	3
400-499	2	2	0	0	0
500 +	5	5	5	5	5
Location					
Hospitals Urban	20	19	20	19	20
Hospitals Rural	76	76	76	77	77
Control					
State and Local Government	45	45	46	47	49
Not for Profit	27	26	28	29	30
Investor owned	24	24	22	20	18
Physician Models					
Independent Practice Association	59	13	11	12	11
Group Practice without Walls	59	9	8	5	4
Open Physician-Hospital Organization	18	22	27	31	30
Closed Physician-Hospital Organization	5	10	9	6	7
Management Service Organization	6	9	8	8	6
Integrated Salary Model	14	16	15	14	15
Equity Model	3	3	3	3	3
Foundation	11	12	13	14	13
Insurance Products					
Health Maintenance Organization	12	13	13	17	16
Preferred Provider Organization	47	48	53	53	57
Indemnity Fee for Service	15	15	15	18	17
Managed Care Contracts					
Health Maintenance Organization	2	0	1	0	26
Preferred Provider Organization	38	3	0	0	74
Affiliations					
Hospitals in a System	36	33	35	36	33
Hospitals in a Network	32	35	32	32	33
Hospitals in a Group Purchasing Organization	1	—	—	—	—

TABLE 6

MISSISSIPPI

U.S. Registered Community Hospitals
(Nonfederal, short-term general and other special hospitals)

Utilization, Personnel, Revenue and Expenses, Community Health Indicators 1997–2001

	2001	2000	1999	1998	1997
TOTAL FACILITY (Includes Hospital and Nursing Home Units)					
Utilization - Inpatient					
Beds	13,670	13,598	13,217	13,005	12,904
Admissions	436,100	424,772	415,776	413,907	413,472
Inpatient Days	2,990,906	2,929,248	2,916,549	2,949,682	2,946,321
Average Length of Stay	6.9	6.9	7.0	7.1	7.1
Inpatient Surgeries	116,292	111,465	120,663	115,790	119,289
Births	42,049	42,199	40,410	39,101	39,213
Utilization - Outpatient					
Emergency Outpatient Visits	1,501,052	1,478,883	1,429,819	1,425,892	1,442,454
Other Outpatient Visits	2,601,447	2,228,914	2,027,658	2,004,076	2,444,738
Total Outpatient Visits	4,102,499	3,707,797	3,457,477	3,429,968	3,887,192
Outpatient Surgeries	154,317	151,832	145,593	129,570	133,990
Personnel					
Full Time RNs	9,467	9,424	9,594	9,488	8,697
Full Time LPNs	2,025	2,001	2,170	2,478	2,613
Part Time RNs	3,636	3,185	2,728	2,701	2,624
Part Time LPNs	648	583	626	598	607
Total Full Time	40,936	39,550	40,398	42,165	41,203
Total Part Time	11,627	11,597	10,122	9,973	9,979
Revenue - Inpatient					
Gross Inpatient Revenue	$5,203,288,483	$4,486,744,256	$4,219,185,699	$3,975,096,989	$3,552,896,622
Revenue - Outpatient					
Gross Outpatient Revenue	$2,891,655,269	$2,471,664,887	$2,196,978,616	$1,932,971,070	$1,749,611,264
Revenue and Expenses - Totals (Includes Inpatient and Outpatient)					
Total Gross Revenue	$8,094,943,752	$6,958,409,143	$6,416,164,315	$5,908,068,059	$5,302,507,886
Deductions from Revenue	4,344,923,458	3,645,598,561	3,165,780,811	2,735,462,519	2,359,786,933
Net Patient Revenue	3,750,020,294	3,312,810,582	3,250,383,504	3,172,605,540	2,942,720,953
Other Operating Revenue	137,215,985	191,115,070	116,160,034	117,184,927	107,098,122
Other Nonoperating Revenue	52,257,480	67,563,680	50,570,163	48,450,755	42,017,449
Total Net Revenue	3,939,493,759	3,571,489,332	3,417,113,701	3,338,241,222	3,091,836,524
Total Expenses	3,614,544,722	3,327,375,432	3,202,825,608	3,138,686,670	2,823,387,183
HOSPITAL UNIT (Excludes Separate Nursing Home Units)					
Utilization - Inpatient					
Beds	12,000	11,995	11,633	11,438	11,403
Admissions	434,827	423,739	414,619	412,755	412,328
Inpatient Days	2,400,974	2,358,912	2,355,643	2,400,129	2,412,368
Average Length of Stay	5.5	5.6	5.7	5.8	5.9
Personnel					
Total Full Time	39,070	38,528	39,375	40,974	40,170
Total Part Time	11,254	11,248	9,815	9,699	9,707
Revenue and Expenses - Totals (Includes Inpatient and Outpatient)					
Total Net Revenue	$3,896,587,199	$3,515,536,637	$3,377,670,317	$3,304,486,181	$3,060,359,483
Total Expenses	3,583,850,640	3,293,094,874	3,174,354,952	3,113,147,029	2,799,995,657
COMMUNITY HEALTH INDICATORS PER 1000 POPULATION					
Total Population (in thousands)	2,858	2,845	2,769	2,751	2,732
Inpatient					
Beds	4.8	4.8	4.8	4.7	4.7
Admissions	152.6	149.3	150.2	150.4	151.4
Inpatient Days	1,046.5	1,029.7	1,053.4	1,072.1	1,078.5
Inpatient Surgeries	40.7	39.2	43.6	42.1	43.7
Births	14.7	14.8	14.6	14.2	14.4
Outpatient					
Emergency Outpatient Visits	525.2	519.9	516.4	518.3	528.0
Other Outpatient Visits	910.2	783.5	732.4	728.4	894.9
Total Outpatient Visits	1,435.4	1,303.4	1,248.8	1,246.7	1,422.9
Outpatient Surgeries	54.0	53.4	52.6	47.1	49.0
Expense per Capita (per person)	$1,264.7	$1,169.7	$1,156.8	$1,140.8	$1,033.5

States

TABLE 6

MISSOURI

U.S. Registered Community Hospitals
(Nonfederal, short-term general and other special hospitals)

Overview 1997–2001

	2001	2000	1999	1998	1997
Total Community Hospitals	**117**	**119**	**118**	**122**	**123**
Bed Size Category					
6-24	4	4	4	3	3
25-49	31	33	29	30	30
50-99	25	24	28	28	30
100-199	22	21	21	25	23
200-299	16	17	13	15	15
300-399	8	9	13	10	10
400-499	5	4	2	3	5
500 +	6	7	8	8	7
Location					
Hospitals Urban	60	61	60	64	64
Hospitals Rural	57	58	58	58	59
Control					
State and Local Government	36	37	35	36	36
Not for Profit	69	71	71	71	73
Investor owned	12	11	12	15	14
Physician Models					
Independent Practice Association	17	22	19	30	28
Group Practice without Walls	4	8	8	9	14
Open Physician-Hospital Organization	26	30	32	35	38
Closed Physician-Hospital Organization	16	17	23	28	28
Management Service Organization	10	9	17	19	26
Integrated Salary Model	50	49	50	44	47
Equity Model	1	3	2	3	6
Foundation	4	3	2	5	9
Insurance Products					
Health Maintenance Organization	31	48	57	56	59
Preferred Provider Organization	22	29	35	48	46
Indemnity Fee for Service	12	11	14	18	15
Managed Care Contracts					
Health Maintenance Organization	99	105	104	107	104
Preferred Provider Organization	106	112	99	108	113
Affiliations					
Hospitals in a System	63	65	63	68	66
Hospitals in a Network	43	44	40	45	40
Hospitals in a Group Purchasing Organization	103	105	100	99	—

States

TABLE 6

MISSOURI

U.S. Registered Community Hospitals
(Nonfederal, short-term general and other special hospitals)

Utilization, Personnel, Revenue and Expenses, Community Health Indicators 1997–2001

	2001	2000	1999	1998	1997
TOTAL FACILITY (Includes Hospital and Nursing Home Units)					
Utilization - Inpatient					
Beds	19,257	20,140	20,253	20,685	20,867
Admissions	800,648	773,261	742,867	741,816	729,914
Inpatient Days	4,219,659	4,269,800	4,247,921	4,325,879	4,311,021
Average Length of Stay	5.3	5.5	5.7	5.8	5.9
Inpatient Surgeries	210,030	207,476	200,706	205,887	198,722
Births	75,350	77,333	75,625	76,031	75,004
Utilization - Outpatient					
Emergency Outpatient Visits	2,443,744	2,326,906	2,411,820	2,115,060	2,036,674
Other Outpatient Visits	11,755,063	12,479,871	12,231,541	8,046,012	7,526,527
Total Outpatient Visits	14,198,807	14,806,777	14,643,361	10,161,072	9,563,201
Outpatient Surgeries	389,098	381,289	362,462	367,983	354,781
Personnel					
Full Time RNs	18,576	18,689	18,685	18,484	18,420
Full Time LPNs	2,881	3,019	2,917	3,432	2,873
Part Time RNs	12,017	11,206	10,562	10,787	10,285
Part Time LPNs	1,171	1,221	1,162	1,380	1,071
Total Full Time	82,978	82,820	79,501	82,902	82,723
Total Part Time	35,676	34,263	31,230	33,394	32,813
Revenue - Inpatient					
Gross Inpatient Revenue	$12,106,385,281	$11,082,223,366	$9,964,294,835	$9,229,915,545	$8,797,770,874
Revenue - Outpatient					
Gross Outpatient Revenue	$7,685,930,325	$6,685,962,437	$5,791,429,121	$5,196,890,359	$4,925,920,580
Revenue and Expenses - Totals (Includes Inpatient and Outpatient)					
Total Gross Revenue	$19,792,315,606	$17,768,185,803	$15,755,723,956	$14,426,805,904	$13,723,691,454
Deductions from Revenue	10,984,983,535	9,652,801,745	8,213,774,013	7,091,069,076	6,499,860,419
Net Patient Revenue	8,807,332,071	8,115,384,058	7,541,949,943	7,335,736,828	7,223,831,035
Other Operating Revenue	486,319,667	440,053,995	484,296,906	457,285,200	407,113,128
Other Nonoperating Revenue	154,063,942	196,916,165	197,565,929	291,564,766	287,764,761
Total Net Revenue	9,447,715,680	8,752,354,218	8,223,812,778	8,081,586,701	7,018,708,024
Total Expenses	9,118,864,692	8,534,174,151	7,953,842,591	7,576,182,640	7,345,773,351
HOSPITAL UNIT (Excludes Separate Nursing Home Units)					
Utilization - Inpatient					
Beds	17,642	18,096	18,003	18,049	18,449
Admissions	779,379	746,131	712,942	703,211	697,823
Inpatient Days	3,781,344	3,724,585	3,599,897	3,573,987	3,618,942
Average Length of Stay	4.9	5.0	5.0	5.1	5.2
Personnel					
Total Full Time	81,903	81,237	77,895	80,127	80,741
Total Part Time	35,092	33,437	30,530	32,565	31,987
Revenue and Expenses - Totals (Includes Inpatient and Outpatient)					
Total Net Revenue	$9,292,053,516	$8,558,718,897	$8,054,357,353	$7,859,783,453	$7,716,401,315
Total Expenses	8,999,337,551	8,392,524,096	7,825,633,137	7,404,638,643	7,198,502,107
COMMUNITY HEALTH INDICATORS PER 1000 POPULATION					
Total Population (in thousands)	5,630	5,595	5,468	5,438	5,407
Inpatient					
Beds	3.4	3.6	3.7	3.8	3.9
Admissions	142.2	138.2	135.8	136.4	135.0
Inpatient Days	749.5	763.1	776.8	795.6	797.3
Inpatient Surgeries	37.3	37.1	36.7	37.9	36.8
Births	13.4	13.8	13.8	14.0	13.9
Outpatient					
Emergency Outpatient Visits	434.1	415.9	441.1	389.0	376.7
Other Outpatient Visits	2,088.0	2,230.5	2,236.8	1,479.7	1,392.0
Total Outpatient Visits	2,522.1	2,646.3	2,677.8	1,868.7	1,768.6
Outpatient Surgeries	69.1	68.1	66.3	67.7	65.6
Expense per Capita (per person)	$1,619.8	$1,525.3	$1,454.5	$1,393.3	$1,358.5

TABLE 6

MONTANA

U.S. Registered Community Hospitals
(Nonfederal, short-term general and other special hospitals)

Overview 1997–2001

	2001	2000	1999	1998	1997
Total Community Hospitals	**53**	**52**	**53**	**53**	**54**
Bed Size Category					
6-24	7	7	7	7	6
25-49	15	14	13	13	15
50-99	17	19	19	20	19
100-199	10	8	9	8	9
200-299	2	2	3	3	4
300-399	1	1	1	1	0
400-499	1	1	1	1	1
500 +	0	0	0	0	0
Location					
Hospitals Urban	5	3	3	3	3
Hospitals Rural	48	49	50	50	51
Control					
State and Local Government	11	10	12	10	14
Not for Profit	42	42	41	43	39
Investor owned	0	0	0	0	1
Physician Models					
Independent Practice Association	7	11	5	6	3
Group Practice without Walls	3	3	1	0	2
Open Physician-Hospital Organization	9	9	9	9	6
Closed Physician-Hospital Organization	1	1	3	0	2
Management Service Organization	6	5	2	5	3
Integrated Salary Model	18	16	16	11	12
Equity Model	1	0	0	0	0
Foundation	2	5	1	2	3
Insurance Products					
Health Maintenance Organization	5	7	7	6	8
Preferred Provider Organization	5	6	3	3	9
Indemnity Fee for Service	2	2	2	4	3
Managed Care Contracts					
Health Maintenance Organization	12	14	15	12	9
Preferred Provider Organization	24	26	20	20	17
Affiliations					
Hospitals in a System	10	10	11	13	10
Hospitals in a Network	23	22	21	16	20
Hospitals in a Group Purchasing Organization	47	48	42	42	—

States

TABLE 6

MONTANA

U.S. Registered Community Hospitals
(Nonfederal, short-term general and other special hospitals)

Utilization, Personnel, Revenue and Expenses, Community Health Indicators 1997–2001

	2001	2000	1999	1998	1997
TOTAL FACILITY (Includes Hospital and Nursing Home Units)					
Utilization - Inpatient					
Beds	4,463	4,255	4,668	4,413	4,482
Admissions	103,346	99,273	97,875	97,345	98,788
Inpatient Days	1,058,079	1,045,460	1,161,334	1,090,989	1,014,709
Average Length of Stay	10.2	10.5	11.9	11.2	10.3
Inpatient Surgeries	31,774	31,365	30,824	30,475	30,093
Births	9,766	9,828	9,826	9,772	9,793
Utilization - Outpatient					
Emergency Outpatient Visits	276,175	270,905	263,239	259,462	254,728
Other Outpatient Visits	2,372,170	2,377,671	2,276,174	2,029,023	1,224,514
Total Outpatient Visits	2,648,345	2,648,576	2,539,413	2,288,485	1,479,242
Outpatient Surgeries	37,544	38,146	38,123	41,027	42,871
Personnel					
Full Time RNs	2,139	2,262	2,206	2,053	2,024
Full Time LPNs	493	520	480	538	525
Part Time RNs	1,695	1,705	1,415	1,643	1,561
Part Time LPNs	347	375	263	435	305
Total Full Time	11,464	11,394	11,578	10,846	10,494
Total Part Time	6,492	6,319	5,676	5,982	6,076
Revenue - Inpatient					
Gross Inpatient Revenue	$1,105,228,828	$999,654,818	$926,618,947	$858,900,634	$852,690,528
Revenue - Outpatient					
Gross Outpatient Revenue	$835,450,580	$737,774,057	$667,505,475	$600,992,951	$552,390,389
Revenue and Expenses - Totals (Includes Inpatient and Outpatient)					
Total Gross Revenue	$1,940,679,408	$1,737,428,875	$1,594,124,422	$1,459,893,585	$1,405,080,917
Deductions from Revenue	727,980,516	625,526,349	527,906,272	448,396,455	443,014,136
Net Patient Revenue	1,212,698,892	1,111,902,526	1,066,218,150	1,011,497,130	962,066,781
Other Operating Revenue	52,002,157	46,591,161	64,179,153	41,278,334	43,356,711
Other Nonoperating Revenue	29,771,646	37,823,173	29,299,977	57,383,432	32,370,187
Total Net Revenue	1,294,472,695	1,196,316,860	1,159,697,280	1,110,158,896	1,037,793,679
Total Expenses	1,216,570,389	1,145,815,779	1,082,320,886	1,002,984,008	972,420,897
HOSPITAL UNIT (Excludes Separate Nursing Home Units)					
Utilization - Inpatient					
Beds	2,591	2,301	2,665	2,479	2,557
Admissions	99,503	95,295	92,995	92,826	94,444
Inpatient Days	466,644	421,283	526,200	460,325	452,570
Average Length of Stay	4.7	4.4	5.7	5.0	4.8
Personnel					
Total Full Time	10,407	10,273	10,632	9,755	9,576
Total Part Time	5,610	5,566	4,994	5,369	5,484
Revenue and Expenses - Totals (Includes Inpatient and Outpatient)					
Total Net Revenue	$1,226,159,560	$1,133,832,079	$1,094,400,649	$1,034,194,455	$987,907,059
Total Expenses	1,149,226,075	1,083,787,392	1,018,250,749	940,693,445	920,720,492
COMMUNITY HEALTH INDICATORS PER 1000 POPULATION					
Total Population (in thousands)	904	902	883	880	879
Inpatient					
Beds	4.9	4.7	5.3	5.0	5.1
Admissions	114.3	110.0	110.9	110.7	112.4
Inpatient Days	1,169.9	1,158.8	1,315.5	1,240.4	1,154.8
Inpatient Surgeries	35.1	34.8	34.9	34.6	34.2
Births	10.8	10.9	11.1	11.1	11.1
Outpatient					
Emergency Outpatient Visits	305.4	300.3	298.2	295.0	289.9
Other Outpatient Visits	2,622.8	2,635.4	2,578.4	2,306.9	1,393.5
Total Outpatient Visits	2,928.2	2,935.7	2,876.6	2,601.9	1,683.4
Outpatient Surgeries	41.5	42.3	43.2	46.6	48.8
Expense per Capita (per person)	$1,345.1	$1,270.0	$1,226.0	$1,140.4	$1,106.7

TABLE 6

NEBRASKA

U.S. Registered Community Hospitals
(Nonfederal, short-term general and other special hospitals)

Overview 1997–2001

	2001	2000	1999	1998	1997
Total Community Hospitals	**84**	**85**	**85**	**86**	**87**
Bed Size Category					
6-24	18	18	18	21	21
25-49	27	28	27	26	27
50-99	17	19	18	16	18
100-199	10	8	10	11	10
200-299	6	6	6	7	7
300-399	2	2	2	1	1
400-499	0	0	0	0	0
500 +	4	4	4	4	3
Location					
Hospitals Urban	14	13	13	13	13
Hospitals Rural	70	72	72	73	74
Control					
State and Local Government	39	41	41	41	42
Not for Profit	43	43	43	43	43
Investor owned	2	1	1	2	2
Physician Models					
Independent Practice Association	6	8	6	6	12
Group Practice without Walls	1	1	1	2	3
Open Physician-Hospital Organization	17	14	16	19	20
Closed Physician-Hospital Organization	0	1	2	1	1
Management Service Organization	0	1	5	5	9
Integrated Salary Model	28	32	34	31	27
Equity Model	0	0	1	1	2
Foundation	1	2	4	4	5
Insurance Products					
Health Maintenance Organization	1	5	5	8	11
Preferred Provider Organization	15	17	21	19	26
Indemnity Fee for Service	2	5	3	3	5
Managed Care Contracts					
Health Maintenance Organization	24	31	28	30	37
Preferred Provider Organization	56	66	64	67	76
Affiliations					
Hospitals in a System	16	22	22	22	22
Hospitals in a Network	40	45	41	42	46
Hospitals in a Group Purchasing Organization	63	73	67	69	—

States

TABLE 6

NEBRASKA

U.S. Registered Community Hospitals
(Nonfederal, short-term general and other special hospitals)

Utilization, Personnel, Revenue and Expenses, Community Health Indicators 1997–2001

	2001	2000	1999	1998	1997
TOTAL FACILITY (Includes Hospital and Nursing Home Units)					
Utilization - Inpatient					
Beds	8,324	8,161	8,326	8,133	7,750
Admissions	206,700	209,498	199,471	192,313	190,960
Inpatient Days	1,826,566	1,760,490	1,821,925	1,779,579	1,683,706
Average Length of Stay	8.8	8.4	9.1	9.3	8.8
Inpatient Surgeries	68,392	68,738	66,997	71,503	69,319
Births	24,313	23,479	21,877	22,770	22,570
Utilization - Outpatient					
Emergency Outpatient Visits	545,607	499,960	491,438	455,953	421,382
Other Outpatient Visits	2,884,235	2,905,439	2,510,386	2,393,171	2,124,635
Total Outpatient Visits	3,429,842	3,405,399	3,001,824	2,849,124	2,546,017
Outpatient Surgeries	129,154	123,042	114,063	115,114	120,015
Personnel					
Full Time RNs	5,456	5,352	5,185	5,149	4,863
Full Time LPNs	1,044	1,041	1,059	1,057	1,206
Part Time RNs	3,695	3,484	3,993	3,703	3,224
Part Time LPNs	649	692	769	749	891
Total Full Time	24,476	23,898	23,412	23,011	22,846
Total Part Time	14,398	13,454	14,887	13,430	11,893
Revenue - Inpatient					
Gross Inpatient Revenue	$3,052,706,197	$2,675,259,869	$2,371,471,871	$2,195,397,641	$1,979,236,890
Revenue - Outpatient					
Gross Outpatient Revenue	$1,898,195,952	$1,561,380,290	$1,344,021,603	$1,162,909,796	$1,095,560,066
Revenue and Expenses - Totals (Includes Inpatient and Outpatient)					
Total Gross Revenue	$4,950,902,149	$4,236,640,159	$3,715,493,474	$3,358,307,437	$3,074,796,956
Deductions from Revenue	2,221,659,602	1,816,852,259	1,523,396,593	1,293,025,623	1,067,106,205
Net Patient Revenue	2,729,242,547	2,419,787,900	2,192,096,881	2,065,281,814	2,007,690,751
Other Operating Revenue	131,134,300	122,358,298	111,258,095	97,728,471	85,168,630
Other Nonoperating Revenue	49,150,380	65,215,309	36,446,213	67,326,888	52,254,051
Total Net Revenue	2,909,527,227	2,607,361,507	2,330,801,180	2,230,337,173	2,145,113,432
Total Expenses	2,645,027,198	2,327,404,184	2,156,055,667	1,988,638,033	1,910,738,003
HOSPITAL UNIT (Excludes Separate Nursing Home Units)					
Utilization - Inpatient					
Beds	6,427	6,144	6,216	6,035	5,702
Admissions	201,225	203,541	191,227	186,219	184,762
Inpatient Days	1,223,636	1,104,318	1,114,416	1,086,543	1,011,387
Average Length of Stay	6.1	5.4	5.8	5.8	5.5
Personnel					
Total Full Time	23,330	22,725	22,230	22,014	21,882
Total Part Time	13,531	12,561	14,016	12,609	11,020
Revenue and Expenses - Totals (Includes Inpatient and Outpatient)					
Total Net Revenue	$2,817,978,178	$2,528,414,477	$2,247,886,654	$2,138,201,381	$2,066,231,742
Total Expenses	2,562,442,544	2,243,914,541	2,078,619,066	1,917,444,766	1,847,693,208
COMMUNITY HEALTH INDICATORS PER 1000 POPULATION					
Total Population (in thousands)	1,713	1,711	1,666	1,661	1,656
Inpatient					
Beds	4.9	4.8	5.0	4.9	4.7
Admissions	120.6	122.4	119.7	115.8	115.3
Inpatient Days	1,066.2	1,028.8	1,093.6	1,071.5	1,016.7
Inpatient Surgeries	39.9	40.2	40.2	43.1	41.9
Births	14.2	13.7	13.1	13.7	13.6
Outpatient					
Emergency Outpatient Visits	318.5	292.2	295.0	274.5	254.5
Other Outpatient Visits	1,683.5	1,697.8	1,506.8	1,441.0	1,283.0
Total Outpatient Visits	2,002.0	1,990.0	1,801.8	1,715.5	1,537.4
Outpatient Surgeries	75.4	71.9	68.5	69.3	72.5
Expense per Capita (per person)	$1,543.9	$1,360.1	$1,294.1	$1,197.4	$1,153.8

TABLE 6

NEVADA

U.S. Registered Community Hospitals
(Nonfederal, short-term general and other special hospitals)

Overview 1997–2001

	2001	2000	1999	1998	1997
Total Community Hospitals	**24**	**22**	**22**	**20**	**19**
Bed Size Category					
6-24	1	1	1	1	1
25-49	5	5	6	5	5
50-99	4	4	3	3	3
100-199	8	6	6	5	3
200-299	2	2	2	2	3
300-399	1	1	1	1	1
400-499	1	1	1	1	1
500 +	2	2	2	2	2
Location					
Hospitals Urban	15	13	14	12	11
Hospitals Rural	9	9	8	8	8
Control					
State and Local Government	7	7	8	7	8
Not for Profit	7	7	6	6	6
Investor owned	10	8	8	7	5
Physician Models					
Independent Practice Association	2	2	4	5	6
Group Practice without Walls	0	0	0	1	1
Open Physician-Hospital Organization	1	1	0	0	1
Closed Physician-Hospital Organization	0	0	0	0	0
Management Service Organization	1	2	3	4	5
Integrated Salary Model	3	2	3	3	3
Equity Model	0	0	0	0	0
Foundation	0	0	1	0	2
Insurance Products					
Health Maintenance Organization	2	3	0	2	3
Preferred Provider Organization	2	3	0	4	5
Indemnity Fee for Service	1	1	0	1	2
Managed Care Contracts					
Health Maintenance Organization	9	8	11	7	6
Preferred Provider Organization	11	9	13	10	10
Affiliations					
Hospitals in a System	11	7	9	9	7
Hospitals in a Network	3	3	4	2	4
Hospitals in a Group Purchasing Organization	14	7	10	7	—

States

TABLE 6

NEVADA

U.S. Registered Community Hospitals
(Nonfederal, short-term general and other special hospitals)

Utilization, Personnel, Revenue and Expenses, Community Health Indicators 1997–2001

	2001	2000	1999	1998	1997
TOTAL FACILITY (Includes Hospital and Nursing Home Units)					
Utilization - Inpatient					
Beds	4,099	3,810	3,706	3,528	3,539
Admissions	207,844	199,455	197,501	171,158	160,770
Inpatient Days	1,019,835	984,845	1,000,369	837,270	869,239
Average Length of Stay	4.9	4.9	5.1	4.9	5.4
Inpatient Surgeries	76,427	72,090	78,969	52,096	56,368
Births	28,040	28,874	30,399	24,799	24,427
Utilization - Outpatient					
Emergency Outpatient Visits	548,798	573,220	527,219	463,706	431,476
Other Outpatient Visits	1,577,315	1,618,898	1,599,270	1,128,937	928,780
Total Outpatient Visits	2,126,113	2,192,118	2,126,489	1,592,643	1,360,256
Outpatient Surgeries	91,748	84,840	111,460	63,138	63,357
Personnel					
Full Time RNs	3,984	4,255	3,992	3,547	3,202
Full Time LPNs	429	455	581	397	435
Part Time RNs	1,523	1,388	1,160	1,252	1,361
Part Time LPNs	101	72	104	87	117
Total Full Time	15,682	16,173	14,846	13,410	12,557
Total Part Time	4,180	3,783	3,671	3,400	3,579
Revenue - Inpatient					
Gross Inpatient Revenue	$3,997,307,168	$3,384,346,250	$3,224,856,025	$2,743,705,642	$2,521,578,934
Revenue - Outpatient					
Gross Outpatient Revenue	$1,486,747,093	$1,175,895,927	$1,120,428,723	$858,030,810	$769,106,724
Revenue and Expenses - Totals (Includes Inpatient and Outpatient)					
Total Gross Revenue	$5,484,054,261	$4,560,242,177	$4,345,284,748	$3,601,736,452	$3,290,685,658
Deductions from Revenue	3,441,708,915	2,795,643,699	2,673,121,276	2,194,873,625	1,892,688,012
Net Patient Revenue	2,042,345,346	1,764,598,478	1,672,163,472	1,406,862,827	1,397,997,646
Other Operating Revenue	95,047,287	77,338,480	45,314,641	58,226,194	67,338,173
Other Nonoperating Revenue	25,143,034	34,250,055	18,599,731	33,553,971	24,191,495
Total Net Revenue	2,162,535,667	1,876,187,013	1,736,077,844	1,498,642,992	1,489,527,314
Total Expenses	2,087,682,180	1,790,079,467	1,623,910,172	1,392,140,547	1,317,288,684
HOSPITAL UNIT (Excludes Separate Nursing Home Units)					
Utilization - Inpatient					
Beds	3,969	3,712	3,600	3,479	3,286
Admissions	207,237	198,904	197,292	170,564	159,553
Inpatient Days	977,487	954,823	959,252	822,289	791,815
Average Length of Stay	4.7	4.8	4.9	4.8	5.0
Personnel					
Total Full Time	15,611	16,039	14,788	13,375	12,327
Total Part Time	4,146	3,755	3,657	3,386	3,448
Revenue and Expenses - Totals (Includes Inpatient and Outpatient)					
Total Net Revenue	$2,156,122,530	$1,870,827,186	$1,731,123,484	$1,495,619,656	$1,471,592,220
Total Expenses	2,083,886,026	1,787,243,271	1,621,429,707	1,390,358,456	1,302,000,569
COMMUNITY HEALTH INDICATORS PER 1000 POPULATION					
Total Population (in thousands)	2,106	1,998	1,809	1,744	1,676
Inpatient					
Beds	1.9	1.9	2.0	2.0	2.1
Admissions	98.7	99.8	109.2	98.2	95.9
Inpatient Days	484.2	492.9	552.9	480.1	518.8
Inpatient Surgeries	36.3	36.1	43.6	29.9	33.6
Births	13.3	14.4	16.8	14.2	14.6
Outpatient					
Emergency Outpatient Visits	260.6	286.9	291.4	265.9	257.5
Other Outpatient Visits	748.9	810.2	883.9	647.4	554.3
Total Outpatient Visits	1,009.5	1,097.0	1,175.3	913.3	811.8
Outpatient Surgeries	43.6	42.5	61.6	36.2	37.8
Expense per Capita (per person)	$991.3	$895.8	$897.6	$798.4	$786.2

States

TABLE 6

NEW HAMPSHIRE

U.S. Registered Community Hospitals
(Nonfederal, short-term general and other special hospitals)

Overview 1997–2001

	2001	2000	1999	1998	1997
Total Community Hospitals	**28**	**28**	**28**	**28**	**28**
Bed Size Category					
6-24	1	1	0	1	1
25-49	6	6	6	6	6
50-99	11	11	12	11	11
100-199	7	7	6	7	7
200-299	2	2	3	2	2
300-399	1	1	1	1	1
400-499	0	0	0	0	0
500 +	0	0	0	0	0
Location					
Hospitals Urban	10	10	10	10	10
Hospitals Rural	18	18	18	18	18
Control					
State and Local Government	0	0	0	0	0
Not for Profit	24	24	24	24	24
Investor owned	4	4	4	4	4
Physician Models					
Independent Practice Association	2	2	2	2	3
Group Practice without Walls	2	2	1	0	0
Open Physician-Hospital Organization	12	14	14	14	15
Closed Physician-Hospital Organization	4	3	2	3	2
Management Service Organization	2	3	3	4	3
Integrated Salary Model	12	11	12	7	9
Equity Model	0	0	0	0	0
Foundation	1	1	3	4	3
Insurance Products					
Health Maintenance Organization	1	1	2	4	6
Preferred Provider Organization	0	0	0	1	2
Indemnity Fee for Service	0	0	0	3	3
Managed Care Contracts					
Health Maintenance Organization	25	26	26	26	27
Preferred Provider Organization	23	22	23	24	25
Affiliations					
Hospitals in a System	14	14	14	12	14
Hospitals in a Network	8	9	7	6	4
Hospitals in a Group Purchasing Organization	25	22	23	22	—

TABLE 6

NEW HAMPSHIRE

U.S. Registered Community Hospitals
(Nonfederal, short-term general and other special hospitals)

Utilization, Personnel, Revenue and Expenses, Community Health Indicators 1997–2001

	2001	2000	1999	1998	1997
TOTAL FACILITY (Includes Hospital and Nursing Home Units)					
Utilization - Inpatient					
Beds	2,853	2,865	2,974	2,841	2,951
Admissions	116,071	111,227	109,110	108,942	110,193
Inpatient Days	637,239	611,919	599,777	658,884	682,841
Average Length of Stay	5.5	5.5	5.5	6.0	6.2
Inpatient Surgeries	33,702	33,595	32,864	31,291	31,078
Births	13,919	13,715	13,470	13,738	13,758
Utilization - Outpatient					
Emergency Outpatient Visits	537,367	526,103	491,840	476,050	450,857
Other Outpatient Visits	2,392,259	2,237,250	1,908,936	1,859,224	1,680,524
Total Outpatient Visits	2,929,626	2,763,353	2,400,776	2,335,274	2,131,381
Outpatient Surgeries	75,467	68,807	60,607	61,163	56,233
Personnel					
Full Time RNs	3,130	2,825	2,643	2,856	2,731
Full Time LPNs	175	172	210	166	200
Part Time RNs	2,087	2,139	2,261	1,994	2,042
Part Time LPNs	135	146	180	160	158
Total Full Time	14,578	12,923	12,681	12,351	11,903
Total Part Time	7,571	7,905	8,186	7,076	6,784
Revenue - Inpatient					
Gross Inpatient Revenue	$1,452,518,894	$1,318,942,481	$1,151,678,573	$1,132,184,877	$1,085,616,496
Revenue - Outpatient					
Gross Outpatient Revenue	$1,422,018,438	$1,189,795,594	$991,577,915	$893,202,730	$807,173,126
Revenue and Expenses - Totals (Includes Inpatient and Outpatient)					
Total Gross Revenue	$2,874,537,332	$2,508,738,075	$2,143,256,488	$2,025,387,607	$1,892,789,622
Deductions from Revenue	1,259,505,490	1,017,348,844	811,801,538	781,467,311	678,816,620
Net Patient Revenue	1,615,031,842	1,491,389,231	1,331,454,950	1,243,920,296	1,213,973,002
Other Operating Revenue	58,806,419	57,582,211	45,891,074	45,890,957	40,154,162
Other Nonoperating Revenue	-2,412,941	60,358,157	88,389,168	53,492,672	78,268,582
Total Net Revenue	1,671,425,320	1,609,329,599	1,465,735,192	1,343,303,925	1,332,395,746
Total Expenses	1,617,994,197	1,466,080,802	1,288,450,986	1,250,170,087	1,182,741,958
HOSPITAL UNIT (Excludes Separate Nursing Home Units)					
Utilization - Inpatient					
Beds	2,665	2,677	2,786	2,661	2,771
Admissions	115,645	110,784	108,741	108,707	109,910
Inpatient Days	574,417	548,348	538,451	597,795	619,816
Average Length of Stay	5.0	4.9	5.0	5.5	5.6
Personnel					
Total Full Time	14,458	12,800	12,559	12,257	11,797
Total Part Time	7,510	7,856	8,107	7,006	6,716
Revenue and Expenses - Totals (Includes Inpatient and Outpatient)					
Total Net Revenue	$1,660,849,124	$1,598,999,933	$1,456,900,913	$1,335,072,570	$1,322,996,011
Total Expenses	1,611,350,879	1,459,873,435	1,283,050,412	1,244,489,322	1,178,410,156
COMMUNITY HEALTH INDICATORS PER 1000 POPULATION					
Total Population (in thousands)	1,259	1,236	1,201	1,186	1,173
Inpatient					
Beds	2.3	2.3	2.5	2.4	2.5
Admissions	92.2	90.0	90.8	91.9	93.9
Inpatient Days	506.1	495.2	499.3	555.6	582.0
Inpatient Surgeries	26.8	27.2	27.4	26.4	26.5
Births	11.1	11.1	11.2	11.6	11.7
Outpatient					
Emergency Outpatient Visits	426.8	425.7	409.5	401.5	384.3
Other Outpatient Visits	1,899.9	1,810.4	1,589.3	1,567.9	1,432.4
Total Outpatient Visits	2,326.6	2,236.1	1,998.8	1,969.3	1,816.7
Outpatient Surgeries	59.9	55.7	50.5	51.6	47.9
Expense per Capita (per person)	$1,285.0	$1,186.4	$1,072.7	$1,054.3	$1,008.1

TABLE 6

NEW JERSEY

U.S. Registered Community Hospitals
(Nonfederal, short-term general and other special hospitals)

Overview 1997–2001

	2001	2000	1999	1998	1997
Total Community Hospitals	**78**	**80**	**81**	**83**	**85**
Bed Size Category					
6-24	0	0	0	0	0
25-49	0	0	1	0	0
50-99	5	5	4	6	5
100-199	20	23	23	23	22
200-299	20	20	20	20	21
300-399	14	13	14	13	14
400-499	9	11	9	11	10
500 +	10	8	10	10	13
Location					
Hospitals Urban	78	80	81	83	85
Hospitals Rural	0	0	0	0	0
Control					
State and Local Government	2	2	2	3	4
Not for Profit	74	76	77	78	80
Investor owned	2	2	2	2	1
Physician Models					
Independent Practice Association	34	27	27	33	39
Group Practice without Walls	2	4	2	5	6
Open Physician-Hospital Organization	14	15	13	16	25
Closed Physician-Hospital Organization	5	7	7	9	8
Management Service Organization	19	16	21	28	34
Integrated Salary Model	16	15	9	13	14
Equity Model	1	1	2	3	2
Foundation	1	0	1	2	3
Insurance Products					
Health Maintenance Organization	7	14	14	17	15
Preferred Provider Organization	11	15	13	20	22
Indemnity Fee for Service	1	1	5	2	3
Managed Care Contracts					
Health Maintenance Organization	65	58	58	63	63
Preferred Provider Organization	63	57	56	60	59
Affiliations					
Hospitals in a System	51	48	22	37	46
Hospitals in a Network	32	21	6	13	23
Hospitals in a Group Purchasing Organization	61	50	19	35	—

States

TABLE 6

NEW JERSEY

U.S. Registered Community Hospitals
(Nonfederal, short-term general and other special hospitals)

Utilization, Personnel, Revenue and Expenses, Community Health Indicators 1997–2001

	2001	2000	1999	1998	1997
TOTAL FACILITY (Includes Hospital and Nursing Home Units)					
Utilization - Inpatient					
Beds	24,580	25,307	24,570	26,353	28,089
Admissions	1,083,798	1,073,619	1,068,664	1,082,668	1,095,897
Inpatient Days	6,165,019	6,340,657	6,150,912	6,790,222	6,969,448
Average Length of Stay	5.7	5.9	5.8	6.3	6.4
Inpatient Surgeries	293,850	313,803	307,971	311,540	313,751
Births	109,870	111,057	109,793	104,533	103,794
Utilization - Outpatient					
Emergency Outpatient Visits	2,936,620	2,853,236	2,882,031	2,675,241	2,443,630
Other Outpatient Visits	15,507,940	13,454,037	13,244,138	12,621,673	11,679,487
Total Outpatient Visits	18,444,560	16,307,273	16,126,169	15,296,914	14,123,117
Outpatient Surgeries	399,564	412,229	414,003	390,589	362,676
Personnel					
Full Time RNs	22,522	23,154	21,826	22,657	22,196
Full Time LPNs	1,931	2,095	2,029	2,272	2,266
Part Time RNs	12,624	14,162	14,232	13,616	12,957
Part Time LPNs	799	955	1,016	1,139	1,222
Total Full Time	98,209	100,557	93,901	99,737	100,086
Total Part Time	42,406	43,732	42,774	41,387	41,911
Revenue - Inpatient					
Gross Inpatient Revenue	$26,602,275,344	$21,827,720,053	$17,817,044,301	$16,318,478,411	$14,739,631,935
Revenue - Outpatient					
Gross Outpatient Revenue	$8,452,299,275	$7,310,430,959	$5,867,036,075	$5,411,483,046	$4,798,078,883
Revenue and Expenses - Totals (Includes Inpatient and Outpatient)					
Total Gross Revenue	$35,054,574,619	$29,138,151,012	$23,684,080,376	$21,729,961,457	$19,537,710,818
Deductions from Revenue	23,885,664,427	18,556,968,225	14,272,643,586	12,181,960,982	10,164,639,651
Net Patient Revenue	11,168,910,192	10,581,182,787	9,411,436,790	9,548,000,475	9,373,071,167
Other Operating Revenue	644,537,713	730,175,554	594,893,499	648,642,263	660,175,115
Other Nonoperating Revenue	77,244,348	226,655,485	205,235,554	286,808,485	242,683,040
Total Net Revenue	11,890,692,253	11,538,013,826	10,211,565,843	10,483,451,223	10,275,929,322
Total Expenses	11,716,951,020	11,253,553,740	10,079,107,532	10,411,039,349	9,968,556,041
HOSPITAL UNIT (Excludes Separate Nursing Home Units)					
Utilization - Inpatient					
Beds	23,716	24,650	23,754	24,756	25,903
Admissions	1,080,365	1,070,105	1,065,294	1,077,264	1,091,672
Inpatient Days	5,885,278	6,136,582	5,878,838	6,293,162	6,217,112
Average Length of Stay	5.4	5.7	5.5	5.8	5.7
Personnel					
Total Full Time	97,533	99,370	92,941	90,011	99,074
Total Part Time	42,140	43,215	42,320	41,009	41,484
Revenue and Expenses - Totals (Includes Inpatient and Outpatient)					
Total Net Revenue	$11,822,055,392	$11,496,256,093	$10,161,679,983	$10,408,979,933	$10,179,562,117
Total Expenses	11,659,210,376	11,210,748,330	10,026,590,107	10,344,410,778	9,880,269,111
COMMUNITY HEALTH INDICATORS PER 1000 POPULATION					
Total Population (in thousands)	8,484	8,414	8,143	8,096	8,054
Inpatient					
Beds	2.9	3.0	3.0	3.3	3.5
Admissions	127.7	127.6	131.2	133.7	136.1
Inpatient Days	726.6	753.6	755.3	838.8	865.3
Inpatient Surgeries	34.6	37.3	37.8	38.5	39.0
Births	12.9	13.2	13.5	12.9	12.9
Outpatient					
Emergency Outpatient Visits	346.1	339.1	353.9	330.5	303.4
Other Outpatient Visits	1,827.8	1,598.9	1,626.4	1,559.1	1,450.1
Total Outpatient Visits	2,173.9	1,938.0	1,980.3	1,889.5	1,753.5
Outpatient Surgeries	47.1	49.0	50.8	48.2	45.0
Expense per Capita (per person)	$1,381.0	$1,337.4	$1,237.7	$1,286.0	$1,237.7

TABLE 6

NEW MEXICO

U.S. Registered Community Hospitals
(Nonfederal, short-term general and other special hospitals)

Overview 1997–2001

	2001	2000	1999	1998	1997
Total Community Hospitals	**35**	**35**	**36**	**36**	**36**
Bed Size Category					
6-24	2	4	5	4	4
25-49	12	9	8	9	9
50-99	8	9	11	10	11
100-199	8	8	9	8	6
200-299	3	4	2	4	5
300-399	2	1	1	1	1
400-499	0	0	0	0	0
500 +	0	0	0	0	0
Location					
Hospitals Urban	13	13	13	13	13
Hospitals Rural	22	22	23	23	23
Control					
State and Local Government	10	9	11	12	11
Not for Profit	19	20	20	18	20
Investor owned	6	6	5	6	5
Physician Models					
Independent Practice Association	5	9	12	11	13
Group Practice without Walls	1	3	4	2	2
Open Physician-Hospital Organization	4	6	6	9	6
Closed Physician-Hospital Organization	1	2	4	2	3
Management Service Organization	0	1	3	1	5
Integrated Salary Model	9	9	5	4	5
Equity Model	0	0	0	1	0
Foundation	3	2	3	4	3
Insurance Products					
Health Maintenance Organization	10	8	8	7	9
Preferred Provider Organization	6	10	11	10	14
Indemnity Fee for Service	4	5	6	4	8
Managed Care Contracts					
Health Maintenance Organization	20	16	22	19	19
Preferred Provider Organization	17	16	18	15	19
Affiliations					
Hospitals in a System	16	14	15	16	15
Hospitals in a Network	5	5	9	8	8
Hospitals in a Group Purchasing Organization	24	21	21	17	—

TABLE 6

NEW MEXICO

U.S. Registered Community Hospitals
(Nonfederal, short-term general and other special hospitals)

Utilization, Personnel, Revenue and Expenses, Community Health Indicators 1997–2001

	2001	2000	1999	1998	1997
TOTAL FACILITY (Includes Hospital and Nursing Home Units)					
Utilization - Inpatient					
Beds	3,584	3,481	3,370	3,489	3,607
Admissions	164,461	173,575	163,700	157,875	163,372
Inpatient Days	758,923	731,708	725,713	707,418	761,888
Average Length of Stay	4.6	4.2	4.4	4.5	4.7
Inpatient Surgeries	45,395	51,466	57,164	54,474	56,536
Births	24,884	24,329	25,526	23,680	24,054
Utilization - Outpatient					
Emergency Outpatient Visits	528,979	532,526	512,645	466,049	489,745
Other Outpatient Visits	2,880,249	2,568,108	2,622,325	2,798,522	2,409,355
Total Outpatient Visits	3,409,228	3,100,634	3,134,970	3,264,571	2,899,100
Outpatient Surgeries	78,047	78,014	86,506	84,918	79,086
Personnel					
Full Time RNs	4,037	3,722	3,467	3,589	4,641
Full Time LPNs	627	487	508	459	706
Part Time RNs	1,330	2,267	2,204	2,860	2,387
Part Time LPNs	150	225	258	311	311
Total Full Time	19,121	15,505	15,616	14,975	20,011
Total Part Time	4,201	6,429	7,608	8,293	7,702
Revenue - Inpatient					
Gross Inpatient Revenue	$2,100,619,929	$2,202,879,494	$2,114,743,157	$1,685,266,585	$1,578,563,236
Revenue - Outpatient					
Gross Outpatient Revenue	$1,530,614,098	$1,280,932,571	$1,235,146,668	$1,381,910,309	$1,188,335,649
Revenue and Expenses - Totals (Includes Inpatient and Outpatient)					
Total Gross Revenue	$3,631,234,027	$3,483,812,065	$3,349,889,825	$3,067,176,894	$2,766,898,885
Deductions from Revenue	1,798,758,901	1,905,810,874	1,454,422,617	1,433,881,000	1,211,547,345
Net Patient Revenue	1,832,475,126	1,578,001,191	1,895,467,208	1,633,295,894	1,555,351,540
Other Operating Revenue	102,566,160	103,866,572	100,671,605	104,122,520	85,133,891
Other Nonoperating Revenue	32,406,351	30,473,501	33,471,257	34,118,361	26,763,686
Total Net Revenue	1,967,447,637	1,712,341,264	2,029,610,070	1,771,536,775	1,667,249,117
Total Expenses	1,868,614,170	1,695,651,227	1,847,553,034	1,599,265,050	1,592,739,008
HOSPITAL UNIT (Excludes Separate Nursing Home Units)					
Utilization - Inpatient					
Beds	3,498	3,426	3,279	3,411	3,514
Admissions	163,080	172,543	161,933	156,490	161,575
Inpatient Days	739,270	715,831	699,736	685,831	739,767
Average Length of Stay	4.5	4.1	4.3	4.4	4.6
Personnel					
Total Full Time	19,094	15,434	15,526	14,954	19,813
Total Part Time	4,196	6,401	7,573	8,292	7,695
Revenue and Expenses - Totals (Includes Inpatient and Outpatient)					
Total Net Revenue	$1,961,248,667	$1,709,281,550	$2,023,848,425	$1,760,937,195	$1,649,131,820
Total Expenses	1,865,267,433	1,693,109,995	1,845,065,340	1,593,743,179	1,582,245,655
COMMUNITY HEALTH INDICATORS PER 1000 POPULATION					
Total Population (in thousands)	1,829	1,819	1,740	1,734	1,723
Inpatient					
Beds	2.0	1.9	1.9	2.0	2.1
Admissions	89.9	95.4	94.1	91.1	94.8
Inpatient Days	414.9	402.2	417.1	408.1	442.2
Inpatient Surgeries	24.8	28.3	32.9	31.4	32.8
Births	13.6	13.4	14.7	13.7	14.0
Outpatient					
Emergency Outpatient Visits	289.2	292.8	294.6	268.8	284.2
Other Outpatient Visits	1,574.6	1,411.8	1,507.2	1,614.3	1,398.4
Total Outpatient Visits	1,863.8	1,704.5	1,801.9	1,883.2	1,682.6
Outpatient Surgeries	42.7	42.9	49.7	49.0	45.9
Expense per Capita (per person)	$1,021.6	$932.2	$1,061.9	$922.5	$924.4

TABLE 6

NEW YORK

U.S. Registered Community Hospitals
(Nonfederal, short-term general and other special hospitals)

Overview 1997–2001

	2001	2000	1999	1998	1997
Total Community Hospitals	**212**	**215**	**218**	**222**	**225**
Bed Size Category					
6-24	4	4	2	3	3
25-49	8	8	12	12	13
50-99	23	25	21	21	19
100-199	51	50	50	53	49
200-299	49	53	54	50	53
300-399	24	23	27	30	28
400-499	21	20	19	19	24
500 +	32	32	33	34	36
Location					
Hospitals Urban	176	180	182	186	189
Hospitals Rural	36	35	36	36	36
Control					
State and Local Government	25	24	25	24	27
Not for Profit	181	183	185	189	187
Investor owned	6	8	8	9	11
Physician Models					
Independent Practice Association	44	70	70	74	74
Group Practice without Walls	6	10	5	6	8
Open Physician-Hospital Organization	28	36	34	41	41
Closed Physician-Hospital Organization	10	11	13	14	15
Management Service Organization	21	32	36	32	35
Integrated Salary Model	30	44	31	35	42
Equity Model	2	2	3	5	1
Foundation	3	5	7	8	9
Insurance Products					
Health Maintenance Organization	38	51	51	61	55
Preferred Provider Organization	30	42	38	48	46
Indemnity Fee for Service	10	10	5	6	14
Managed Care Contracts					
Health Maintenance Organization	115	140	140	141	157
Preferred Provider Organization	108	128	117	111	111
Affiliations					
Hospitals in a System	81	92	90	84	79
Hospitals in a Network	71	77	87	86	81
Hospitals in a Group Purchasing Organization	138	133	133	121	—

States

TABLE 6

NEW YORK

U.S. Registered Community Hospitals
(Nonfederal, short-term general and other special hospitals)

Utilization, Personnel, Revenue and Expenses, Community Health Indicators 1997–2001

	2001	2000	1999	1998	1997
TOTAL FACILITY (Includes Hospital and Nursing Home Units)					
Utilization - Inpatient					
Beds	67,296	66,434	68,924	68,511	70,973
Admissions	2,410,906	2,416,112	2,406,327	2,364,608	2,371,164
Inpatient Days	19,021,960	19,074,063	19,349,127	19,176,323	19,652,565
Average Length of Stay	7.9	7.9	8.0	8.1	8.3
Inpatient Surgeries	692,769	722,083	710,183	725,774	704,528
Births	249,035	254,165	256,910	249,782	257,455
Utilization - Outpatient					
Emergency Outpatient Visits	7,452,574	7,275,122	7,141,070	6,785,222	6,768,851
Other Outpatient Visits	38,193,199	39,096,732	38,601,503	36,888,203	34,150,928
Total Outpatient Visits	45,645,773	46,371,854	45,742,573	43,673,425	40,919,779
Outpatient Surgeries	1,254,924	1,263,783	1,176,107	1,224,017	1,059,079
Personnel					
Full Time RNs	63,798	63,283	62,747	61,620	61,029
Full Time LPNs	7,538	7,424	7,318	7,282	7,659
Part Time RNs	18,869	20,945	19,568	19,064	18,576
Part Time LPNs	2,094	2,208	2,188	2,102	2,237
Total Full Time	308,267	301,182	305,163	298,813	299,373
Total Part Time	65,664	70,536	66,143	62,730	66,833
Revenue - Inpatient					
Gross Inpatient Revenue	$42,992,186,646	$37,492,283,644	$34,644,592,681	$33,644,430,383	$30,966,531,656
Revenue - Outpatient					
Gross Outpatient Revenue	$19,539,156,438	$16,875,958,120	$15,564,285,898	$14,046,961,332	$13,082,687,637
Revenue and Expenses - Totals (Includes Inpatient and Outpatient)					
Total Gross Revenue	$62,531,343,084	$54,368,241,764	$50,208,878,579	$47,691,391,715	$44,049,219,293
Deductions from Revenue	31,905,296,191	25,694,206,309	22,649,391,683	21,019,392,047	17,713,533,999
Net Patient Revenue	30,626,046,893	28,674,035,455	27,559,486,896	26,671,999,668	26,335,685,294
Other Operating Revenue	3,163,011,300	2,641,649,037	2,645,639,145	2,248,627,300	2,286,104,739
Other Nonoperating Revenue	482,220,705	500,659,020	587,485,474	663,053,669	699,415,663
Total Net Revenue	34,271,278,898	31,816,343,512	30,792,611,515	29,583,680,637	29,321,205,696
Total Expenses	34,352,757,050	31,963,065,624	31,023,119,426	29,269,407,269	28,875,239,979
HOSPITAL UNIT (Excludes Separate Nursing Home Units)					
Utilization - Inpatient					
Beds	60,609	58,655	61,313	61,617	64,059
Admissions	2,398,757	2,404,711	2,395,003	2,355,270	2,362,989
Inpatient Days	16,630,275	16,229,578	16,680,325	16,782,177	17,194,456
Average Length of Stay	6.9	6.7	7.0	7.1	7.3
Personnel					
Total Full Time	302,901	294,588	300,691	294,622	295,089
Total Part Time	63,968	68,570	64,730	61,220	65,175
Revenue and Expenses - Totals (Includes Inpatient and Outpatient)					
Total Net Revenue	$33,722,096,947	$31,324,367,381	$30,300,120,420	$29,118,978,713	$28,879,649,305
Total Expenses	33,937,745,908	31,557,256,923	30,613,692,890	28,898,772,886	28,549,579,217
COMMUNITY HEALTH INDICATORS PER 1000 POPULATION					
Total Population (in thousands)	19,011	18,976	18,197	18,159	18,143
Inpatient					
Beds	3.5	3.5	3.8	3.8	3.9
Admissions	126.8	127.3	132.2	130.2	130.7
Inpatient Days	1,000.6	1,005.1	1,063.3	1,056.0	1,083.2
Inpatient Surgeries	36.4	38.1	39.0	40.0	38.8
Births	13.1	13.4	14.1	13.8	14.2
Outpatient					
Emergency Outpatient Visits	392.0	383.4	392.4	373.7	373.1
Other Outpatient Visits	2,009.0	2,060.3	2,121.4	2,031.4	1,882.3
Total Outpatient Visits	2,401.0	2,443.7	2,513.8	2,405.0	2,255.4
Outpatient Surgeries	66.0	66.6	64.6	67.4	58.4
Expense per Capita (per person)	$1,807.0	$1,684.4	$1,704.9	$1,611.8	$1,591.5

TABLE 6

NORTH CAROLINA

U.S. Registered Community Hospitals
(Nonfederal, short-term general and other special hospitals)

Overview 1997–2001

	2001	2000	1999	1998	1997
Total Community Hospitals	**111**	**113**	**114**	**116**	**118**
Bed Size Category					
6-24	2	2	2	3	2
25-49	11	12	12	11	13
50-99	23	22	22	24	24
100-199	38	41	43	42	42
200-299	14	14	14	16	18
300-399	8	9	9	7	7
400-499	3	1	0	1	1
500 +	12	12	12	12	11
Location					
Hospitals Urban	50	51	52	54	54
Hospitals Rural	61	62	62	62	64
Control					
State and Local Government	32	32	33	33	35
Not for Profit	70	71	72	72	70
Investor owned	9	10	9	11	13
Physician Models					
Independent Practice Association	10	14	24	19	15
Group Practice without Walls	3	2	1	3	6
Open Physician-Hospital Organization	24	25	31	24	20
Closed Physician-Hospital Organization	5	3	7	17	15
Management Service Organization	14	17	16	21	22
Integrated Salary Model	31	27	31	30	27
Equity Model	0	1	1	4	1
Foundation	6	5	9	13	15
Insurance Products					
Health Maintenance Organization	11	21	31	31	25
Preferred Provider Organization	19	28	39	40	46
Indemnity Fee for Service	4	5	10	8	12
Managed Care Contracts					
Health Maintenance Organization	67	71	73	76	77
Preferred Provider Organization	82	83	88	90	92
Affiliations					
Hospitals in a System	45	46	47	47	44
Hospitals in a Network	42	42	55	63	64
Hospitals in a Group Purchasing Organization	86	86	96	88	—

TABLE 6

NORTH CAROLINA

U.S. Registered Community Hospitals
(Nonfederal, short-term general and other special hospitals)

Utilization, Personnel, Revenue and Expenses, Community Health Indicators 1997–2001

	2001	2000	1999	1998	1997
TOTAL FACILITY (Includes Hospital and Nursing Home Units)					
Utilization - Inpatient					
Beds	23,755	23,081	23,391	23,297	23,244
Admissions	973,451	970,742	930,747	907,911	874,389
Inpatient Days	5,959,143	5,859,282	5,726,618	5,813,321	5,783,489
Average Length of Stay	6.1	6.0	6.2	6.4	6.6
Inpatient Surgeries	289,260	278,532	279,057	267,831	281,840
Births	110,585	112,885	107,946	104,193	99,251
Utilization - Outpatient					
Emergency Outpatient Visits	3,230,198	2,983,548	2,844,680	2,885,802	2,816,826
Other Outpatient Visits	10,200,478	9,395,105	8,695,722	8,181,231	7,239,982
Total Outpatient Visits	13,430,676	12,378,653	11,540,402	11,067,033	10,056,808
Outpatient Surgeries	460,545	435,210	442,859	398,481	383,345
Personnel					
Full Time RNs	25,892	25,047	25,390	24,800	23,403
Full Time LPNs	2,381	2,393	2,441	2,515	2,731
Part Time RNs	10,855	10,575	9,506	8,517	7,907
Part Time LPNs	711	829	778	828	852
Total Full Time	105,994	104,926	102,981	102,539	100,198
Total Part Time	30,745	31,480	29,055	27,862	26,307
Revenue - Inpatient					
Gross Inpatient Revenue	$12,324,492,251	$11,353,688,447	$10,061,207,112	$9,313,486,463	$8,834,342,163
Revenue - Outpatient					
Gross Outpatient Revenue	$7,225,934,040	$6,225,077,316	$5,345,769,802	$4,754,725,497	$4,242,919,421
Revenue and Expenses - Totals (Includes Inpatient and Outpatient)					
Total Gross Revenue	$19,550,426,291	$17,578,765,763	$15,406,976,914	$14,068,211,960	$13,077,261,584
Deductions from Revenue	8,934,901,143	7,748,738,093	6,466,123,700	5,495,522,936	4,953,479,568
Net Patient Revenue	10,615,525,148	9,830,027,670	8,940,853,214	8,572,689,024	8,123,782,016
Other Operating Revenue	651,522,219	604,076,521	516,615,284	411,891,798	384,033,882
Other Nonoperating Revenue	181,114,779	376,862,714	311,116,988	362,764,227	492,654,986
Total Net Revenue	11,448,162,146	10,810,966,905	9,768,585,486	9,347,345,049	9,000,470,884
Total Expenses	10,625,022,294	10,028,178,236	8,980,841,368	8,364,935,329	7,974,179,402
HOSPITAL UNIT (Excludes Separate Nursing Home Units)					
Utilization - Inpatient					
Beds	21,040	20,047	20,130	20,119	20,411
Admissions	964,357	961,312	919,616	897,079	864,790
Inpatient Days	5,064,097	4,881,713	4,623,084	4,756,240	4,813,602
Average Length of Stay	5.3	5.1	5.0	5.3	5.6
Personnel					
Total Full Time	103,658	102,369	100,023	100,191	97,815
Total Part Time	29,819	30,453	28,139	27,031	25,445
Revenue and Expenses - Totals (Includes Inpatient and Outpatient)					
Total Net Revenue	$11,322,622,945	$10,665,778,056	$9,617,095,929	$9,189,418,129	$8,862,240,575
Total Expenses	10,504,024,494	9,896,919,542	8,840,059,827	8,223,397,759	7,836,671,723
COMMUNITY HEALTH INDICATORS PER 1000 POPULATION					
Total Population (in thousands)	8,186	8,049	7,651	7,546	7,429
Inpatient					
Beds	2.9	2.9	3.1	3.1	3.1
Admissions	118.9	120.6	121.7	120.3	117.7
Inpatient Days	727.9	727.9	748.5	770.4	778.5
Inpatient Surgeries	35.3	34.6	36.5	35.5	37.9
Births	13.5	14.0	14.1	13.8	13.4
Outpatient					
Emergency Outpatient Visits	394.6	370.7	371.8	382.4	379.2
Other Outpatient Visits	1,246.0	1,167.2	1,136.6	1,084.2	974.6
Total Outpatient Visits	1,640.6	1,537.9	1,508.4	1,466.6	1,353.8
Outpatient Surgeries	56.3	54.1	57.9	52.8	51.6
Expense per Capita (per person)	$1,297.9	$1,245.8	$1,173.8	$1,108.6	$1,073.4

TABLE 6

NORTH DAKOTA

U.S. Registered Community Hospitals
(Nonfederal, short-term general and other special hospitals)

Overview 1997–2001

	2001	2000	1999	1998	1997
Total Community Hospitals	**40**	**42**	**41**	**43**	**41**
Bed Size Category					
6-24	7	7	6	6	5
25-49	11	10	11	12	12
50-99	14	15	13	14	13
100-199	1	3	4	4	4
200-299	5	5	5	5	5
300-399	1	1	1	1	1
400-499	0	1	1	1	1
500 +	1	0	0	0	0
Location					
Hospitals Urban	7	6	6	6	5
Hospitals Rural	33	36	35	37	36
Control					
State and Local Government	0	0	0	0	0
Not for Profit	39	40	39	41	40
Investor owned	1	2	2	2	1
Physician Models					
Independent Practice Association	4	5	7	7	9
Group Practice without Walls	0	1	1	2	2
Open Physician-Hospital Organization	1	1	2	2	3
Closed Physician-Hospital Organization	3	1	1	1	2
Management Service Organization	0	1	1	1	1
Integrated Salary Model	13	15	10	12	13
Equity Model	0	0	1	1	1
Foundation	1	0	1	2	3
Insurance Products					
Health Maintenance Organization	0	1	1	1	3
Preferred Provider Organization	3	4	5	6	8
Indemnity Fee for Service	1	2	1	1	0
Managed Care Contracts					
Health Maintenance Organization	7	8	9	9	13
Preferred Provider Organization	21	21	19	16	20
Affiliations					
Hospitals in a System	13	15	14	18	18
Hospitals in a Network	10	8	7	9	9
Hospitals in a Group Purchasing Organization	28	28	28	28	—

TABLE 6

NORTH DAKOTA

U.S. Registered Community Hospitals
(Nonfederal, short-term general and other special hospitals)

Utilization, Personnel, Revenue and Expenses, Community Health Indicators 1997–2001

	2001	2000	1999	1998	1997
TOTAL FACILITY (Includes Hospital and Nursing Home Units)					
Utilization - Inpatient					
Beds	3,717	3,865	3,884	3,978	3,900
Admissions	91,530	89,219	86,931	85,176	83,688
Inpatient Days	787,722	841,256	852,457	873,623	877,085
Average Length of Stay	8.6	9.4	9.8	10.3	10.5
Inpatient Surgeries	23,814	25,052	29,603	29,012	30,496
Births	8,691	8,282	8,366	8,523	8,721
Utilization - Outpatient					
Emergency Outpatient Visits	259,673	248,562	249,955	221,797	201,721
Other Outpatient Visits	1,599,065	1,446,407	1,381,484	1,200,140	1,137,849
Total Outpatient Visits	1,858,738	1,694,969	1,631,439	1,421,937	1,339,570
Outpatient Surgeries	45,718	43,764	42,656	46,070	44,530
Personnel					
Full Time RNs	1,734	2,075	1,634	1,931	1,746
Full Time LPNs	524	458	438	405	481
Part Time RNs	2,409	1,910	2,191	2,523	2,166
Part Time LPNs	524	376	560	542	535
Total Full Time	11,343	10,921	9,831	9,946	9,933
Total Part Time	8,618	7,529	7,749	8,620	7,895
Revenue - Inpatient					
Gross Inpatient Revenue	$1,068,649,264	$1,003,041,889	$919,295,692	$947,292,506	$822,222,174
Revenue - Outpatient					
Gross Outpatient Revenue	$879,815,286	$766,845,547	$759,586,932	$752,533,518	$605,009,944
Revenue and Expenses - Totals (Includes Inpatient and Outpatient)					
Total Gross Revenue	$1,948,464,550	$1,769,887,436	$1,678,882,624	$1,699,826,024	$1,427,232,118
Deductions from Revenue	798,865,633	705,636,353	648,667,094	667,836,387	462,722,491
Net Patient Revenue	1,149,598,917	1,064,251,083	1,030,215,530	1,031,989,637	964,509,627
Other Operating Revenue	65,081,910	66,992,430	66,044,016	60,404,086	45,576,800
Other Nonoperating Revenue	20,055,117	32,833,000	20,696,900	35,634,346	28,095,809
Total Net Revenue	1,234,735,944	1,164,076,513	1,116,956,446	1,128,020,069	1,038,182,236
Total Expenses	1,220,687,431	1,111,495,262	1,063,751,582	1,052,697,761	961,130,975
HOSPITAL UNIT (Excludes Separate Nursing Home Units)					
Utilization - Inpatient					
Beds	2,762	3,099	2,935	3,069	2,865
Admissions	90,169	87,453	84,780	83,464	81,942
Inpatient Days	479,300	606,974	536,949	566,947	513,824
Average Length of Stay	5.3	6.9	6.3	6.8	6.3
Personnel					
Total Full Time	10,726	10,496	9,077	9,315	9,411
Total Part Time	8,119	7,126	7,134	7,921	7,306
Revenue and Expenses - Totals (Includes Inpatient and Outpatient)					
Total Net Revenue	$1,196,091,770	$1,136,148,987	$1,075,514,346	$1,090,055,879	$998,922,083
Total Expenses	1,188,642,681	1,088,906,965	1,032,134,787	1,022,248,824	929,872,861
COMMUNITY HEALTH INDICATORS PER 1000 POPULATION					
Total Population (in thousands)	634	642	634	638	641
Inpatient					
Beds	5.9	6.0	6.1	6.2	6.1
Admissions	144.3	138.9	137.2	133.5	130.6
Inpatient Days	1,241.6	1,310.0	1,345.3	1,369.7	1,368.4
Inpatient Surgeries	37.5	39.0	46.7	45.5	47.6
Births	13.7	12.9	13.2	13.4	13.6
Outpatient					
Emergency Outpatient Visits	409.3	387.0	394.5	347.7	314.7
Other Outpatient Visits	2,520.4	2,252.3	2,180.1	1,881.7	1,775.3
Total Outpatient Visits	2,929.7	2,639.3	2,574.6	2,229.4	2,090.0
Outpatient Surgeries	72.1	68.1	67.3	72.2	69.5
Expense per Capita (per person)	$1,924.0	$1,730.8	$1,678.7	$1,650.5	$1,499.6

States

TABLE 6

OHIO

U.S. Registered Community Hospitals
(Nonfederal, short-term general and other special hospitals)

Overview 1997–2001

	2001	2000	1999	1998	1997
Total Community Hospitals	**166**	**163**	**167**	**172**	**170**
Bed Size Category					
6-24	2	2	3	3	2
25-49	22	21	21	20	19
50-99	33	31	33	33	32
100-199	50	50	52	50	49
200-299	26	24	23	32	32
300-399	14	15	14	14	13
400-499	9	9	10	10	12
500 +	10	11	11	10	11
Location					
Hospitals Urban	114	111	114	120	117
Hospitals Rural	52	52	53	52	53
Control					
State and Local Government	23	22	23	23	23
Not for Profit	139	137	139	139	138
Investor owned	4	4	5	10	9
Physician Models					
Independent Practice Association	23	15	19	16	20
Group Practice without Walls	12	10	11	10	7
Open Physician-Hospital Organization	46	51	63	66	54
Closed Physician-Hospital Organization	26	19	20	22	18
Management Service Organization	33	39	44	44	43
Integrated Salary Model	53	44	52	47	40
Equity Model	9	7	7	8	8
Foundation	21	18	21	26	22
Insurance Products					
Health Maintenance Organization	32	38	45	44	50
Preferred Provider Organization	36	37	44	46	58
Indemnity Fee for Service	12	11	12	13	15
Managed Care Contracts					
Health Maintenance Organization	110	110	112	123	118
Preferred Provider Organization	115	116	118	126	123
Affiliations					
Hospitals in a System	84	75	79	78	71
Hospitals in a Network	68	52	54	56	53
Hospitals in a Group Purchasing Organization	134	130	133	124	—

TABLE 6

OHIO

U.S. Registered Community Hospitals
(Nonfederal, short-term general and other special hospitals)

Utilization, Personnel, Revenue and Expenses, Community Health Indicators 1997–2001

	2001	2000	1999	1998	1997
TOTAL FACILITY (Includes Hospital and Nursing Home Units)					
Utilization - Inpatient					
Beds	33,310	33,849	34,164	35,187	36,079
Admissions	1,439,252	1,404,467	1,358,662	1,355,186	1,376,291
Inpatient Days	7,483,873	7,556,261	7,362,468	7,289,259	7,674,238
Average Length of Stay	5.2	5.4	5.4	5.4	5.6
Inpatient Surgeries	417,023	400,999	390,732	409,404	435,576
Births	151,371	149,565	147,506	151,247	154,259
Utilization - Outpatient					
Emergency Outpatient Visits	5,124,561	5,133,276	4,906,178	5,003,406	4,732,151
Other Outpatient Visits	23,252,713	21,724,028	19,980,036	19,794,816	19,250,824
Total Outpatient Visits	28,377,274	26,857,304	24,886,214	24,798,222	23,982,975
Outpatient Surgeries	793,989	798,907	765,459	790,645	793,420
Personnel					
Full Time RNs	34,676	33,921	34,424	35,530	34,178
Full Time LPNs	3,961	3,644	4,039	4,019	4,307
Part Time RNs	22,713	22,568	19,371	18,419	19,497
Part Time LPNs	2,123	2,028	2,140	2,031	2,223
Total Full Time	159,239	151,382	151,875	154,471	155,443
Total Part Time	66,944	66,769	60,642	56,449	58,973
Revenue - Inpatient					
Gross Inpatient Revenue	$20,613,914,515	$17,881,757,694	$15,806,982,496	$15,196,210,325	$15,028,331,988
Revenue - Outpatient					
Gross Outpatient Revenue	$14,224,448,482	$11,888,253,297	$10,278,820,338	$9,119,353,937	$8,656,505,506
Revenue and Expenses - Totals (Includes Inpatient and Outpatient)					
Total Gross Revenue	$34,838,362,997	$29,770,010,991	$26,085,802,834	$24,315,564,262	$23,684,837,494
Deductions from Revenue	17,753,807,229	14,553,540,678	11,859,000,198	10,533,346,817	9,768,130,576
Net Patient Revenue	17,084,555,768	15,216,470,313	14,226,802,636	13,782,217,445	13,916,706,918
Other Operating Revenue	1,084,169,641	727,705,267	834,560,047	781,078,239	826,078,209
Other Nonoperating Revenue	132,770,316	558,247,388	446,576,015	506,628,141	544,072,306
Total Net Revenue	18,301,495,725	16,502,422,968	15,507,938,698	15,069,923,825	15,286,857,433
Total Expenses	17,866,114,856	15,550,349,910	14,881,546,876	14,354,350,789	14,070,575,469
HOSPITAL UNIT (Excludes Separate Nursing Home Units)					
Utilization - Inpatient					
Beds	31,471	31,413	31,118	33,036	33,358
Admissions	1,421,435	1,381,778	1,328,866	1,329,828	1,350,491
Inpatient Days	6,925,175	6,775,436	6,471,288	6,632,608	6,817,721
Average Length of Stay	4.9	4.9	4.9	5.0	5.0
Personnel					
Total Full Time	157,884	149,237	149,246	152,222	152,854
Total Part Time	66,306	65,817	59,403	55,358	57,621
Revenue and Expenses - Totals (Includes Inpatient and Outpatient)					
Total Net Revenue	$18,146,551,602	$16,331,999,691	$15,247,381,253	$14,860,887,528	$15,065,563,596
Total Expenses	17,752,957,340	15,427,132,070	14,660,321,444	14,197,589,490	13,897,461,267
COMMUNITY HEALTH INDICATORS PER 1000 POPULATION					
Total Population (in thousands)	11,374	11,353	11,257	11,238	11,212
Inpatient					
Beds	2.9	3.0	3.0	3.1	3.2
Admissions	126.5	123.7	120.7	120.6	122.7
Inpatient Days	658.0	665.6	654.1	648.6	684.4
Inpatient Surgeries	36.7	35.3	34.7	36.4	38.8
Births	13.3	13.2	13.1	13.5	13.8
Outpatient					
Emergency Outpatient Visits	450.6	452.1	435.8	445.2	422.0
Other Outpatient Visits	2,044.5	1,913.5	1,775.0	1,761.5	1,716.9
Total Outpatient Visits	2,495.0	2,365.6	2,210.8	2,206.7	2,139.0
Outpatient Surgeries	69.8	70.4	68.0	70.4	70.8
Expense per Capita (per person)	$1,570.8	$1,369.7	$1,322.0	$1,277.3	$1,254.9

TABLE 6

OKLAHOMA

U.S. Registered Community Hospitals
(Nonfederal, short-term general and other special hospitals)

Overview 1997–2001

	2001	2000	1999	1998	1997
Total Community Hospitals	**108**	**108**	**109**	**109**	**111**
Bed Size Category					
6-24	15	14	15	16	13
25-49	38	41	40	40	43
50-99	22	22	21	21	21
100-199	18	15	17	16	19
200-299	7	8	8	7	7
300-399	2	2	3	3	4
400-499	3	3	1	2	2
500 +	3	3	4	4	2
Location					
Hospitals Urban	40	40	41	41	42
Hospitals Rural	68	68	68	68	69
Control					
State and Local Government	45	45	50	49	53
Not for Profit	48	49	44	41	40
Investor owned	15	14	15	19	18
Physician Models					
Independent Practice Association	12	16	16	16	14
Group Practice without Walls	1	3	3	4	4
Open Physician-Hospital Organization	14	22	23	24	23
Closed Physician-Hospital Organization	10	6	8	14	14
Management Service Organization	11	15	11	17	19
Integrated Salary Model	16	16	19	18	13
Equity Model	1	2	1	2	2
Foundation	4	4	2	3	3
Insurance Products					
Health Maintenance Organization	18	26	28	28	33
Preferred Provider Organization	18	32	32	34	41
Indemnity Fee for Service	5	6	6	10	11
Managed Care Contracts					
Health Maintenance Organization	40	42	55	48	58
Preferred Provider Organization	61	65	82	68	82
Affiliations					
Hospitals in a System	33	39	42	42	40
Hospitals in a Network	18	22	29	30	33
Hospitals in a Group Purchasing Organization	67	63	—	—	—

OKLAHOMA

U.S. Registered Community Hospitals
(Nonfederal, short-term general and other special hospitals)

Utilization, Personnel, Revenue and Expenses, Community Health Indicators 1997–2001

	2001	2000	1999	1998	1997
TOTAL FACILITY (Includes Hospital and Nursing Home Units)					
Utilization - Inpatient					
Beds	11,207	11,112	11,075	11,022	10,882
Admissions	434,831	428,927	411,025	391,243	377,776
Inpatient Days	2,360,979	2,280,050	2,273,850	2,169,379	2,148,426
Average Length of Stay	5.4	5.3	5.5	5.5	5.7
Inpatient Surgeries	120,417	117,785	123,765	107,628	108,679
Births	43,053	43,461	44,295	38,639	40,894
Utilization - Outpatient					
Emergency Outpatient Visits	1,226,716	1,134,337	1,172,259	1,101,327	1,037,970
Other Outpatient Visits	3,343,188	3,567,619	3,452,578	3,285,675	3,127,034
Total Outpatient Visits	4,569,904	4,701,956	4,624,837	4,387,002	4,165,004
Outpatient Surgeries	173,752	182,488	186,624	165,150	161,443
Personnel					
Full Time RNs	8,403	8,194	8,054	8,184	8,604
Full Time LPNs	2,422	2,087	2,312	2,253	2,595
Part Time RNs	3,708	3,453	3,041	2,801	2,884
Part Time LPNs	758	618	701	574	725
Total Full Time	43,342	41,964	39,901	40,712	42,910
Total Part Time	12,815	11,583	11,864	11,276	11,172
Revenue - Inpatient					
Gross Inpatient Revenue	$5,478,614,594	$5,218,973,104	$4,678,294,998	$4,207,669,067	$3,829,921,644
Revenue - Outpatient					
Gross Outpatient Revenue	$2,830,596,281	$2,560,162,792	$2,337,006,164	$2,103,831,457	$1,980,939,855
Revenue and Expenses - Totals (Includes Inpatient and Outpatient)					
Total Gross Revenue	$8,309,210,875	$7,779,135,896	$7,015,301,162	$6,311,500,524	$5,810,861,499
Deductions from Revenue	4,548,324,907	4,263,955,656	3,677,580,563	3,167,902,504	2,700,586,218
Net Patient Revenue	3,760,885,968	3,515,180,240	3,337,720,599	3,143,598,020	3,110,275,281
Other Operating Revenue	234,843,029	268,105,178	238,136,668	190,021,268	201,556,987
Other Nonoperating Revenue	39,695,513	28,871,537	64,910,590	33,155,610	43,824,283
Total Net Revenue	4,035,424,510	3,812,156,955	3,640,767,857	3,366,774,898	3,355,656,551
Total Expenses	3,722,315,467	3,689,668,282	3,433,636,312	3,217,517,307	3,178,796,604
HOSPITAL UNIT (Excludes Separate Nursing Home Units)					
Utilization - Inpatient					
Beds	10,857	10,788	10,577	10,615	10,400
Admissions	431,093	423,287	406,459	385,731	373,150
Inpatient Days	2,248,489	2,179,541	2,123,082	2,051,482	2,000,460
Average Length of Stay	5.2	5.1	5.2	5.3	5.4
Personnel					
Total Full Time	42,873	41,541	39,636	40,498	42,315
Total Part Time	12,693	11,436	11,809	11,239	11,062
Revenue and Expenses - Totals (Includes Inpatient and Outpatient)					
Total Net Revenue	$4,008,168,171	$3,774,861,696	$3,624,098,673	$3,336,083,870	$3,326,504,422
Total Expenses	3,697,330,894	3,669,710,412	3,421,100,441	3,105,565,729	3,159,552,806
COMMUNITY HEALTH INDICATORS PER 1000 POPULATION					
Total Population (in thousands)	3,460	3,451	3,358	3,339	3,314
Inpatient					
Beds	3.2	3.2	3.3	3.3	3.3
Admissions	125.7	124.3	122.4	117.2	114.0
Inpatient Days	682.3	660.8	677.1	649.6	648.2
Inpatient Surgeries	34.8	34.1	36.9	32.2	32.8
Births	12.4	12.6	13.2	11.6	12.3
Outpatient					
Emergency Outpatient Visits	354.5	328.7	349.1	329.8	313.2
Other Outpatient Visits	966.2	1,033.9	1,028.2	983.9	943.5
Total Outpatient Visits	1,320.7	1,362.6	1,377.2	1,313.7	1,256.7
Outpatient Surgeries	50.2	52.9	55.6	49.5	48.7
Expense per Capita (per person)	$1,075.8	$1,069.3	$1,022.5	$963.5	$959.1

TABLE 6

OREGON

U.S. Registered Community Hospitals
(Nonfederal, short-term general and other special hospitals)

Overview 1997–2001

	2001	2000	1999	1998	1997
Total Community Hospitals	**60**	**59**	**59**	**60**	**61**
Bed Size Category					
6-24	5	5	5	4	5
25-49	19	21	21	20	19
50-99	17	13	11	12	17
100-199	10	10	12	14	10
200-299	3	4	4	4	2
300-399	3	3	4	5	6
400-499	3	3	2	1	2
500 +	0	0	0	0	0
Location					
Hospitals Urban	28	27	27	27	27
Hospitals Rural	32	32	32	33	34
Control					
State and Local Government	12	15	15	15	15
Not for Profit	44	41	41	41	42
Investor owned	4	3	3	4	4
Physician Models					
Independent Practice Association	26	22	19	22	30
Group Practice without Walls	3	0	1	1	2
Open Physician-Hospital Organization	7	3	7	6	8
Closed Physician-Hospital Organization	5	3	4	4	6
Management Service Organization	8	7	6	5	6
Integrated Salary Model	24	23	21	14	16
Equity Model	0	0	0	0	0
Foundation	2	1	1	0	2
Insurance Products					
Health Maintenance Organization	13	12	17	17	20
Preferred Provider Organization	12	12	13	9	12
Indemnity Fee for Service	2	1	1	1	5
Managed Care Contracts					
Health Maintenance Organization	44	40	41	41	48
Preferred Provider Organization	49	43	42	40	46
Affiliations					
Hospitals in a System	35	28	29	27	28
Hospitals in a Network	21	16	17	21	17
Hospitals in a Group Purchasing Organization	56	48	49	46	—

States

TABLE 6

OREGON

U.S. Registered Community Hospitals
(Nonfederal, short-term general and other special hospitals)

Utilization, Personnel, Revenue and Expenses, Community Health Indicators 1997–2001

	2001	2000	1999	1998	1997
TOTAL FACILITY (Includes Hospital and Nursing Home Units)					
Utilization - Inpatient					
Beds	6,660	6,631	6,643	6,809	6,986
Admissions	334,862	329,932	317,808	313,350	308,512
Inpatient Days	1,449,556	1,435,545	1,409,906	1,401,720	1,347,809
Average Length of Stay	4.3	4.4	4.4	4.5	4.4
Inpatient Surgeries	108,024	105,967	103,162	104,239	105,951
Births	45,279	46,065	45,328	44,610	43,679
Utilization - Outpatient					
Emergency Outpatient Visits	1,098,201	1,008,428	921,414	958,415	928,641
Other Outpatient Visits	6,559,929	6,264,342	5,736,216	4,830,333	4,653,491
Total Outpatient Visits	7,658,130	7,272,770	6,657,630	5,788,748	5,582,132
Outpatient Surgeries	172,400	167,938	163,147	164,553	158,308
Personnel					
Full Time RNs	7,975	8,054	6,426	6,692	6,494
Full Time LPNs	420	448	409	524	390
Part Time RNs	6,588	6,224	6,315	5,983	7,119
Part Time LPNs	314	285	349	348	322
Total Full Time	32,473	31,121	26,971	29,348	27,060
Total Part Time	18,793	17,828	17,324	17,885	18,591
Revenue - Inpatient					
Gross Inpatient Revenue	$3,859,967,211	$3,485,892,570	$3,113,689,297	$2,933,384,377	$2,662,409,673
Revenue - Outpatient					
Gross Outpatient Revenue	$2,728,455,375	$2,350,061,380	$2,048,806,236	$1,829,620,648	$1,661,204,135
Revenue and Expenses - Totals (Includes Inpatient and Outpatient)					
Total Gross Revenue	$6,588,422,586	$5,835,953,950	$5,162,495,533	$4,763,005,025	$4,323,613,808
Deductions from Revenue	2,617,704,367	2,306,496,669	1,947,905,128	1,730,229,358	1,437,006,138
Net Patient Revenue	3,970,718,219	3,529,457,281	3,214,590,405	3,032,775,667	2,886,607,670
Other Operating Revenue	225,753,818	233,238,786	201,378,271	181,708,607	133,227,121
Other Nonoperating Revenue	63,051,233	69,416,016	75,147,493	102,764,290	76,098,231
Total Net Revenue	4,259,523,270	3,832,112,083	3,491,116,169	3,317,248,564	3,095,933,022
Total Expenses	3,951,387,339	3,600,487,783	3,286,343,045	3,095,154,279	2,867,526,498
HOSPITAL UNIT (Excludes Separate Nursing Home Units)					
Utilization - Inpatient					
Beds	6,184	6,111	6,027	6,288	6,412
Admissions	331,985	326,453	313,845	309,453	305,380
Inpatient Days	1,325,563	1,294,908	1,251,063	1,269,063	1,196,478
Average Length of Stay	4.0	4.0	4.0	4.1	3.9
Personnel					
Total Full Time	32,229	30,783	26,646	29,039	26,705
Total Part Time	18,651	17,669	17,145	17,733	18,359
Revenue and Expenses - Totals (Includes Inpatient and Outpatient)					
Total Net Revenue	$4,234,725,706	$3,810,739,241	$3,469,658,693	$3,295,734,830	$3,073,839,843
Total Expenses	3,927,287,050	3,582,438,850	3,271,980,437	3,075,675,635	2,849,678,837
COMMUNITY HEALTH INDICATORS PER 1000 POPULATION					
Total Population (in thousands)	3,473	3,421	3,316	3,282	3,243
Inpatient					
Beds	1.9	1.9	2.0	2.1	2.2
Admissions	96.4	96.4	95.8	95.5	95.1
Inpatient Days	417.4	419.6	425.2	427.1	415.6
Inpatient Surgeries	31.1	31.0	31.1	31.8	32.7
Births	13.0	13.5	13.7	13.6	13.5
Outpatient					
Emergency Outpatient Visits	316.2	294.7	277.9	292.0	286.3
Other Outpatient Visits	1,888.9	1,830.9	1,729.8	1,471.7	1,434.8
Total Outpatient Visits	2,205.1	2,125.7	2,007.6	1,763.8	1,721.2
Outpatient Surgeries	49.6	49.1	49.2	50.1	48.8
Expense per Capita (per person)	$1,137.8	$1,052.3	$991.0	$943.1	$884.2

TABLE 6

PENNSYLVANIA

U.S. Registered Community Hospitals
(Nonfederal, short-term general and other special hospitals)

Overview 1997–2001

	2001	2000	1999	1998	1997
Total Community Hospitals	**205**	**207**	**210**	**212**	**217**
Bed Size Category					
6-24	3	4	5	4	4
25-49	14	12	12	11	10
50-99	33	34	34	33	39
100-199	74	79	78	82	79
200-299	42	39	42	40	42
300-399	14	11	11	12	11
400-499	12	15	13	14	15
500 +	13	13	15	16	17
Location					
Hospitals Urban	161	163	165	167	172
Hospitals Rural	44	44	45	45	45
Control					
State and Local Government	2	2	1	1	1
Not for Profit	189	194	199	203	208
Investor owned	14	11	10	8	8
Physician Models					
Independent Practice Association	20	23	29	29	39
Group Practice without Walls	12	12	13	11	11
Open Physician-Hospital Organization	39	53	54	63	69
Closed Physician-Hospital Organization	10	15	24	25	27
Management Service Organization	32	41	39	40	40
Integrated Salary Model	53	53	53	52	53
Equity Model	3	11	8	3	6
Foundation	5	9	9	18	18
Insurance Products					
Health Maintenance Organization	25	32	36	47	48
Preferred Provider Organization	38	41	46	55	67
Indemnity Fee for Service	6	4	5	13	13
Managed Care Contracts					
Health Maintenance Organization	150	153	153	150	169
Preferred Provider Organization	144	147	148	145	163
Affiliations					
Hospitals in a System	104	108	108	103	100
Hospitals in a Network	45	57	53	61	70
Hospitals in a Group Purchasing Organization	151	151	137	131	—

States

TABLE 6

PENNSYLVANIA

U.S. Registered Community Hospitals
(Nonfederal, short-term general and other special hospitals)

Utilization, Personnel, Revenue and Expenses, Community Health Indicators 1997–2001

	2001	2000	1999	1998	1997
TOTAL FACILITY (Includes Hospital and Nursing Home Units)					
Utilization - Inpatient					
Beds	42,131	42,303	42,999	44,739	45,723
Admissions	1,808,531	1,796,081	1,755,029	1,752,298	1,756,446
Inpatient Days	10,395,360	10,558,152	10,652,791	10,927,224	11,165,571
Average Length of Stay	5.7	5.9	6.1	6.2	6.4
Inpatient Surgeries	544,254	534,894	555,367	578,008	563,834
Births	143,463	139,408	139,888	142,896	142,396
Utilization - Outpatient					
Emergency Outpatient Visits	4,873,595	4,727,149	4,615,588	4,620,945	4,620,241
Other Outpatient Visits	27,189,829	27,122,027	24,653,538	25,959,042	23,047,489
Total Outpatient Visits	32,063,424	31,849,176	29,269,126	30,579,987	27,667,730
Outpatient Surgeries	1,034,191	997,911	969,895	983,299	962,836
Personnel					
Full Time RNs	39,444	39,290	39,819	39,327	40,024
Full Time LPNs	4,962	4,807	5,287	5,306	5,576
Part Time RNs	23,733	22,678	22,707	23,391	23,802
Part Time LPNs	2,515	2,541	2,735	2,929	3,123
Total Full Time	181,276	178,775	179,851	180,604	181,714
Total Part Time	71,386	68,530	70,841	74,102	75,426
Revenue - Inpatient					
Gross Inpatient Revenue	$33,160,635,367	$29,235,892,623	$27,097,518,634	$25,636,639,265	$25,478,284,460
Revenue - Outpatient					
Gross Outpatient Revenue	$17,751,314,945	$15,605,206,965	$13,919,316,631	$12,554,243,341	$11,514,554,797
Revenue and Expenses - Totals (Includes Inpatient and Outpatient)					
Total Gross Revenue	$50,911,950,312	$44,841,099,588	$41,016,835,265	$38,190,882,606	$36,992,839,257
Deductions from Revenue	31,902,707,556	27,167,023,083	24,081,858,092	21,495,641,201	20,250,575,794
Net Patient Revenue	19,009,242,756	17,674,076,505	16,934,977,173	16,695,241,405	16,742,263,463
Other Operating Revenue	1,050,625,699	1,001,303,780	918,424,356	871,307,419	831,704,815
Other Nonoperating Revenue	320,138,109	473,372,882	436,390,618	604,119,011	486,026,161
Total Net Revenue	20,380,006,564	19,148,753,167	18,289,792,147	18,170,667,835	18,059,994,439
Total Expenses	19,668,618,568	18,449,395,399	17,762,016,623	17,561,776,794	17,055,231,614
HOSPITAL UNIT (Excludes Separate Nursing Home Units)					
Utilization - Inpatient					
Beds	38,652	38,642	38,320	40,334	41,214
Admissions	1,772,168	1,753,702	1,704,806	1,707,740	1,718,124
Inpatient Days	9,322,503	9,424,533	9,224,935	9,514,173	9,804,292
Average Length of Stay	5.3	5.4	5.4	5.6	5.7
Personnel					
Total Full Time	178,633	175,754	176,561	177,072	178,061
Total Part Time	69,755	66,833	69,104	72,322	73,322
Revenue and Expenses - Totals (Includes Inpatient and Outpatient)					
Total Net Revenue	$20,087,923,397	$18,857,929,952	$17,920,002,342	$17,747,827,775	$17,691,928,660
Total Expenses	19,453,873,721	18,267,250,601	17,508,949,084	17,276,532,062	16,801,066,293
COMMUNITY HEALTH INDICATORS PER 1000 POPULATION					
Total Population (in thousands)	12,287	12,281	11,994	12,002	12,016
Inpatient					
Beds	3.4	3.4	3.6	3.7	3.8
Admissions	147.2	146.2	146.3	146.0	146.2
Inpatient Days	846.0	859.7	888.2	910.4	929.2
Inpatient Surgeries	44.3	43.6	46.3	48.2	46.9
Births	11.7	11.4	11.7	11.9	11.9
Outpatient					
Emergency Outpatient Visits	396.6	384.9	384.8	385.0	384.5
Other Outpatient Visits	2,212.9	2,208.4	2,055.5	2,162.8	1,918.1
Total Outpatient Visits	2,609.5	2,593.4	2,440.3	2,547.8	2,302.6
Outpatient Surgeries	84.2	81.3	80.9	81.9	80.1
Expense per Capita (per person)	$1,600.7	$1,502.3	$1,480.9	$1,463.2	$1,419.4

TABLE 6

RHODE ISLAND

U.S. Registered Community Hospitals
(Nonfederal, short-term general and other special hospitals)

Overview 1997–2001

	2001	2000	1999	1998	1997
Total Community Hospitals	**11**	**11**	**11**	**12**	**11**
Bed Size Category					
6-24	0	0	0	0	0
25-49	0	0	0	0	0
50-99	1	1	1	1	1
100-199	5	5	6	8	6
200-299	3	3	2	1	1
300-399	1	1	1	1	2
400-499	0	0	0	0	0
500 +	1	1	1	1	1
Location					
Hospitals Urban	10	10	10	11	10
Hospitals Rural	1	1	1	1	1
Control					
State and Local Government	0	0	0	0	0
Not for Profit	11	11	11	12	11
Investor owned	0	0	0	0	0
Physician Models					
Independent Practice Association	7	3	3	5	5
Group Practice without Walls	1	0	0	0	2
Open Physician-Hospital Organization	6	7	8	8	8
Closed Physician-Hospital Organization	3	2	1	1	1
Management Service Organization	3	2	3	3	5
Integrated Salary Model	5	4	5	5	6
Equity Model	1	1	0	0	0
Foundation	4	4	4	4	4
Insurance Products					
Health Maintenance Organization	2	0	0	0	1
Preferred Provider Organization	2	0	0	2	4
Indemnity Fee for Service	1	0	0	0	0
Managed Care Contracts					
Health Maintenance Organization	11	11	11	12	10
Preferred Provider Organization	9	10	10	10	8
Affiliations					
Hospitals in a System	7	7	6	6	5
Hospitals in a Network	1	3	2	2	2
Hospitals in a Group Purchasing Organization	11	11	9	10	—

TABLE 6

RHODE ISLAND

U.S. Registered Community Hospitals
(Nonfederal, short-term general and other special hospitals)

Utilization, Personnel, Revenue and Expenses, Community Health Indicators 1997–2001

	2001	2000	1999	1998	1997
TOTAL FACILITY (Includes Hospital and Nursing Home Units)					
Utilization - Inpatient					
Beds	2,449	2,400	2,400	2,581	2,544
Admissions	120,901	119,070	117,163	117,320	116,354
Inpatient Days	638,571	625,939	623,306	659,966	658,143
Average Length of Stay	5.3	5.3	5.3	5.6	5.7
Inpatient Surgeries	35,543	35,483	35,116	35,232	36,964
Births	13,375	13,064	13,320	13,398	13,335
Utilization - Outpatient					
Emergency Outpatient Visits	451,325	440,098	421,667	407,366	415,173
Other Outpatient Visits	1,699,915	1,640,847	1,489,890	1,762,581	1,570,313
Total Outpatient Visits	2,151,240	2,080,945	1,911,557	2,169,947	1,985,486
Outpatient Surgeries	99,423	94,146	86,783	80,546	74,088
Personnel					
Full Time RNs	1,539	1,630	1,545	1,588	1,796
Full Time LPNs	184	183	161	192	211
Part Time RNs	3,056	3,087	3,145	2,748	2,706
Part Time LPNs	221	206	197	220	222
Total Full Time	10,793	10,894	10,491	11,224	11,696
Total Part Time	8,620	8,409	8,558	8,733	7,840
Revenue - Inpatient					
Gross Inpatient Revenue	$1,738,042,664	$1,512,132,670	$1,415,053,397	$1,393,271,369	$1,312,485,143
Revenue - Outpatient					
Gross Outpatient Revenue	$1,342,251,100	$1,154,392,267	$1,041,727,122	$933,791,131	$827,526,372
Revenue and Expenses - Totals (Includes Inpatient and Outpatient)					
Total Gross Revenue	$3,080,293,764	$2,666,524,937	$2,456,780,519	$2,327,062,500	$2,140,011,515
Deductions from Revenue	1,626,498,267	1,338,811,208	1,230,336,909	1,098,641,571	939,127,474
Net Patient Revenue	1,453,795,497	1,327,713,729	1,226,443,610	1,228,420,929	1,200,884,041
Other Operating Revenue	97,199,257	101,392,569	84,757,555	86,452,618	67,571,663
Other Nonoperating Revenue	18,363,394	48,479,673	28,358,285	30,473,011	54,631,917
Total Net Revenue	1,569,358,148	1,477,585,971	1,339,559,450	1,345,346,558	1,323,087,621
Total Expenses	1,592,333,629	1,488,194,792	1,362,140,752	1,278,223,306	1,268,181,214
HOSPITAL UNIT (Excludes Separate Nursing Home Units)					
Utilization - Inpatient					
Beds	2,405	2,337	2,361	2,542	2,525
Admissions	119,649	117,446	116,370	116,611	116,071
Inpatient Days	622,075	604,416	612,307	648,796	653,483
Average Length of Stay	5.2	5.1	5.3	5.6	5.6
Personnel					
Total Full Time	10,718	10,811	10,485	11,210	11,671
Total Part Time	8,538	8,315	8,520	8,692	7,832
Revenue and Expenses - Totals (Includes Inpatient and Outpatient)					
Total Net Revenue	$1,557,628,889	$1,465,522,013	$1,333,633,000	$1,337,590,292	$1,318,047,080
Total Expenses	1,582,522,184	1,479,990,940	1,356,396,823	1,271,503,480	1,264,670,728
COMMUNITY HEALTH INDICATORS PER 1000 POPULATION					
Total Population (in thousands)	1,050	1,048	991	988	987
Inpatient					
Beds	2.3	2.3	2.4	2.6	2.6
Admissions	114.2	113.6	118.2	118.8	117.9
Inpatient Days	603.0	597.1	629.1	668.2	666.8
Inpatient Surgeries	33.6	33.8	35.4	35.7	37.5
Births	12.6	12.5	13.4	13.6	13.5
Outpatient					
Emergency Outpatient Visits	426.2	419.8	425.6	412.4	420.7
Other Outpatient Visits	1,605.3	1,565.2	1,503.7	1,784.5	1,591.1
Total Outpatient Visits	2,031.5	1,985.0	1,929.3	2,197.0	2,011.7
Outpatient Surgeries	93.9	89.8	87.6	81.5	75.1
Expense per Capita (per person)	$1,503.7	$1,419.6	$1,374.8	$1,294.1	$1,284.9

TABLE 6

SOUTH CAROLINA

U.S. Registered Community Hospitals
(Nonfederal, short-term general and other special hospitals)

Overview 1997–2001

	2001	2000	1999	1998	1997
Total Community Hospitals	**62**	**63**	**64**	**65**	**65**
Bed Size Category					
6-24	1	1	1	1	2
25-49	9	11	9	12	10
50-99	13	12	13	12	12
100-199	16	15	18	18	17
200-299	14	14	12	12	14
300-399	4	4	6	5	5
400-499	2	3	2	2	2
500 +	3	3	3	3	3
Location					
Hospitals Urban	35	35	36	37	37
Hospitals Rural	27	28	28	28	28
Control					
State and Local Government	22	23	24	24	23
Not for Profit	20	20	20	20	22
Investor owned	20	20	20	21	20
Physician Models					
Independent Practice Association	6	6	4	4	11
Group Practice without Walls	0	0	0	1	9
Open Physician-Hospital Organization	13	13	11	21	4
Closed Physician-Hospital Organization	1	4	7	2	8
Management Service Organization	9	9	4	7	3
Integrated Salary Model	6	9	8	5	3
Equity Model	1	7	6	5	10
Foundation	1	1	1	0	6
Insurance Products					
Health Maintenance Organization	4	8	10	11	10
Preferred Provider Organization	11	11	14	20	18
Indemnity Fee for Service	1	1	1	3	8
Managed Care Contracts					
Health Maintenance Organization	34	38	41	40	35
Preferred Provider Organization	38	41	46	46	42
Affiliations					
Hospitals in a System	35	34	34	33	30
Hospitals in a Network	20	22	23	29	25
Hospitals in a Group Purchasing Organization	0	0	—	—	—

TABLE 6

SOUTH CAROLINA

U.S. Registered Community Hospitals
(Nonfederal, short-term general and other special hospitals)

Utilization, Personnel, Revenue and Expenses, Community Health Indicators 1997–2001

	2001	2000	1999	1998	1997
TOTAL FACILITY (Includes Hospital and Nursing Home Units)					
Utilization - Inpatient					
Beds	11,282	11,520	11,629	11,518	11,974
Admissions	505,294	495,410	478,936	457,347	443,355
Inpatient Days	2,940,707	2,916,386	2,816,481	2,763,146	2,802,382
Average Length of Stay	5.8	5.9	5.9	6.0	6.3
Inpatient Surgeries	173,046	173,645	150,556	140,781	140,962
Births	50,304	51,355	48,875	47,634	46,531
Utilization - Outpatient					
Emergency Outpatient Visits	1,840,819	1,831,462	1,675,252	1,531,231	1,466,495
Other Outpatient Visits	5,788,476	5,947,571	4,684,820	4,327,410	4,429,214
Total Outpatient Visits	7,629,295	7,779,033	6,360,072	5,858,641	5,895,709
Outpatient Surgeries	262,308	253,389	220,015	218,676	205,761
Personnel					
Full Time RNs	11,674	10,921	11,437	11,276	10,584
Full Time LPNs	1,689	1,623	1,687	1,662	1,969
Part Time RNs	5,366	4,911	5,061	3,927	4,609
Part Time LPNs	622	585	599	613	681
Total Full Time	48,615	45,230	46,006	45,568	46,025
Total Part Time	15,342	14,772	13,878	12,808	14,385
Revenue - Inpatient					
Gross Inpatient Revenue	$7,754,863,580	$6,462,086,026	$6,267,433,167	$5,599,831,497	$5,362,505,085
Revenue - Outpatient					
Gross Outpatient Revenue	$4,036,284,822	$3,446,830,663	$3,111,764,599	$2,700,429,264	$2,548,577,785
Revenue and Expenses - Totals (Includes Inpatient and Outpatient)					
Total Gross Revenue	$11,791,148,402	$9,908,916,689	$9,379,197,766	$8,300,260,761	$7,911,082,870
Deductions from Revenue	6,352,960,698	4,892,874,213	4,637,273,635	3,895,425,584	3,637,925,886
Net Patient Revenue	5,438,187,704	5,016,042,476	4,741,924,131	4,404,835,177	4,273,156,984
Other Operating Revenue	214,469,378	198,031,960	206,800,122	225,359,463	214,022,581
Other Nonoperating Revenue	60,313,151	85,852,895	55,842,812	98,172,230	135,310,015
Total Net Revenue	5,712,970,233	5,299,927,331	5,004,567,065	4,728,300,870	4,622,489,580
Total Expenses	5,211,814,991	5,017,991,441	4,714,616,676	4,348,407,394	4,068,825,946
HOSPITAL UNIT (Excludes Separate Nursing Home Units)					
Utilization - Inpatient					
Beds	10,229	10,411	10,676	10,640	10,972
Admissions	499,396	488,626	472,693	451,827	438,704
Inpatient Days	2,600,069	2,570,557	2,512,213	2,487,633	2,475,272
Average Length of Stay	5.2	5.3	5.3	5.5	5.6
Personnel					
Total Full Time	47,744	44,175	45,228	44,814	45,135
Total Part Time	15,057	14,394	13,615	12,538	14,089
Revenue and Expenses - Totals (Includes Inpatient and Outpatient)					
Total Net Revenue	$5,647,774,666	$4,478,643,578	$4,912,849,352	$4,655,195,598	$4,548,510,736
Total Expenses	5,160,720,870	4,960,782,656	4,658,570,962	4,301,557,086	4,022,549,793
COMMUNITY HEALTH INDICATORS PER 1000 POPULATION					
Total Population (in thousands)	4,063	4,012	3,886	3,840	3,790
Inpatient					
Beds	2.8	2.9	3.0	3.0	3.2
Admissions	124.4	123.5	123.3	119.1	117.0
Inpatient Days	723.8	726.9	724.8	719.6	739.4
Inpatient Surgeries	42.6	43.3	38.7	36.7	37.2
Births	12.4	12.8	12.6	12.4	12.3
Outpatient					
Emergency Outpatient Visits	453.1	456.5	431.1	398.8	386.9
Other Outpatient Visits	1,424.7	1,482.4	1,205.6	1,127.1	1,168.6
Total Outpatient Visits	1,877.7	1,938.9	1,636.8	1,525.9	1,555.6
Outpatient Surgeries	64.6	63.2	56.6	57.0	54.3
Expense per Capita (per person)	$1,282.7	$1,250.7	$1,213.3	$1,132.5	$1,073.6

TABLE 6

SOUTH DAKOTA

U.S. Registered Community Hospitals
(Nonfederal, short-term general and other special hospitals)

Overview 1997–2001

	2001	2000	1999	1998	1997
Total Community Hospitals	**50**	**48**	**48**	**49**	**49**
Bed Size Category					
6-24	13	13	13	13	13
25-49	10	10	10	8	10
50-99	13	11	11	16	13
100-199	8	9	9	7	8
200-299	3	1	2	2	2
300-399	1	2	1	1	1
400-499	1	1	1	0	0
500 +	1	1	1	2	2
Location					
Hospitals Urban	6	5	5	5	5
Hospitals Rural	44	43	43	44	44
Control					
State and Local Government	6	7	8	7	7
Not for Profit	43	41	40	42	42
Investor owned	1	0	0	0	0
Physician Models					
Independent Practice Association	11	9	7	5	5
Group Practice without Walls	2	3	2	4	2
Open Physician-Hospital Organization	4	6	5	3	2
Closed Physician-Hospital Organization	2	4	3	3	2
Management Service Organization	3	4	4	7	6
Integrated Salary Model	13	14	12	13	11
Equity Model	1	1	0	0	0
Foundation	1	0	2	2	2
Insurance Products					
Health Maintenance Organization	13	13	13	13	7
Preferred Provider Organization	17	17	14	11	12
Indemnity Fee for Service	6	5	6	7	5
Managed Care Contracts					
Health Maintenance Organization	21	21	22	22	22
Preferred Provider Organization	34	35	36	32	26
Affiliations					
Hospitals in a System	33	32	28	26	26
Hospitals in a Network	17	17	15	20	18
Hospitals in a Group Purchasing Organization	46	43	38	35	—

States

TABLE 6

SOUTH DAKOTA

U.S. Registered Community Hospitals
(Nonfederal, short-term general and other special hospitals)

Utilization, Personnel, Revenue and Expenses, Community Health Indicators 1997–2001

	2001	2000	1999	1998	1997
TOTAL FACILITY (Includes Hospital and Nursing Home Units)					
Utilization - Inpatient					
Beds	4,465	4,339	4,344	4,401	4,416
Admissions	103,907	98,508	97,316	96,055	94,101
Inpatient Days	1,046,760	1,035,027	1,052,039	1,032,566	1,047,494
Average Length of Stay	10.1	10.5	10.8	10.7	11.1
Inpatient Surgeries	32,462	32,993	32,627	32,976	34,734
Births	10,261	10,006	9,363	9,445	9,350
Utilization - Outpatient					
Emergency Outpatient Visits	211,200	196,054	192,035	183,556	175,193
Other Outpatient Visits	1,616,898	1,522,147	1,361,718	1,324,908	1,081,044
Total Outpatient Visits	1,828,098	1,718,201	1,553,753	1,508,464	1,256,237
Outpatient Surgeries	44,596	43,642	46,065	43,081	40,333
Personnel					
Full Time RNs	2,719	2,486	2,147	2,029	2,086
Full Time LPNs	267	226	186	209	293
Part Time RNs	1,508	1,822	2,058	1,915	2,043
Part Time LPNs	142	201	197	196	296
Total Full Time	12,093	10,774	9,989	9,510	9,274
Total Part Time	6,074	7,124	7,034	6,658	6,724
Revenue - Inpatient					
Gross Inpatient Revenue	$1,134,749,973	$1,000,043,131	$925,396,063	$863,704,037	$813,611,896
Revenue - Outpatient					
Gross Outpatient Revenue	$613,055,802	$550,896,116	$457,270,200	$415,256,677	$370,359,780
Revenue and Expenses - Totals (Includes Inpatient and Outpatient)					
Total Gross Revenue	$1,747,805,775	$1,550,939,247	$1,382,666,263	$1,278,960,714	$1,183,971,676
Deductions from Revenue	647,480,234	527,471,606	434,728,043	377,142,751	328,291,929
Net Patient Revenue	1,100,325,541	1,023,467,641	947,938,220	901,817,963	855,679,747
Other Operating Revenue	77,627,200	60,933,637	57,779,801	51,660,847	49,136,279
Other Nonoperating Revenue	11,008,624	43,912,340	28,755,729	29,569,700	47,752,507
Total Net Revenue	1,188,961,365	1,128,313,618	1,034,473,750	983,048,510	952,568,533
Total Expenses	1,106,276,599	1,058,129,155	942,471,403	923,990,512	847,774,854
HOSPITAL UNIT (Excludes Separate Nursing Home Units)					
Utilization - Inpatient					
Beds	2,763	2,619	2,659	2,802	2,896
Admissions	102,468	97,152	96,048	94,853	92,844
Inpatient Days	503,878	475,240	485,592	495,477	502,290
Average Length of Stay	4.9	4.9	5.1	5.2	5.4
Personnel					
Total Full Time	11,146	9,803	9,299	8,789	8,571
Total Part Time	5,249	6,324	6,271	5,865	5,992
Revenue and Expenses - Totals (Includes Inpatient and Outpatient)					
Total Net Revenue	$1,129,594,457	$1,075,161,508	$979,061,301	$932,540,100	$908,748,583
Total Expenses	1,048,181,427	1,010,362,656	895,701,751	878,640,302	803,694,025
COMMUNITY HEALTH INDICATORS PER 1000 POPULATION					
Total Population (in thousands)	757	755	733	731	701
Inpatient					
Beds	5.9	5.7	5.9	6.0	6.0
Admissions	137.3	130.5	132.7	131.4	128.8
Inpatient Days	1,383.5	1,371.2	1,435.0	1,412.9	1,433.2
Inpatient Surgeries	42.9	43.7	44.5	45.1	47.5
Births	13.6	13.3	12.8	12.9	12.8
Outpatient					
Emergency Outpatient Visits	279.1	259.7	261.9	251.2	239.7
Other Outpatient Visits	2,137.1	2,016.5	1,857.4	1,813.0	1,479.1
Total Outpatient Visits	2,416.2	2,276.2	2,119.3	2,064.2	1,718.9
Outpatient Surgeries	58.9	57.8	62.8	59.0	55.2
Expense per Capita (per person)	$1,462.2	$1,401.8	$1,285.5	$1,264.4	$1,160.0

TABLE 6

TENNESSEE

U.S. Registered Community Hospitals
(Nonfederal, short-term general and other special hospitals)

Overview 1997–2001

	2001	2000	1999	1998	1997
Total Community Hospitals	**123**	**121**	**121**	**122**	**124**
Bed Size Category					
6-24	1	0	0	2	1
25-49	26	25	20	23	22
50-99	30	33	39	35	38
100-199	36	34	33	33	31
200-299	11	10	11	13	14
300-399	6	7	5	4	6
400-499	5	3	3	3	3
500 +	8	9	10	9	9
Location					
Hospitals Urban	60	58	58	59	61
Hospitals Rural	63	63	63	63	63
Control					
State and Local Government	26	27	27	30	31
Not for Profit	61	57	56	58	50
Investor owned	36	37	38	34	43
Physician Models					
Independent Practice Association	21	19	22	21	23
Group Practice without Walls	1	0	1	4	6
Open Physician-Hospital Organization	25	15	19	24	26
Closed Physician-Hospital Organization	5	4	3	6	11
Management Service Organization	31	23	24	27	40
Integrated Salary Model	18	11	12	10	14
Equity Model	0	0	2	3	6
Foundation	3	4	4	1	5
Insurance Products					
Health Maintenance Organization	17	16	21	19	29
Preferred Provider Organization	35	27	36	34	54
Indemnity Fee for Service	11	10	10	8	17
Managed Care Contracts					
Health Maintenance Organization	80	62	65	63	82
Preferred Provider Organization	92	70	71	73	95
Affiliations					
Hospitals in a System	73	52	53	51	67
Hospitals in a Network	44	24	30	26	37
Hospitals in a Group Purchasing Organization	90	69	69	57	—

Table 6

TENNESSEE

U.S. Registered Community Hospitals
(Nonfederal, short-term general and other special hospitals)

Utilization, Personnel, Revenue and Expenses, Community Health Indicators 1997–2001

	2001	2000	1999	1998	1997
TOTAL FACILITY (Includes Hospital and Nursing Home Units)					
Utilization - Inpatient					
Beds	20,600	20,561	20,627	20,682	21,077
Admissions	751,495	737,313	751,523	744,913	762,758
Inpatient Days	4,122,419	4,225,812	4,296,679	4,292,500	4,523,889
Average Length of Stay	5.5	5.7	5.7	5.8	5.9
Inpatient Surgeries	238,914	241,938	236,298	228,702	233,055
Births	76,722	71,854	76,194	74,433	73,571
Utilization - Outpatient					
Emergency Outpatient Visits	2,710,481	2,601,659	2,589,171	2,443,232	2,325,632
Other Outpatient Visits	6,826,446	7,673,605	6,890,695	6,787,328	6,094,857
Total Outpatient Visits	9,536,927	10,275,264	9,479,866	9,230,560	8,420,489
Outpatient Surgeries	406,248	399,184	378,646	372,857	337,320
Personnel					
Full Time RNs	16,806	18,265	19,220	18,900	18,738
Full Time LPNs	3,799	3,273	3,388	3,581	4,186
Part Time RNs	6,683	6,880	5,037	4,430	4,524
Part Time LPNs	1,070	916	723	854	1,024
Total Full Time	79,904	78,784	80,276	81,263	80,620
Total Part Time	18,899	20,550	15,446	15,274	15,152
Revenue - Inpatient					
Gross Inpatient Revenue	$11,374,599,693	$10,080,668,101	$9,327,573,723	$8,743,361,839	$8,345,188,739
Revenue - Outpatient					
Gross Outpatient Revenue	$6,608,725,588	$5,810,556,366	$5,004,878,950	$4,463,657,836	$4,175,307,396
Revenue and Expenses - Totals (Includes Inpatient and Outpatient)					
Total Gross Revenue	$17,983,325,281	$15,891,224,467	$14,332,452,673	$13,207,019,675	$12,520,496,135
Deductions from Revenue	10,088,328,741	8,531,972,395	7,456,932,016	6,508,958,847	5,785,628,639
Net Patient Revenue	7,894,996,540	7,359,252,072	6,875,520,657	6,698,060,828	6,734,867,496
Other Operating Revenue	395,634,694	361,920,349	419,276,199	383,930,905	291,399,372
Other Nonoperating Revenue	310,696,758	328,615,366	163,624,734	134,814,577	184,378,772
Total Net Revenue	8,601,327,992	8,049,787,787	7,458,421,590	7,216,806,310	7,210,645,640
Total Expenses	8,143,131,226	7,554,623,035	7,233,873,814	6,530,695,662	6,563,092,641
HOSPITAL UNIT (Excludes Separate Nursing Home Units)					
Utilization - Inpatient					
Beds	19,170	19,273	19,104	19,310	19,280
Admissions	739,360	726,271	738,689	734,223	751,154
Inpatient Days	3,621,415	3,801,360	3,827,904	3,862,873	3,953,878
Average Length of Stay	4.9	5.2	5.2	5.3	5.3
Personnel					
Total Full Time	78,783	77,416	78,259	79,829	79,172
Total Part Time	18,561	20,230	15,095	15,065	14,799
Revenue and Expenses - Totals (Includes Inpatient and Outpatient)					
Total Net Revenue	$8,500,355,125	$7,950,369,293	$7,321,010,015	$7,116,607,493	$7,095,028,299
Total Expenses	8,058,017,723	7,475,659,236	7,128,551,841	6,446,647,305	6,464,612,830
COMMUNITY HEALTH INDICATORS PER 1000 POPULATION					
Total Population (in thousands)	5,740	5,689	5,484	5,133	5,378
Inpatient					
Beds	3.6	3.6	3.8	3.8	3.9
Admissions	130.9	129.6	137.1	137.1	141.8
Inpatient Days	718.2	742.8	783.6	790.1	841.1
Inpatient Surgeries	41.6	42.5	43.1	42.1	43.3
Births	13.4	12.6	13.9	13.7	13.7
Outpatient					
Emergency Outpatient Visits	472.2	457.3	472.2	449.7	432.4
Other Outpatient Visits	1,189.3	1,348.8	1,256.6	1,249.4	1,133.2
Total Outpatient Visits	1,661.5	1,806.1	1,728.8	1,699.1	1,565.6
Outpatient Surgeries	70.8	70.2	69.1	68.6	62.7
Expense per Capita (per person)	$1,418.7	$1,327.9	$1,319.2	$1,202.1	$1,220.3

TABLE 6

TEXAS

U.S. Registered Community Hospitals
(Nonfederal, short-term general and other special hospitals)

Overview 1997–2001

	2001	2000	1999	1998	1997
Total Community Hospitals	**411**	**403**	**408**	**400**	**407**
Bed Size Category					
6-24	48	48	54	47	48
25-49	111	108	101	104	101
50-99	75	68	70	69	74
100-199	88	86	91	88	97
200-299	34	41	40	40	37
300-399	31	28	26	22	23
400-499	8	7	9	14	13
500 +	16	17	17	16	14
Location					
Hospitals Urban	250	241	245	238	244
Hospitals Rural	161	162	163	162	163
Control					
State and Local Government	128	130	131	133	138
Not for Profit	146	142	143	138	137
Investor owned	137	131	134	129	132
Physician Models					
Independent Practice Association	76	82	103	107	102
Group Practice without Walls	18	20	18	23	23
Open Physician-Hospital Organization	96	104	109	124	117
Closed Physician-Hospital Organization	21	23	30	31	42
Management Service Organization	53	79	98	105	128
Integrated Salary Model	58	55	64	68	52
Equity Model	8	15	22	30	12
Foundation	34	41	50	59	61
Insurance Products					
Health Maintenance Organization	60	73	100	101	97
Preferred Provider Organization	76	95	118	126	151
Indemnity Fee for Service	22	27	39	44	41
Managed Care Contracts					
Health Maintenance Organization	311	309	330	316	318
Preferred Provider Organization	351	350	370	350	367
Affiliations					
Hospitals in a System	233	226	228	217	215
Hospitals in a Network	93	102	121	136	151
Hospitals in a Group Purchasing Organization	335	326	306	280	—

States

TABLE 6

TEXAS

U.S. Registered Community Hospitals
(Nonfederal, short-term general and other special hospitals)

Utilization, Personnel, Revenue and Expenses, Community Health Indicators 1997–2001

	2001	2000	1999	1998	1997
TOTAL FACILITY (Includes Hospital and Nursing Home Units)					
Utilization - Inpatient					
Beds	56,354	55,877	56,824	56,573	55,759
Admissions	2,461,016	2,366,652	2,302,892	2,227,166	2,125,610
Inpatient Days	12,650,063	12,122,361	12,015,612	11,732,621	11,355,612
Average Length of Stay	5.1	5.1	5.2	5.3	5.3
Inpatient Surgeries	725,998	716,990	695,394	709,815	629,108
Births	366,373	357,906	339,105	332,825	320,542
Utilization - Outpatient					
Emergency Outpatient Visits	7,806,334	7,375,580	7,071,236	6,722,059	6,296,427
Other Outpatient Visits	23,647,614	22,017,896	21,187,640	20,616,924	19,560,947
Total Outpatient Visits	31,453,948	29,393,476	28,258,876	27,338,983	25,857,374
Outpatient Surgeries	1,049,923	1,043,853	1,033,349	986,411	882,821
Personnel					
Full Time RNs	55,139	52,889	53,028	51,559	49,680
Full Time LPNs	11,908	11,420	12,738	12,681	12,574
Part Time RNs	18,430	17,165	16,782	17,951	16,139
Part Time LPNs	3,484	3,197	3,199	3,610	3,835
Total Full Time	235,495	227,471	231,401	225,409	220,417
Total Part Time	57,901	53,904	53,137	57,372	54,459
Revenue - Inpatient					
Gross Inpatient Revenue	$42,086,234,028	$36,110,028,792	$32,577,994,295	$29,472,655,033	$26,887,624,884
Revenue - Outpatient					
Gross Outpatient Revenue	$20,856,680,055	$17,722,021,020	$15,630,753,126	$13,914,506,461	$12,347,895,974
Revenue and Expenses - Totals (Includes Inpatient and Outpatient)					
Total Gross Revenue	$62,942,914,083	$53,832,049,812	$48,168,747,421	$43,387,161,494	$39,235,520,858
Deductions from Revenue	37,784,174,261	31,935,698,552	27,344,870,806	23,349,445,508	20,256,858,453
Net Patient Revenue	25,158,739,822	21,896,351,260	20,823,876,615	20,037,715,986	18,978,662,405
Other Operating Revenue	2,466,963,729	2,311,583,837	2,071,860,033	2,000,853,453	1,788,881,717
Other Nonoperating Revenue	397,849,826	476,653,999	457,181,324	418,580,724	467,141,627
Total Net Revenue	28,023,553,377	24,684,589,096	23,352,917,972	22,457,150,163	21,234,685,749
Total Expenses	25,906,399,927	23,494,693,306	21,811,587,994	20,578,760,550	19,229,224,055
HOSPITAL UNIT (Excludes Separate Nursing Home Units)					
Utilization - Inpatient					
Beds	54,430	53,335	53,570	53,128	52,504
Admissions	2,427,696	2,323,817	2,246,168	2,165,772	2,070,866
Inpatient Days	12,142,510	11,498,881	11,180,783	10,839,457	10,520,117
Average Length of Stay	5.0	4.9	5.0	5.0	5.1
Personnel					
Total Full Time	233,563	225,255	228,566	221,876	217,228
Total Part Time	57,471	53,479	52,351	56,306	52,591
Revenue and Expenses - Totals (Includes Inpatient and Outpatient)					
Total Net Revenue	$27,788,903,511	$24,508,683,378	$23,037,586,558	$22,070,657,603	$20,855,004,177
Total Expenses	25,757,452,142	23,374,693,756	21,595,696,612	20,334,411,518	18,989,938,094
COMMUNITY HEALTH INDICATORS PER 1000 POPULATION					
Total Population (in thousands)	21,325	20,852	20,044	19,712	19,355
Inpatient					
Beds	2.6	2.7	2.8	2.9	2.9
Admissions	115.4	113.5	114.9	113.0	109.8
Inpatient Days	593.2	581.4	599.5	595.2	586.7
Inpatient Surgeries	34.0	34.4	34.7	36.0	32.5
Births	17.2	17.2	16.9	16.9	16.6
Outpatient					
Emergency Outpatient Visits	366.1	353.7	352.8	341.0	325.3
Other Outpatient Visits	1,108.9	1,055.9	1,057.0	1,045.9	1,010.6
Total Outpatient Visits	1,475.0	1,409.6	1,409.8	1,386.9	1,335.9
Outpatient Surgeries	49.2	50.1	51.6	50.0	45.6
Expense per Capita (per person)	$1,214.8	$1,126.7	$1,088.2	$1,044.0	$993.5

TABLE 6

UTAH

U.S. Registered Community Hospitals
(Nonfederal, short-term general and other special hospitals)

Overview 1997–2001

	2001	2000	1999	1998	1997
Total Community Hospitals	**42**	**42**	**42**	**41**	**41**
Bed Size Category					
6-24	8	7	7	7	7
25-49	11	14	12	12	12
50-99	8	5	7	7	6
100-199	9	10	11	10	10
200-299	3	3	2	2	3
300-399	1	2	2	2	2
400-499	2	1	1	1	1
500 +	0	0	0	0	0
Location					
Hospitals Urban	21	20	20	19	19
Hospitals Rural	21	22	22	22	22
Control					
State and Local Government	7	7	9	9	9
Not for Profit	22	22	20	20	20
Investor owned	13	13	13	12	12
Physician Models					
Independent Practice Association	11	16	15	16	14
Group Practice without Walls	1	1	1	3	4
Open Physician-Hospital Organization	4	5	3	4	6
Closed Physician-Hospital Organization	0	0	1	0	1
Management Service Organization	2	4	5	8	9
Integrated Salary Model	17	18	16	18	20
Equity Model	0	0	0	0	0
Foundation	0	0	1	3	4
Insurance Products					
Health Maintenance Organization	18	19	15	22	25
Preferred Provider Organization	20	20	16	25	28
Indemnity Fee for Service	12	11	6	15	16
Managed Care Contracts					
Health Maintenance Organization	21	25	24	24	27
Preferred Provider Organization	23	28	26	27	32
Affiliations					
Hospitals in a System	28	32	26	30	33
Hospitals in a Network	11	14	8	8	9
Hospitals in a Group Purchasing Organization	33	32	24	30	—

States

TABLE 6

UTAH

U.S. Registered Community Hospitals
(Nonfederal, short-term general and other special hospitals)

Utilization, Personnel, Revenue and Expenses, Community Health Indicators 1997–2001

	2001	2000	1999	1998	1997
TOTAL FACILITY (Includes Hospital and Nursing Home Units)					
Utilization - Inpatient					
Beds	4,437	4,330	4,170	4,010	4,134
Admissions	203,037	194,047	189,430	192,357	186,393
Inpatient Days	902,313	886,846	871,864	885,746	820,872
Average Length of Stay	4.4	4.6	4.6	4.6	4.4
Inpatient Surgeries	59,425	58,729	56,992	60,493	56,126
Births	47,319	47,389	45,831	44,259	42,105
Utilization - Outpatient					
Emergency Outpatient Visits	699,934	697,703	687,822	625,879	632,366
Other Outpatient Visits	3,718,415	3,771,285	3,677,904	3,598,412	2,931,899
Total Outpatient Visits	4,418,349	4,468,988	4,365,726	4,224,291	3,564,265
Outpatient Surgeries	122,692	125,430	120,031	128,033	111,654
Personnel					
Full Time RNs	4,442	4,143	4,405	5,078	4,495
Full Time LPNs	566	413	493	856	667
Part Time RNs	2,749	3,426	3,134	2,604	3,133
Part Time LPNs	387	359	326	330	403
Total Full Time	20,005	18,807	18,880	19,692	18,467
Total Part Time	10,822	11,987	9,052	8,223	9,890
Revenue - Inpatient					
Gross Inpatient Revenue	$2,559,345,455	$2,168,015,062	$2,124,901,031	$1,888,753,714	$1,799,080,954
Revenue - Outpatient					
Gross Outpatient Revenue	$1,582,419,304	$1,347,153,458	$1,328,671,681	$1,104,236,886	$1,047,590,217
Revenue and Expenses - Totals (Includes Inpatient and Outpatient)					
Total Gross Revenue	$4,141,764,759	$3,515,168,520	$3,453,572,712	$2,992,990,600	$2,846,671,171
Deductions from Revenue	1,865,061,006	1,391,174,618	1,439,113,434	1,144,878,464	1,064,131,695
Net Patient Revenue	2,276,703,753	2,123,993,902	2,014,459,278	1,848,112,136	1,782,539,476
Other Operating Revenue	158,563,665	115,758,563	105,790,033	119,057,672	105,900,795
Other Nonoperating Revenue	21,198,879	12,177,408	16,489,703	5,226,424	1,863,175
Total Net Revenue	2,456,466,297	2,251,929,873	2,136,739,014	1,972,396,232	1,890,303,746
Total Expenses	2,242,551,322	2,069,630,397	1,927,577,263	1,826,222,339	1,680,391,312
HOSPITAL UNIT (Excludes Separate Nursing Home Units)					
Utilization - Inpatient					
Beds	4,283	4,187	3,967	3,737	3,882
Admissions	200,838	191,941	187,940	189,316	183,718
Inpatient Days	857,332	844,301	825,693	807,010	755,616
Average Length of Stay	4.3	4.4	4.4	4.3	4.1
Personnel					
Total Full Time	19,858	18,739	18,803	19,433	18,218
Total Part Time	10,609	11,891	9,772	7,958	9,791
Revenue and Expenses - Totals (Includes Inpatient and Outpatient)					
Total Net Revenue	$2,435,680,792	$2,239,569,389	$2,124,836,350	$1,957,383,056	$1,870,536,641
Total Expenses	2,230,611,574	2,064,796,222	1,921,753,908	1,818,502,949	1,672,235,198
COMMUNITY HEALTH INDICATORS PER 1000 POPULATION					
Total Population (in thousands)	2,270	2,233	2,130	2,101	2,065
Inpatient					
Beds	2.0	1.9	2.0	1.9	2.0
Admissions	89.5	86.9	88.9	91.6	90.2
Inpatient Days	397.5	397.1	409.4	421.7	397.4
Inpatient Surgeries	26.2	26.3	26.8	28.8	27.2
Births	20.8	21.2	21.5	21.1	20.4
Outpatient					
Emergency Outpatient Visits	308.4	312.4	322.9	298.0	306.2
Other Outpatient Visits	1,638.2	1,688.8	1,726.8	1,713.1	1,419.5
Total Outpatient Visits	1,946.6	2,001.2	2,049.8	2,011.0	1,725.7
Outpatient Surgeries	54.1	56.2	56.4	61.0	54.1
Expense per Capita (per person)	$988.0	$926.8	$905.0	$869.4	$813.6

TABLE 6

VERMONT

U.S. Registered Community Hospitals
(Nonfederal, short-term general and other special hospitals)

Overview 1997–2001

	2001	2000	1999	1998	1997
Total Community Hospitals	**14**	**14**	**14**	**14**	**14**
Bed Size Category					
6-24	0	0	0	0	0
25-49	5	5	5	4	3
50-99	5	4	5	6	8
100-199	2	3	2	2	1
200-299	1	1	1	1	1
300-399	0	0	0	0	1
400-499	0	0	0	1	0
500 +	1	1	1	0	0
Location					
Hospitals Urban	2	2	2	2	2
Hospitals Rural	12	12	12	12	12
Control					
State and Local Government	0	0	0	0	0
Not for Profit	14	14	14	14	14
Investor owned	0	0	0	0	0
Physician Models					
Independent Practice Association	1	1	1	1	2
Group Practice without Walls	2	0	1	1	2
Open Physician-Hospital Organization	6	5	5	5	6
Closed Physician-Hospital Organization	1	2	2	2	1
Management Service Organization	3	2	3	2	3
Integrated Salary Model	8	5	6	6	5
Equity Model	0	0	0	0	0
Foundation	1	0	0	0	1
Insurance Products					
Health Maintenance Organization	6	6	6	7	5
Preferred Provider Organization	3	2	2	2	3
Indemnity Fee for Service	1	2	1	1	2
Managed Care Contracts					
Health Maintenance Organization	11	8	11	11	11
Preferred Provider Organization	9	8	10	7	8
Affiliations					
Hospitals in a System	7	5	3	3	2
Hospitals in a Network	3	3	4	4	5
Hospitals in a Group Purchasing Organization	13	9	7	7	—

States

TABLE 6

VERMONT

U.S. Registered Community Hospitals
(Nonfederal, short-term general and other special hospitals)

Utilization, Personnel, Revenue and Expenses, Community Health Indicators 1997–2001

	2001	2000	1999	1998	1997
TOTAL FACILITY (Includes Hospital and Nursing Home Units)					
Utilization - Inpatient					
Beds	1,694	1,674	1,669	1,671	1,565
Admissions	54,701	52,413	50,820	50,076	52,275
Inpatient Days	403,993	407,915	394,752	393,539	406,985
Average Length of Stay	7.4	7.8	7.8	7.9	7.8
Inpatient Surgeries	14,507	14,677	15,890	15,763	16,893
Births	5,982	6,086	6,521	6,366	6,733
Utilization - Outpatient					
Emergency Outpatient Visits	237,773	236,337	220,500	213,367	221,636
Other Outpatient Visits	1,053,731	1,006,715	1,193,334	938,260	641,952
Total Outpatient Visits	1,291,504	1,243,052	1,413,834	1,151,627	863,588
Outpatient Surgeries	37,983	34,739	33,443	32,198	31,354
Personnel					
Full Time RNs	939	977	948	868	1,113
Full Time LPNs	202	167	170	183	236
Part Time RNs	1,201	1,651	1,505	1,491	1,437
Part Time LPNs	216	265	222	233	250
Total Full Time	7,317	5,977	5,911	5,594	6,280
Total Part Time	4,134	5,307	4,058	4,351	4,102
Revenue - Inpatient					
Gross Inpatient Revenue	$594,629,834	$574,346,167	$518,323,168	$554,981,205	$462,487,247
Revenue - Outpatient					
Gross Outpatient Revenue	$583,052,967	$496,200,352	$435,098,015	$399,689,481	$319,256,386
Revenue and Expenses - Totals (Includes Inpatient and Outpatient)					
Total Gross Revenue	$1,177,682,801	$1,070,546,519	$953,421,183	$954,670,686	$781,743,633
Deductions from Revenue	406,248,096	373,526,131	321,690,952	404,255,939	243,480,058
Net Patient Revenue	771,434,705	697,020,388	631,730,231	550,414,747	538,263,575
Other Operating Revenue	16,049,961	15,403,343	15,793,813	24,695,865	15,909,216
Other Nonoperating Revenue	-17,559,247	27,208,270	15,736,174	13,200,342	34,243,422
Total Net Revenue	769,925,419	739,632,001	663,260,218	588,310,954	588,416,213
Total Expenses	771,202,476	696,036,667	646,945,630	572,807,035	550,684,461
HOSPITAL UNIT (Excludes Separate Nursing Home Units)					
Utilization - Inpatient					
Beds	1,318	1,425	1,302	1,263	1,156
Admissions	54,016	52,048	50,270	49,593	51,838
Inpatient Days	275,686	320,624	270,279	251,889	264,802
Average Length of Stay	5.1	6.2	5.4	5.1	5.1
Personnel					
Total Full Time	7,062	5,844	5,712	5,358	6,006
Total Part Time	3,936	5,192	4,753	4,112	3,879
Revenue and Expenses - Totals (Includes Inpatient and Outpatient)					
Total Net Revenue	$749,316,386	$727,972,770	$645,310,922	$569,552,051	$574,266,741
Total Expenses	751,409,578	685,479,802	629,980,592	554,130,892	536,594,221
COMMUNITY HEALTH INDICATORS PER 1000 POPULATION					
Total Population (in thousands)	613	609	594	591	589
Inpatient					
Beds	2.8	2.7	2.8	2.8	2.7
Admissions	89.2	86.1	85.6	84.8	88.8
Inpatient Days	658.9	670.0	664.9	666.4	691.4
Inpatient Surgeries	23.7	24.1	26.8	26.7	28.7
Births	9.8	10.0	11.0	10.8	11.4
Outpatient					
Emergency Outpatient Visits	387.8	388.2	371.4	361.3	376.5
Other Outpatient Visits	1,718.7	1,653.5	2,009.9	1,588.7	1,090.5
Total Outpatient Visits	2,106.5	2,041.7	2,381.2	1,950.0	1,467.0
Outpatient Surgeries	62.0	57.1	56.3	54.5	53.3
Expense per Capita (per person)	$1,257.9	$1,143.2	$1,089.6	$969.9	$935.5

TABLE 6

VIRGINIA

U.S. Registered Community Hospitals
(Nonfederal, short-term general and other special hospitals)

Overview 1997–2001

	2001	2000	1999	1998	1997
Total Community Hospitals	**87**	**88**	**89**	**93**	**93**
Bed Size Category					
6-24	2	4	2	2	1
25-49	10	7	7	8	8
50-99	18	17	20	18	16
100-199	25	29	28	33	34
200-299	17	15	16	15	17
300-399	5	7	8	8	8
400-499	3	3	2	2	2
500 +	7	6	6	7	7
Location					
Hospitals Urban	52	53	54	58	57
Hospitals Rural	35	35	35	35	36
Control					
State and Local Government	5	5	5	5	6
Not for Profit	67	66	68	70	70
Investor owned	15	17	16	18	17
Physician Models					
Independent Practice Association	6	11	11	14	22
Group Practice without Walls	1	6	10	8	11
Open Physician-Hospital Organization	22	24	30	30	35
Closed Physician-Hospital Organization	2	4	8	12	15
Management Service Organization	9	11	21	21	26
Integrated Salary Model	23	28	32	26	24
Equity Model	1	3	6	6	5
Foundation	3	4	4	5	4
Insurance Products					
Health Maintenance Organization	23	25	31	28	24
Preferred Provider Organization	30	37	41	42	41
Indemnity Fee for Service	7	13	17	19	22
Managed Care Contracts					
Health Maintenance Organization	51	55	55	60	51
Preferred Provider Organization	57	64	64	72	70
Affiliations					
Hospitals in a System	45	48	51	51	54
Hospitals in a Network	28	32	29	38	38
Hospitals in a Group Purchasing Organization	60	65	62	60	—

TABLE 6

VIRGINIA

U.S. Registered Community Hospitals
(Nonfederal, short-term general and other special hospitals)

Utilization, Personnel, Revenue and Expenses, Community Health Indicators 1997–2001

	2001	2000	1999	1998	1997
TOTAL FACILITY (Includes Hospital and Nursing Home Units)					
Utilization - Inpatient					
Beds	16,775	16,869	17,295	17,890	18,179
Admissions	743,992	726,772	723,803	716,976	705,038
Inpatient Days	4,239,227	4,161,981	4,133,834	4,090,018	4,216,773
Average Length of Stay	5.7	5.7	5.7	5.7	6.0
Inpatient Surgeries	235,109	221,837	215,568	219,878	213,556
Births	90,043	88,419	87,384	85,573	83,925
Utilization - Outpatient					
Emergency Outpatient Visits	2,482,380	2,476,006	2,291,867	2,255,094	2,126,854
Other Outpatient Visits	7,266,153	7,067,468	6,439,017	6,068,901	5,903,915
Total Outpatient Visits	9,748,533	9,543,474	8,730,884	8,323,995	8,030,769
Outpatient Surgeries	468,427	424,570	399,995	373,869	344,801
Personnel					
Full Time RNs	17,572	17,875	17,243	17,657	16,766
Full Time LPNs	2,690	2,704	2,778	2,872	2,970
Part Time RNs	7,902	7,432	6,990	6,952	6,393
Part Time LPNs	865	861	1,090	1,006	1,021
Total Full Time	72,228	71,430	68,276	68,914	66,572
Total Part Time	24,196	23,153	22,200	21,451	21,105
Revenue - Inpatient					
Gross Inpatient Revenue	$10,850,288,232	$9,441,736,067	$8,879,124,657	$8,168,485,435	$7,614,491,161
Revenue - Outpatient					
Gross Outpatient Revenue	$6,253,409,826	$5,348,095,706	$4,761,310,776	$4,098,142,024	$3,740,875,479
Revenue and Expenses - Totals (Includes Inpatient and Outpatient)					
Total Gross Revenue	$17,103,698,058	$14,789,831,773	$13,640,435,433	$12,266,627,459	$11,355,366,640
Deductions from Revenue	8,992,877,116	7,349,786,545	6,565,622,328	5,636,877,770	4,870,341,879
Net Patient Revenue	8,110,820,942	7,440,045,228	7,074,813,105	6,629,749,689	6,485,024,761
Other Operating Revenue	302,761,541	273,304,634	261,032,965	197,884,519	182,048,475
Other Nonoperating Revenue	131,168,071	126,490,381	226,795,432	117,590,421	134,389,720
Total Net Revenue	8,544,750,554	7,839,840,243	7,562,641,502	6,945,224,629	6,801,462,956
Total Expenses	7,961,019,921	7,109,751,133	6,637,854,513	6,294,405,851	6,138,915,405
HOSPITAL UNIT (Excludes Separate Nursing Home Units)					
Utilization - Inpatient					
Beds	15,866	15,709	15,872	16,430	16,673
Admissions	740,997	723,853	720,497	712,640	699,303
Inpatient Days	3,927,254	3,769,912	3,653,766	3,595,253	3,647,353
Average Length of Stay	5.3	5.2	5.1	5.0	5.2
Personnel					
Total Full Time	71,289	70,525	67,346	67,693	65,319
Total Part Time	23,845	22,889	21,770	21,131	20,660
Revenue and Expenses - Totals (Includes Inpatient and Outpatient)					
Total Net Revenue	$8,501,564,931	$7,795,125,327	$7,500,435,588	$6,874,805,160	$6,731,561,708
Total Expenses	7,921,569,817	7,069,123,980	6,592,027,665	6,233,864,195	6,058,698,443
COMMUNITY HEALTH INDICATORS PER 1000 POPULATION					
Total Population (in thousands)	7,100	7,079	6,873	6,789	6,733
Inpatient					
Beds	2.3	2.4	2.5	2.6	2.7
Admissions	103.5	102.7	105.3	105.6	104.7
Inpatient Days	589.8	588.0	601.5	602.4	626.3
Inpatient Surgeries	32.7	31.3	31.4	32.4	31.7
Births	12.5	12.5	12.7	12.6	12.5
Outpatient					
Emergency Outpatient Visits	345.4	349.8	333.5	332.2	315.9
Other Outpatient Visits	1,010.9	998.4	936.9	893.9	876.9
Total Outpatient Visits	1,356.3	1,348.2	1,270.3	1,226.1	1,192.8
Outpatient Surgeries	65.2	60.0	58.2	55.1	51.2
Expense per Capita (per person)	$1,107.6	$1,004.4	$965.8	$927.1	$911.8

TABLE 6

WASHINGTON

U.S. Registered Community Hospitals
(Nonfederal, short-term general and other special hospitals)

Overview 1997–2001

	2001	2000	1999	1998	1997
Total Community Hospitals	**84**	**84**	**86**	**86**	**88**
Bed Size Category					
6-24	5	6	8	6	5
25-49	22	22	22	25	26
50-99	18	17	17	17	19
100-199	17	16	18	19	18
200-299	12	15	13	10	13
300-399	7	6	6	7	5
400-499	1	0	0	0	0
500 +	2	2	2	2	2
Location					
Hospitals Urban	44	44	46	46	49
Hospitals Rural	40	40	40	40	39
Control					
State and Local Government	39	38	40	41	40
Not for Profit	41	42	43	42	44
Investor owned	4	4	3	3	4
Physician Models					
Independent Practice Association	9	9	11	10	16
Group Practice without Walls	5	2	2	2	3
Open Physician-Hospital Organization	10	13	14	10	20
Closed Physician-Hospital Organization	3	3	6	5	4
Management Service Organization	7	7	9	9	10
Integrated Salary Model	22	22	20	17	24
Equity Model	1	2	2	1	0
Foundation	2	3	3	3	4
Insurance Products					
Health Maintenance Organization	6	7	13	11	19
Preferred Provider Organization	9	11	17	16	21
Indemnity Fee for Service	3	4	6	6	7
Managed Care Contracts					
Health Maintenance Organization	35	37	43	35	49
Preferred Provider Organization	39	43	48	38	51
Affiliations					
Hospitals in a System	27	24	24	21	32
Hospitals in a Network	19	15	17	11	19
Hospitals in a Group Purchasing Organization	53	49	52	47	—

TABLE 6 — WASHINGTON

U.S. Registered Community Hospitals
(Nonfederal, short-term general and other special hospitals)

Utilization, Personnel, Revenue and Expenses, Community Health Indicators 1997–2001

	2001	2000	1999	1998	1997
TOTAL FACILITY (Includes Hospital and Nursing Home Units)					
Utilization - Inpatient					
Beds	11,382	11,136	11,092	10,739	10,845
Admissions	522,624	504,836	490,659	474,394	477,874
Inpatient Days	2,501,066	2,432,089	2,375,711	2,295,333	2,254,232
Average Length of Stay	4.8	4.8	4.8	4.8	4.7
Inpatient Surgeries	163,263	163,298	164,275	144,499	157,710
Births	74,134	73,816	72,814	72,506	71,382
Utilization - Outpatient					
Emergency Outpatient Visits	2,063,313	1,932,238	1,887,881	1,602,826	1,493,542
Other Outpatient Visits	7,369,191	7,656,940	8,072,113	7,118,236	6,238,083
Total Outpatient Visits	9,432,504	9,589,178	9,959,994	8,721,062	7,731,625
Outpatient Surgeries	312,357	261,219	247,937	239,312	225,713
Personnel					
Full Time RNs	10,991	10,083	8,427	9,154	9,024
Full Time LPNs	1,098	1,175	932	1,026	1,159
Part Time RNs	9,567	11,165	11,467	9,579	9,017
Part Time LPNs	595	1,155	1,176	992	946
Total Full Time	54,672	50,106	45,373	42,071	46,361
Total Part Time	27,551	33,201	33,715	28,849	26,643
Revenue - Inpatient					
Gross Inpatient Revenue	$7,463,136,201	$6,558,652,349	$5,936,579,978	$5,037,900,244	$4,721,702,626
Revenue - Outpatient					
Gross Outpatient Revenue	$5,100,762,752	$4,446,084,034	$3,979,924,518	$3,089,214,485	$2,917,813,045
Revenue and Expenses - Totals (Includes Inpatient and Outpatient)					
Total Gross Revenue	$12,563,898,953	$11,004,736,383	$9,916,504,496	$8,127,114,729	$7,639,515,671
Deductions from Revenue	5,870,547,412	4,776,586,811	3,981,377,196	3,055,762,073	2,647,296,774
Net Patient Revenue	6,693,351,541	6,228,149,572	5,935,127,300	5,071,352,656	4,992,218,897
Other Operating Revenue	438,253,314	344,678,358	329,844,922	289,826,305	225,617,125
Other Nonoperating Revenue	81,540,504	160,620,397	127,455,356	117,022,748	100,133,517
Total Net Revenue	7,213,145,359	6,733,448,327	6,392,427,578	5,479,101,709	5,317,969,539
Total Expenses	6,971,690,572	6,384,423,283	6,091,763,363	5,240,148,977	5,200,081,887
HOSPITAL UNIT (Excludes Separate Nursing Home Units)					
Utilization - Inpatient					
Beds	10,696	10,326	10,217	10,148	10,228
Admissions	516,955	501,157	484,728	470,529	474,096
Inpatient Days	2,292,820	2,211,500	2,125,679	2,107,302	2,067,673
Average Length of Stay	4.4	4.4	4.4	4.5	4.4
Personnel					
Total Full Time	54,120	49,627	44,769	41,514	45,026
Total Part Time	27,177	32,905	33,403	28,527	26,363
Revenue and Expenses - Totals (Includes Inpatient and Outpatient)					
Total Net Revenue	$7,171,721,867	$6,697,390,270	$6,346,757,006	$5,449,820,746	$5,275,631,849
Total Expenses	6,932,850,141	6,352,247,750	6,054,313,545	5,215,161,786	5,170,853,087
COMMUNITY HEALTH INDICATORS PER 1000 POPULATION					
Total Population (in thousands)	5,900	5,894	5,756	5,688	5,604
Inpatient					
Beds	1.9	1.9	1.9	1.9	1.9
Admissions	87.3	85.7	85.2	83.4	85.3
Inpatient Days	417.7	412.6	412.7	403.6	402.2
Inpatient Surgeries	27.3	27.7	28.5	25.4	28.1
Births	12.4	12.5	12.6	12.7	12.7
Outpatient					
Emergency Outpatient Visits	344.6	327.8	328.0	281.8	266.5
Other Outpatient Visits	1,230.7	1,299.1	1,402.3	1,251.5	1,113.1
Total Outpatient Visits	1,575.2	1,626.9	1,730.3	1,533.3	1,379.6
Outpatient Surgeries	52.2	44.3	43.1	42.1	40.3
Expense per Capita (per person)	$1,164.3	$1,083.2	$1,058.3	$921.3	$927.9

WEST VIRGINIA

U.S. Registered Community Hospitals
(Nonfederal, short-term general and other special hospitals)

Overview 1997–2001

	2001	2000	1999	1998	1997
Total Community Hospitals	**57**	**57**	**58**	**58**	**58**
Bed Size Category					
6-24	3	3	3	3	4
25-49	13	13	13	13	12
50-99	16	16	16	16	16
100-199	10	10	10	10	10
200-299	10	10	10	11	10
300-399	3	2	3	2	4
400-499	1	2	2	2	1
500 +	1	1	1	1	1
Location					
Hospitals Urban	18	18	18	18	18
Hospitals Rural	39	39	40	40	40
Control					
State and Local Government	10	10	10	10	10
Not for Profit	33	33	34	33	33
Investor owned	14	14	14	15	15
Physician Models					
Independent Practice Association	3	3	0	2	1
Group Practice without Walls	2	2	3	6	5
Open Physician-Hospital Organization	17	17	19	20	16
Closed Physician-Hospital Organization	1	3	1	1	2
Management Service Organization	4	7	10	13	11
Integrated Salary Model	20	17	14	11	12
Equity Model	1	1	1	1	1
Foundation	0	0	1	3	2
Insurance Products					
Health Maintenance Organization	4	8	7	8	12
Preferred Provider Organization	8	12	12	15	17
Indemnity Fee for Service	4	6	4	5	9
Managed Care Contracts					
Health Maintenance Organization	35	37	38	35	40
Preferred Provider Organization	45	47	46	42	41
Affiliations					
Hospitals in a System	29	30	28	24	22
Hospitals in a Network	28	28	26	21	18
Hospitals in a Group Purchasing Organization	52	48	45	42	—

TABLE 6

WEST VIRGINIA

U.S. Registered Community Hospitals
(Nonfederal, short-term general and other special hospitals)

Utilization, Personnel, Revenue and Expenses, Community Health Indicators 1997–2001

	2001	2000	1999	1998	1997
TOTAL FACILITY (Includes Hospital and Nursing Home Units)					
Utilization - Inpatient					
Beds	7,906	7,966	8,109	8,117	8,155
Admissions	297,079	288,095	289,427	280,729	277,257
Inpatient Days	1,806,411	1,772,580	1,792,038	1,778,264	1,745,689
Average Length of Stay	6.1	6.2	6.2	6.3	6.3
Inpatient Surgeries	82,783	81,969	100,693	77,859	81,717
Births	20,775	20,917	20,785	21,030	20,572
Utilization - Outpatient					
Emergency Outpatient Visits	1,057,155	1,007,028	1,002,071	1,020,060	994,710
Other Outpatient Visits	4,705,105	4,188,510	4,093,375	3,987,301	3,561,954
Total Outpatient Visits	5,762,260	5,195,538	5,095,446	5,007,361	4,556,664
Outpatient Surgeries	203,775	185,222	196,421	189,507	160,716
Personnel					
Full Time RNs	7,005	7,013	6,869	7,049	6,471
Full Time LPNs	1,656	1,639	1,599	1,603	1,625
Part Time RNs	3,019	2,435	2,426	2,327	2,597
Part Time LPNs	452	512	468	514	459
Total Full Time	29,730	29,191	29,397	29,089	28,378
Total Part Time	9,679	8,528	8,212	8,421	8,157
Revenue - Inpatient					
Gross Inpatient Revenue	$3,059,121,057	$2,738,379,228	$2,558,226,357	$2,414,070,698	$2,393,269,392
Revenue - Outpatient					
Gross Outpatient Revenue	$2,108,241,241	$1,896,927,001	$1,702,148,428	$1,624,810,990	$1,449,838,341
Revenue and Expenses - Totals (Includes Inpatient and Outpatient)					
Total Gross Revenue	$5,167,362,298	$4,635,306,229	$4,260,374,785	$4,038,881,688	$3,843,107,733
Deductions from Revenue	2,318,812,349	2,018,286,724	1,717,929,145	1,534,687,947	1,441,283,622
Net Patient Revenue	2,848,549,949	2,617,019,505	2,542,445,640	2,504,193,741	2,401,824,111
Other Operating Revenue	94,610,622	83,958,168	67,331,452	54,616,020	60,218,228
Other Nonoperating Revenue	42,442,849	62,118,544	73,508,215	72,933,826	58,170,701
Total Net Revenue	2,985,603,420	2,763,096,217	2,683,285,307	2,631,743,587	2,520,213,040
Total Expenses	2,867,459,406	2,672,667,972	2,569,940,576	2,476,492,231	2,345,608,928
HOSPITAL UNIT (Excludes Separate Nursing Home Units)					
Utilization - Inpatient					
Beds	6,835	6,904	7,063	7,022	7,227
Admissions	288,941	279,560	280,887	270,905	269,819
Inpatient Days	1,475,652	1,442,082	1,463,906	1,428,662	1,443,594
Average Length of Stay	5.1	5.2	5.2	5.3	5.4
Personnel					
Total Full Time	28,817	28,286	28,402	28,173	27,281
Total Part Time	9,398	8,251	7,907	8,130	7,750
Revenue and Expenses - Totals (Includes Inpatient and Outpatient)					
Total Net Revenue	$2,917,661,986	$2,707,349,521	$2,628,108,392	$2,562,192,400	$2,463,438,048
Total Expenses	2,818,658,157	2,625,906,089	2,521,864,295	2,419,075,794	2,306,234,702
COMMUNITY HEALTH INDICATORS PER 1000 POPULATION					
Total Population (in thousands)	1,802	1,808	1,807	1,812	1,816
Inpatient					
Beds	4.4	4.4	4.5	4.5	4.5
Admissions	164.9	159.3	160.2	155.0	152.7
Inpatient Days	1,002.5	980.2	991.8	981.6	961.5
Inpatient Surgeries	45.9	45.3	55.7	43.0	45.0
Births	11.5	11.6	11.5	11.6	11.3
Outpatient					
Emergency Outpatient Visits	586.7	556.9	554.6	563.0	547.9
Other Outpatient Visits	2,611.2	2,316.2	2,265.4	2,200.9	1,961.9
Total Outpatient Visits	3,197.9	2,873.1	2,819.9	2,763.9	2,509.7
Outpatient Surgeries	113.1	102.4	108.7	104.6	88.5
Expense per Capita (per person)	$1,591.3	$1,478.0	$1,422.3	$1,367.0	$1,291.9

TABLE 6

WISCONSIN

U.S. Registered Community Hospitals
(Nonfederal, short-term general and other special hospitals)

Overview 1997–2001

	2001	2000	1999	1998	1997
Total Community Hospitals	**121**	**118**	**123**	**123**	**124**
Bed Size Category					
6-24	5	5	6	6	6
25-49	30	27	26	24	25
50-99	29	26	29	30	29
100-199	35	40	40	39	42
200-299	15	13	15	15	12
300-399	2	2	2	4	5
400-499	3	3	3	2	2
500 +	2	2	2	3	3
Location					
Hospitals Urban	56	56	57	57	57
Hospitals Rural	65	62	66	66	67
Control					
State and Local Government	2	2	2	2	2
Not for Profit	118	115	120	120	121
Investor owned	1	1	1	1	1
Physician Models					
Independent Practice Association	12	16	14	15	21
Group Practice without Walls	10	8	11	6	7
Open Physician-Hospital Organization	12	17	14	14	17
Closed Physician-Hospital Organization	6	8	5	3	3
Management Service Organization	6	9	7	6	8
Integrated Salary Model	36	35	38	36	36
Equity Model	3	7	3	3	3
Foundation	2	6	2	1	1
Insurance Products					
Health Maintenance Organization	30	22	25	29	26
Preferred Provider Organization	20	27	35	31	28
Indemnity Fee for Service	5	7	10	10	10
Managed Care Contracts					
Health Maintenance Organization	106	93	112	111	110
Preferred Provider Organization	113	101	115	111	110
Affiliations					
Hospitals in a System	69	58	66	62	61
Hospitals in a Network	39	38	41	40	40
Hospitals in a Group Purchasing Organization	107	93	61	—	—

States

TABLE 6

WISCONSIN

U.S. Registered Community Hospitals
(Nonfederal, short-term general and other special hospitals)

Utilization, Personnel, Revenue and Expenses, Community Health Indicators 1997–2001

	2001	2000	1999	1998	1997
TOTAL FACILITY (Includes Hospital and Nursing Home Units)					
Utilization - Inpatient					
Beds	15,597	15,329	15,870	16,693	16,695
Admissions	579,089	558,357	553,337	553,810	551,436
Inpatient Days	3,455,633	3,331,095	3,394,502	3,442,860	3,471,636
Average Length of Stay	6.0	6.0	6.1	6.2	6.3
Inpatient Surgeries	184,704	181,028	179,457	180,783	188,936
Births	67,772	66,406	65,961	65,751	65,864
Utilization - Outpatient					
Emergency Outpatient Visits	1,866,201	1,785,771	1,723,490	1,608,391	1,604,779
Other Outpatient Visits	9,163,082	9,068,481	8,787,589	8,025,131	7,709,946
Total Outpatient Visits	11,029,283	10,854,252	10,511,079	9,633,522	9,314,725
Outpatient Surgeries	358,874	346,742	329,008	309,459	304,151
Personnel					
Full Time RNs	9,873	9,982	10,002	10,297	9,628
Full Time LPNs	751	689	712	919	821
Part Time RNs	13,772	13,399	12,989	13,169	13,479
Part Time LPNs	1,114	1,139	1,163	1,307	1,263
Total Full Time	51,379	49,099	50,249	49,216	47,043
Total Part Time	43,352	41,266	42,222	40,726	40,703
Revenue - Inpatient					
Gross Inpatient Revenue	$6,991,429,425	$6,098,946,220	$5,948,871,964	$5,786,700,159	$5,466,760,983
Revenue - Outpatient					
Gross Outpatient Revenue	$5,291,918,670	$4,468,653,347	$4,013,180,391	$3,539,897,672	$3,200,682,591
Revenue and Expenses - Totals (Includes Inpatient and Outpatient)					
Total Gross Revenue	$12,283,348,095	$10,567,599,567	$9,962,052,355	$9,326,597,831	$8,667,443,574
Deductions from Revenue	5,054,991,610	3,975,769,894	3,784,662,896	3,476,564,635	3,034,174,544
Net Patient Revenue	7,228,356,485	6,591,829,673	6,177,389,459	5,850,033,196	5,633,269,030
Other Operating Revenue	330,549,912	318,938,842	308,659,328	310,750,930	270,272,029
Other Nonoperating Revenue	132,446,055	153,176,880	139,860,357	166,270,056	146,801,901
Total Net Revenue	7,691,352,452	7,063,945,395	6,625,909,144	6,327,054,182	6,050,342,960
Total Expenses	7,182,972,349	6,662,561,165	6,232,856,297	5,899,798,976	5,608,593,105
HOSPITAL UNIT (Excludes Separate Nursing Home Units)					
Utilization - Inpatient					
Beds	13,124	13,069	13,455	14,210	14,147
Admissions	575,849	555,586	549,946	550,790	548,059
Inpatient Days	2,656,174	2,587,690	2,596,699	2,611,012	2,632,209
Average Length of Stay	4.6	4.7	4.7	4.7	4.8
Personnel					
Total Full Time	50,535	47,730	49,158	48,254	46,205
Total Part Time	42,513	40,098	41,046	39,547	39,557
Revenue and Expenses - Totals (Includes Inpatient and Outpatient)					
Total Net Revenue	$7,614,643,256	$7,003,452,628	$6,535,271,256	$6,247,192,029	$5,971,842,495
Total Expenses	7,116,127,111	6,570,298,128	6,157,416,203	5,833,422,569	5,550,117,960
COMMUNITY HEALTH INDICATORS PER 1000 POPULATION					
Total Population (in thousands)	5,402	5,364	5,250	5,222	5,200
Inpatient					
Beds	2.9	2.9	3.0	3.2	3.2
Admissions	107.2	104.1	105.4	106.1	106.0
Inpatient Days	639.7	621.0	646.5	659.3	667.6
Inpatient Surgeries	34.2	33.8	34.2	34.6	36.3
Births	12.5	12.4	12.6	12.6	12.7
Outpatient					
Emergency Outpatient Visits	345.5	332.9	328.3	308.0	308.6
Other Outpatient Visits	1,696.3	1,690.7	1,673.7	1,536.8	1,482.6
Total Outpatient Visits	2,041.7	2,023.7	2,001.9	1,844.8	1,791.2
Outpatient Surgeries	66.4	64.6	62.7	59.3	58.5
Expense per Capita (per person)	$1,329.7	$1,242.2	$1,187.1	$1,129.8	$1,078.5

Table 6

WYOMING

U.S. Registered Community Hospitals
(Nonfederal, short-term general and other special hospitals)

Overview 1997–2001

	2001	2000	1999	1998	1997
Total Community Hospitals	**24**	**24**	**23**	**25**	**25**
Bed Size Category					
6-24	0	0	0	1	1
25-49	9	9	9	9	9
50-99	10	9	8	8	8
100-199	4	4	5	7	7
200-299	1	2	1	0	0
300-399	0	0	0	0	0
400-499	0	0	0	0	0
500 +	0	0	0	0	0
Location					
Hospitals Urban	2	2	2	2	2
Hospitals Rural	22	22	21	23	23
Control					
State and Local Government	16	16	15	17	16
Not for Profit	5	5	5	6	7
Investor owned	3	3	3	2	2
Physician Models					
Independent Practice Association	2	2	3	3	2
Group Practice without Walls	0	0	0	0	1
Open Physician-Hospital Organization	1	1	2	3	2
Closed Physician-Hospital Organization	1	1	1	1	1
Management Service Organization	1	1	1	2	2
Integrated Salary Model	5	4	3	3	4
Equity Model	0	0	0	0	0
Foundation	0	1	0	0	1
Insurance Products					
Health Maintenance Organization	0	1	1	3	3
Preferred Provider Organization	3	4	4	5	2
Indemnity Fee for Service	1	1	0	0	0
Managed Care Contracts					
Health Maintenance Organization	3	2	3	3	4
Preferred Provider Organization	10	10	10	8	8
Affiliations					
Hospitals in a System	6	5	6	7	6
Hospitals in a Network	2	2	0	1	2
Hospitals in a Group Purchasing Organization	22	20	17	17	—

TABLE 6

WYOMING

U.S. Registered Community Hospitals
(Nonfederal, short-term general and other special hospitals)

Utilization, Personnel, Revenue and Expenses, Community Health Indicators 1997–2001

	2001	2000	1999	1998	1997
TOTAL FACILITY (Includes Hospital and Nursing Home Units)					
Utilization - Inpatient					
Beds	1,920	1,920	1,830	1,935	1,966
Admissions	47,587	47,852	45,212	43,833	44,170
Inpatient Days	379,674	392,856	350,011	380,351	376,111
Average Length of Stay	8.0	8.2	7.7	8.7	8.5
Inpatient Surgeries	13,020	13,277	13,788	13,237	12,476
Births	5,779	5,668	5,376	5,396	5,712
Utilization - Outpatient					
Emergency Outpatient Visits	196,723	198,691	184,370	173,155	165,863
Other Outpatient Visits	621,299	679,917	681,309	676,373	663,842
Total Outpatient Visits	818,022	878,608	865,679	849,528	829,705
Outpatient Surgeries	27,168	26,600	24,333	23,230	23,379
Personnel					
Full Time RNs	1,385	1,250	1,346	1,255	1,257
Full Time LPNs	251	254	237	157	161
Part Time RNs	440	461	339	588	490
Part Time LPNs	86	78	56	53	48
Total Full Time	6,265	5,693	5,719	5,651	5,642
Total Part Time	1,905	2,075	1,532	2,085	1,639
Revenue - Inpatient					
Gross Inpatient Revenue	$490,186,370	$459,146,586	$391,557,628	$373,737,424	$359,469,662
Revenue - Outpatient					
Gross Outpatient Revenue	$370,431,371	$341,692,739	$286,160,208	$265,896,402	$254,926,423
Revenue and Expenses - Totals (Includes Inpatient and Outpatient)					
Total Gross Revenue	$860,617,741	$800,839,325	$677,717,836	$639,633,826	$614,396,085
Deductions from Revenue	307,942,802	270,948,291	213,650,230	197,412,034	189,684,330
Net Patient Revenue	552,674,939	529,891,034	464,067,606	442,221,792	424,711,755
Other Operating Revenue	26,930,485	26,084,236	23,737,455	23,324,074	22,413,356
Other Nonoperating Revenue	16,580,965	17,942,529	12,176,866	16,335,608	11,979,842
Total Net Revenue	596,186,389	573,917,799	499,981,927	481,881,474	459,104,953
Total Expenses	558,590,503	514,916,805	445,760,593	430,470,596	409,252,037
HOSPITAL UNIT (Excludes Separate Nursing Home Units)					
Utilization - Inpatient					
Beds	1,298	1,296	1,275	1,306	1,404
Admissions	46,489	46,687	44,283	43,021	43,570
Inpatient Days	183,768	194,293	175,560	186,006	208,391
Average Length of Stay	4.0	4.2	4.0	4.3	4.8
Personnel					
Total Full Time	5,740	5,248	5,351	5,233	5,300
Total Part Time	1,743	1,937	1,440	1,948	1,504
Revenue and Expenses - Totals (Includes Inpatient and Outpatient)					
Total Net Revenue	$568,830,781	$548,439,718	$480,479,888	$461,481,640	$443,021,288
Total Expenses	533,736,510	494,194,490	427,158,396	410,789,054	394,200,425
COMMUNITY HEALTH INDICATORS PER 1000 POPULATION					
Total Population (in thousands)	494	494	480	480	480
Inpatient					
Beds	3.9	3.9	3.8	4.0	4.1
Admissions	96.2	96.9	94.3	91.3	92.0
Inpatient Days	767.9	795.6	729.8	792.3	783.5
Inpatient Surgeries	26.3	26.9	28.7	27.6	26.0
Births	11.7	11.5	11.2	11.2	11.9
Outpatient					
Emergency Outpatient Visits	397.9	402.4	384.4	360.7	345.5
Other Outpatient Visits	1,256.6	1,377.0	1,420.6	1,409.0	1,382.9
Total Outpatient Visits	1,654.5	1,779.3	1,805.0	1,769.7	1,728.4
Outpatient Surgeries	54.9	53.9	50.7	48.4	48.7
Expense per Capita (per person)	$1,129.8	$1,042.8	$929.4	$896.7	$852.6

Table 7

The facilities and services presented in Table 7 are listed below in alphabetical order by major heading (where applicable).

Table

7

2001 Facilities and Services in the U.S. Census Divisions and States

These data include only hospital-based facilities and services as reported by responding hospitals in Section C of the 2001 AHA Annual Survey, beginning on page 197. All hospitals are represented with Community Hospitals listed separately under United States. No estimates have been made for nonresponding hospitals. Definitions of facilities and services are listed in the Glossary, page 187.

CLASSIFICATION	HOSPITALS REPORTING	GENERAL MEDICAL SURGICAL CARE				OBSTETRICS INPATIENT CARE		NEONATAL INTERMEDIATE CARE		INTENSIVE CARE									
		ADULT UNITS		PEDIATRIC UNITS		UNITS		UNITS		NEONATAL UNITS		PEDIATRIC UNITS		CARDIAC UNITS		MEDICAL SURGICAL UNITS		OTHER UNITS	
		Number	Percent	Number	Percent	Number	Percent	Number	Percent	Number	Percent	Number	Percent	Number	Percent	Number	Percent	Number	Percent
UNITED STATES	4,728	4,149	87.8	2,209	46.7	2,938	62.1	610	12.9	825	17.4	413	8.7	1,543	32.6	3,120	66.0	392	8.3
COMMUNITY HOSPITALS	4,150	3,952	95.2	2,162	52.1	2,900	69.9	604	14.6	815	19.6	408	9.8	1,498	36.1	2,993	72.1	375	9.0
CENSUS DIVISION 1, NEW ENGLAND	218	178	81.7	118	54.1	143	65.6	23	10.6	31	14.2	14	6.4	67	30.7	161	73.9	11	5.0
Connecticut	35	29	82.9	23	65.7	27	77.1	4	11.4	13	37.1	2	5.7	17	48.6	28	80.0	3	8.6
Maine	38	34	89.5	13	34.2	29	76.3	1	2.6	2	5.3	2	5.3	7	18.4	31	81.6	1	2.6
Massachusetts	82	61	74.4	48	58.5	42	51.2	14	17.1	10	12.2	6	7.3	24	29.3	54	65.9	3	3.7
New Hampshire	30	26	86.7	17	56.7	25	83.3	1	3.3	4	13.3	2	6.7	7	23.3	24	80.0	1	3.3
Rhode Island	16	13	81.3	7	43.8	7	43.8	2	12.5	1	6.3	1	6.3	5	31.3	10	62.5	3	18.8
Vermont	17	15	88.2	10	58.8	13	76.5	1	5.9	1	5.9	1	5.9	7	41.2	14	82.4	0	0.0
CENSUS DIVISION 2, MIDDLE ATLANTIC	438	382	87.2	248	56.6	287	65.5	89	20.3	98	22.4	42	9.6	201	45.9	348	79.5	43	9.8
New Jersey	76	66	86.8	49	64.5	50	65.8	34	44.7	19	25.0	9	11.8	40	52.6	64	84.2	10	13.2
New York	177	155	87.6	110	62.1	115	65.0	29	16.4	38	21.5	25	14.1	89	50.3	140	79.1	16	9.0
Pennsylvania	185	161	87.0	89	48.1	122	65.9	26	14.1	41	22.2	8	4.3	72	38.9	144	77.8	17	9.2
CENSUS DIVISION 3, SOUTH ATLANTIC	721	621	86.1	344	47.7	421	58.4	116	16.1	149	20.7	69	9.6	275	38.1	520	72.1	71	9.8
Delaware	7	6	85.7	4	57.1	5	71.4	1	14.3	4	57.1	2	28.6	3	42.9	6	85.7	3	42.9
District of Columbia	12	9	75.0	5	41.7	7	58.3	3	25.0	7	58.3	3	25.0	7	58.3	9	75.0	1	8.3
Florida	174	151	86.8	71	40.8	88	50.6	21	12.1	45	25.9	22	12.6	83	47.7	137	78.7	18	10.3
Georgia	147	128	87.1	70	47.6	87	59.2	29	19.7	29	19.7	8	5.4	39	26.5	97	66.0	6	4.1
Maryland	65	49	75.4	35	53.8	35	53.8	7	10.8	15	23.1	4	6.2	28	43.1	47	72.3	5	7.7
North Carolina	102	96	94.1	48	47.1	72	70.6	21	20.6	18	17.6	10	9.8	35	34.3	78	76.5	17	16.7
South Carolina	72	61	84.7	48	66.7	44	61.1	18	25.0	9	12.5	9	12.5	36	50.0	50	69.4	9	12.5
Virginia	78	66	84.6	36	46.2	50	64.1	10	12.8	17	21.8	7	9.0	25	32.1	59	75.6	8	10.3
West Virginia	64	55	85.9	27	42.2	33	51.6	6	9.4	5	7.8	4	6.3	19	29.7	37	57.8	4	6.3
CENSUS DIVISION 4, EAST NORTH CENTRAL	687	629	91.6	425	61.9	502	73.1	75	10.9	113	16.4	88	12.8	282	41.0	522	76.0	114	16.6
Illinois	174	161	92.5	111	63.8	126	72.4	32	18.4	28	16.1	20	11.5	50	28.7	139	79.9	5	2.9
Indiana	90	81	90.0	53	58.9	72	80.0	13	14.4	16	17.8	7	7.8	31	34.4	71	78.9	7	7.8
Michigan	146	132	90.4	81	55.5	94	64.4	7	4.8	23	15.8	13	8.9	57	39.0	97	66.4	10	6.8
Ohio	148	140	94.6	74	50.0	110	74.3	23	15.5	25	16.9	8	5.4	59	39.9	126	85.1	13	8.8
Wisconsin	129	115	89.1	106	82.2	100	77.5	0	0.0	21	16.3	40	31.0	85	65.9	89	69.0	79	61.2
CENSUS DIVISION 5, EAST SOUTH CENTRAL	399	351	88.0	193	48.4	217	54.4	62	15.5	61	15.3	41	10.3	141	35.3	247	61.9	36	9.0
Alabama	74	67	90.5	33	44.6	42	56.8	7	9.5	12	16.2	9	12.2	26	35.1	51	68.9	7	9.5
Kentucky	99	87	87.9	38	38.4	51	51.5	15	15.2	14	14.1	4	4.0	33	33.3	67	67.7	7	7.1
Mississippi	97	90	92.8	80	82.5	52	53.6	29	29.9	18	18.6	19	19.6	50	51.5	51	52.6	8	8.2
Tennessee	129	107	82.9	42	32.6	72	55.8	11	8.5	17	13.2	9	7.0	32	24.8	78	60.5	14	10.9
CENSUS DIVISION 6, WEST NORTH CENTRAL	686	636	92.7	288	42.0	422	61.5	58	8.5	72	10.5	36	5.2	164	23.9	373	54.4	26	3.8
Iowa	123	118	95.9	53	43.1	89	72.4	8	6.5	15	12.2	7	5.7	26	21.1	77	62.6	3	2.4
Kansas	144	132	91.7	41	28.5	68	47.2	6	4.2	10	6.9	5	3.5	16	11.1	56	38.9	2	1.4
Minnesota	120	112	93.3	60	50.0	93	77.5	12	10.0	9	7.5	8	6.7	39	32.5	63	52.5	8	6.7
Missouri	139	121	87.1	66	47.5	78	56.1	17	12.2	19	13.7	8	5.8	36	25.9	95	68.3	10	7.2
Nebraska	70	66	94.3	28	40.0	46	65.7	7	10.0	9	12.9	2	2.9	18	25.7	37	52.9	2	2.9
North Dakota	33	32	97.0	19	57.6	19	57.6	5	15.2	7	21.2	3	9.1	16	48.5	20	60.6	0	0.0
South Dakota	57	55	96.5	21	36.8	29	50.9	3	5.3	3	5.3	3	5.3	13	22.8	25	43.9	1	1.8
CENSUS DIVISION 7, WEST SOUTH CENTRAL	762	609	79.9	237	31.1	393	51.6	91	11.9	115	15.1	49	6.4	154	20.2	408	53.5	43	5.6
Arkansas	95	78	82.1	28	29.5	51	53.7	13	13.7	11	11.6	1	1.1	33	34.7	50	52.6	6	6.3
Louisiana	107	93	86.9	45	42.1	48	44.9	11	10.3	27	25.2	13	12.1	22	20.6	67	62.6	6	5.6
Oklahoma	93	83	89.2	32	34.4	49	52.7	7	7.5	5	5.4	4	4.3	23	24.7	42	45.2	3	3.2
Texas	467	355	76.0	132	28.3	245	52.5	60	12.8	72	15.4	31	6.6	76	16.3	249	53.3	28	6.0
CENSUS DIVISION 8, MOUNTAIN	337	298	88.4	149	44.2	214	63.5	44	13.1	44	13.1	22	6.5	77	22.8	194	57.6	15	4.5
Arizona	54	45	83.3	21	38.9	30	55.6	7	13.0	5	9.3	4	7.4	15	27.8	34	63.0	3	5.6
Colorado	64	57	89.1	31	48.4	43	67.2	13	20.3	12	18.8	3	4.7	10	15.6	40	62.5	5	7.8
Idaho	34	30	88.2	13	38.2	22	64.7	3	8.8	4	11.8	3	8.8	8	23.5	19	55.9	3	8.8
Montana	54	52	96.3	20	37.0	30	55.6	3	5.6	5	9.3	3	5.6	17	31.5	26	48.1	2	3.7
Nevada	28	24	85.7	13	46.4	15	53.6	3	10.7	6	21.4	3	10.7	7	25.0	18	64.3	0	0.0
New Mexico	38	29	76.3	18	47.4	23	60.5	5	13.2	2	5.3	2	5.3	3	7.9	18	47.4	1	2.6
Utah	37	34	91.9	23	62.2	31	83.8	7	18.9	10	27.0	3	8.1	10	27.0	21	56.8	1	2.7
Wyoming	28	27	96.4	10	35.7	20	71.4	3	10.7	0	0.0	1	3.6	7	25.0	18	64.3	0	0.0
CENSUS DIVISION 9, PACIFIC	480	445	92.7	207	43.1	339	70.6	52	10.8	142	29.6	52	10.8	182	37.9	347	72.3	33	6.9
Alaska	13	13	100.0	8	61.5	13	100.0	2	15.4	3	23.1	2	15.4	4	30.8	6	46.2	0	0.0
California	305	282	92.5	136	44.6	201	65.9	28	9.2	115	37.7	39	12.8	127	41.6	225	73.8	19	6.2
Hawaii	22	18	81.8	5	22.7	11	50.0	1	4.5	2	9.1	1	4.5	8	36.4	12	54.5	1	4.5
Oregon	61	61	100.0	24	39.3	55	90.2	5	8.2	6	9.8	2	3.3	17	27.9	50	82.0	7	11.5
Washington	79	71	89.9	34	43.0	59	74.7	16	20.3	16	20.3	8	10.1	26	32.9	54	68.4	6	7.6

Table 7 (Continued)

These data include only hospital-based facilities and services as reported by responding hospitals in Section C of the 2001 AHA Annual Survey, beginning on page 197. All hospitals are represented with Community Hospitals listed separately under United States. No estimates have been made for nonresponding hospitals. Definitions of facilities and services are listed in the Glossary, page 187.

CLASSIFICATION	HOSPITALS REPORTING	BURN CARE UNITS		LONG-TERM CARE: ACUTE LONG-TERM CARE UNITS		LONG-TERM CARE: SKILLED NURSING CARE UNITS		LONG-TERM CARE: INTERMEDIATE CARE UNITS		LONG-TERM CARE: OTHER LONG-TERM CARE UNITS		PSYCHIATRIC INPATIENT CARE UNITS		ALCOHOL/DRUG ABUSE OR DEPENDENCY INPATIENT CARE UNITS		OTHER SPECIAL CARE UNITS		PHYSICAL REHABILITATION INPATIENT CARE UNITS	
		Number	Percent	Number	Percent	Number	Percent	Number	Percent	Number	Percent	Number	Percent	Number	Percent	Number	Percent	Number	Percent
UNITED STATES	4,728	147	3.1	203	4.3	1,722	36.4	450	9.5	653	13.8	1,778	37.6	564	11.9	664	14.0	1,266	26.8
COMMUNITY HOSPITALS	4,150	144	3.5	127	3.1	1,620	39.0	379	9.1	565	13.6	1,410	34.0	423	10.2	631	15.2	1,195	28.8
CENSUS DIVISION 1, NEW ENGLAND	218	5	2.3	4	1.8	62	28.4	25	11.5	31	14.2	117	53.7	26	11.9	17	7.8	53	24.3
Connecticut	35	1	2.9	1	2.9	3	8.6	4	11.4	6	17.1	28	80.0	8	22.9	4	11.4	11	31.4
Maine	38	0	0.0	0	0.0	13	34.2	7	18.4	4	10.5	12	31.6	6	15.8	1	2.6	6	15.8
Massachusetts	82	3	3.7	3	3.7	28	34.1	2	2.4	12	14.6	44	53.7	9	11.0	9	11.0	15	18.3
New Hampshire	30	0	0.0	0	0.0	9	30.0	8	26.7	6	20.0	15	50.0	1	3.3	1	3.3	7	23.3
Rhode Island	16	0	0.0	0	0.0	3	18.8	1	6.3	1	6.3	10	62.5	1	6.3	2	12.5	7	43.8
Vermont	17	1	5.9	0	0.0	6	35.3	3	17.6	2	11.8	8	47.1	1	5.9	0	0.0	7	41.2
CENSUS DIVISION 2, MIDDLE ATLANTIC	438	15	3.4	7	1.6	151	34.5	21	4.8	69	15.8	247	56.4	79	18.0	58	13.2	131	29.9
New Jersey	76	2	2.6	1	1.3	15	19.7	8	10.5	8	10.5	45	59.2	11	14.5	7	9.2	11	14.5
New York	177	7	4.0	2	1.1	55	31.1	2	1.1	38	21.5	99	55.9	45	25.4	25	14.1	52	29.4
Pennsylvania	185	6	3.2	4	2.2	81	43.8	11	5.9	23	12.4	103	55.7	23	12.4	26	14.1	68	36.8
CENSUS DIVISION 3, SOUTH ATLANTIC	721	17	2.4	32	4.4	236	32.7	78	10.8	137	19.0	281	39.0	90	12.5	131	18.2	186	25.8
Delaware	7	0	0.0	0	0.0	5	71.4	3	42.9	2	28.6	3	42.9	1	14.3	2	28.6	4	57.1
District of Columbia	12	1	8.3	0	0.0	4	33.3	3	25.0	5	41.7	10	83.3	1	8.3	3	25.0	4	33.3
Florida	174	5	2.9	7	4.0	48	27.6	18	10.3	24	13.8	66	37.9	22	12.6	35	20.1	40	23.0
Georgia	147	2	1.4	10	6.8	47	32.0	16	10.9	25	17.0	43	29.3	13	8.8	17	11.6	38	25.9
Maryland	65	1	1.5	0	0.0	21	32.3	3	4.6	14	21.5	42	64.6	8	12.3	16	24.6	14	21.5
North Carolina	102	3	2.9	2	2.0	42	41.2	17	16.7	20	19.6	46	45.1	14	13.7	19	18.6	23	22.5
South Carolina	72	1	1.4	12	16.7	13	18.1	0	0.0	26	36.1	21	29.2	11	15.3	21	29.2	35	48.6
Virginia	78	3	3.8	1	1.3	21	26.9	11	14.1	14	17.9	33	42.3	14	17.9	13	16.7	19	24.4
West Virginia	64	1	1.6	0	0.0	35	54.7	7	10.9	7	10.9	17	26.6	6	9.4	5	7.8	9	14.1
CENSUS DIVISION 4, EAST NORTH CENTRAL	687	38	5.5	21	3.1	261	38.0	72	10.5	89	13.0	308	44.8	128	18.6	175	25.5	249	36.2
Illinois	174	6	3.4	6	3.4	79	45.4	15	8.6	14	8.0	76	43.7	23	13.2	20	11.5	48	27.6
Indiana	90	3	3.3	1	1.1	44	48.9	12	13.3	15	16.7	35	38.9	16	17.8	12	13.3	23	25.6
Michigan	146	7	4.8	5	3.4	35	24.0	6	4.1	16	11.0	62	42.5	15	10.3	15	10.3	53	36.3
Ohio	148	7	4.7	2	1.4	65	43.9	11	7.4	28	18.9	82	55.4	25	16.9	21	14.2	58	39.2
Wisconsin	129	15	11.6	7	5.4	38	29.5	28	21.7	16	12.4	53	41.1	49	38.0	107	82.9	67	51.9
CENSUS DIVISION 5, EAST SOUTH CENTRAL	399	14	3.5	12	3.0	148	37.1	21	5.3	61	15.3	163	40.9	49	12.3	64	16.0	102	25.6
Alabama	74	3	4.1	5	6.8	11	14.9	3	4.1	9	12.2	26	35.1	8	10.8	9	12.2	14	18.9
Kentucky	99	3	3.0	2	2.0	49	49.5	5	5.1	14	14.1	38	38.4	7	7.1	15	15.2	16	16.2
Mississippi	97	5	5.2	0	0.0	42	43.3	0	0.0	21	21.6	55	56.7	19	19.6	21	21.6	43	44.3
Tennessee	129	3	2.3	5	3.9	46	35.7	13	10.1	17	13.2	44	34.1	15	11.6	19	14.7	29	22.5
CENSUS DIVISION 6, WEST NORTH CENTRAL	686	18	2.6	22	3.2	352	51.3	140	20.4	107	15.6	186	27.1	54	7.9	61	8.9	137	20.0
Iowa	123	4	3.3	2	1.6	54	43.9	38	30.9	21	17.1	36	29.3	11	8.9	11	8.9	16	13.0
Kansas	144	3	2.1	4	2.8	78	54.2	46	31.9	18	12.5	33	22.9	3	2.1	5	3.5	23	16.0
Minnesota	120	3	2.5	5	4.2	64	53.3	5	4.2	11	9.2	31	25.8	17	14.2	9	7.5	22	18.3
Missouri	139	5	3.6	4	2.9	71	51.1	18	12.9	25	18.0	61	43.9	15	10.8	27	19.4	50	36.0
Nebraska	70	2	2.9	3	4.3	40	57.1	15	21.4	10	14.3	11	15.7	4	5.7	3	4.3	9	12.9
North Dakota	33	0	0.0	0	0.0	15	45.5	4	12.1	5	15.2	7	21.2	3	9.1	1	3.0	8	24.2
South Dakota	57	1	1.8	4	7.0	30	52.6	14	24.6	17	29.8	7	12.3	1	1.8	5	8.8	9	15.8
CENSUS DIVISION 7, WEST SOUTH CENTRAL	762	13	1.7	65	8.5	180	23.6	19	2.5	67	8.8	232	30.4	66	8.7	82	10.8	208	27.3
Arkansas	95	1	1.1	3	3.2	23	24.2	2	2.1	15	15.8	38	40.0	4	4.2	4	4.2	32	33.7
Louisiana	107	5	4.7	13	12.1	41	38.3	7	6.5	16	15.0	57	53.3	12	11.2	15	14.0	31	29.0
Oklahoma	93	1	1.1	3	3.2	25	26.9	3	3.2	14	15.1	31	33.3	3	3.2	7	7.5	24	25.8
Texas	467	6	1.3	46	9.9	91	19.5	7	1.5	22	4.7	106	22.7	47	10.1	56	12.0	121	25.9
CENSUS DIVISION 8, MOUNTAIN	337	7	2.1	17	5.0	145	43.0	44	13.1	39	11.6	85	25.2	28	8.3	27	8.0	91	27.0
Arizona	54	1	1.9	2	3.7	12	22.2	5	9.3	4	7.4	14	25.9	4	7.4	2	3.7	19	35.2
Colorado	64	3	4.7	3	4.7	22	34.4	7	10.9	9	14.1	19	29.7	5	7.8	6	9.4	24	37.5
Idaho	34	0	0.0	1	2.9	21	61.8	3	8.8	3	8.8	7	20.6	2	5.9	1	2.9	6	17.6
Montana	54	0	0.0	5	9.3	42	77.8	6	11.1	9	16.7	9	16.7	3	5.6	1	1.9	6	11.1
Nevada	28	1	3.6	3	10.7	11	39.3	5	17.9	3	10.7	6	21.4	2	7.1	5	17.9	10	35.7
New Mexico	38	1	2.6	1	2.6	9	23.7	2	5.3	6	15.8	11	28.9	5	13.2	5	13.2	9	23.7
Utah	37	1	2.7	1	2.7	18	48.6	9	24.3	2	5.4	12	32.4	3	8.1	4	10.8	12	32.4
Wyoming	28	0	0.0	1	3.6	10	35.7	7	25.0	3	10.7	7	25.0	4	14.3	3	10.7	5	17.9
CENSUS DIVISION 9, PACIFIC	480	20	4.2	23	4.8	187	39.0	30	6.3	53	11.0	159	33.1	44	9.2	49	10.2	109	22.7
Alaska	13	1	7.7	0	0.0	6	46.2	3	23.1	0	0.0	5	38.5	2	15.4	1	7.7	2	15.4
California	305	15	4.9	18	5.9	137	44.9	7	2.3	27	8.9	105	34.4	24	7.9	29	9.5	75	24.6
Hawaii	22	1	4.5	0	0.0	11	50.0	7	31.8	10	45.5	7	31.8	1	4.5	2	9.1	1	4.5
Oregon	61	1	1.6	2	3.3	12	19.7	9	14.8	5	8.2	18	29.5	6	9.8	8	13.1	9	14.8
Washington	79	2	2.5	3	3.8	21	26.6	4	5.1	11	13.9	24	30.4	11	13.9	9	11.4	22	27.8

Table 7 (Continued)

These data include only hospital-based facilities and services as reported by responding hospitals in Section C of the 2001 AHA Annual Survey, beginning on page 197. All hospitals are represented with Community Hospitals listed separately under United States. No estimates have been made for nonresponding hospitals. Definitions of facilities and services are listed in the Glossary, page 187.

CLASSIFICATION	HOSPITALS REPORTING	ADULT DAY CARE PROGRAM		ALCOHOL/DRUG ABUSE OR DEPENDENCY OUTPATIENT SERVICES		AMBULANCE SERVICES		ANGIOPLASTY		ARTHRITIS TREATMENT CENTER		ASSISTED LIVING		AUXILIARY		BIRTHING/LDR/ LDRP ROOM		BREAST CANCER SCREENING	
		Number	Percent	Number	Percent	Number	Percent	Number	Percent	Number	Percent	Number	Percent	Number	Percent	Number	Percent	Number	Percent
UNITED STATES	4,728	435	9.2	918	19.4	806	17.0	1,150	24.3	292	6.2	269	5.7	2,858	60.4	2,871	60.7	3,444	72.8
COMMUNITY HOSPITALS	4,150	375	9.0	704	17.0	756	18.2	1,102	26.6	265	6.4	235	5.7	2,780	67.0	2,836	68.3	3,344	80.6
CENSUS DIVISION 1, NEW ENGLAND	218	31	14.2	71	32.6	27	12.4	38	17.4	16	7.3	12	5.5	125	57.3	139	63.8	167	76.6
Connecticut	35	4	11.4	18	51.4	2	5.7	8	22.9	2	5.7	2	5.7	22	62.9	27	77.1	29	82.9
Maine	38	1	2.6	13	34.2	8	21.1	5	13.2	0	0.0	1	2.6	20	52.6	29	76.3	32	84.2
Massachusetts	82	15	18.3	30	36.6	5	6.1	13	15.9	9	11.0	3	3.7	47	57.3	39	47.6	57	69.5
New Hampshire	30	6	20.0	2	6.7	7	23.3	7	23.3	1	3.3	2	6.7	16	53.3	25	83.3	25	83.3
Rhode Island	16	2	12.5	4	25.0	2	12.5	3	18.8	2	12.5	2	12.5	9	56.3	7	43.8	11	68.8
Vermont	17	3	17.6	4	23.5	3	17.6	2	11.8	2	11.8	2	11.8	11	64.7	12	70.6	13	76.5
CENSUS DIVISION 2, MIDDLE ATLANTIC	438	53	12.1	134	30.6	75	17.1	114	26.0	49	11.2	23	5.3	278	63.5	279	63.7	356	81.3
New Jersey	76	18	23.7	32	42.1	16	21.1	17	22.4	10	13.2	5	6.6	56	73.7	49	64.5	65	85.5
New York	177	25	14.1	65	36.7	30	16.9	42	23.7	18	10.2	5	2.8	97	54.8	109	61.6	141	79.7
Pennsylvania	185	10	5.4	37	20.0	29	15.7	55	29.7	21	11.4	13	7.0	125	67.6	121	65.4	150	81.1
CENSUS DIVISION 3, SOUTH ATLANTIC	721	43	6.0	142	19.7	99	13.7	180	25.0	53	7.4	34	4.7	438	60.7	406	56.3	547	75.9
Delaware	7	2	28.6	2	28.6	1	14.3	3	42.9	1	14.3	0	0.0	5	71.4	5	71.4	5	71.4
District of Columbia	12	0	0.0	6	50.0	3	25.0	7	58.3	5	41.7	1	8.3	4	33.3	6	50.0	8	66.7
Florida	174	11	6.3	26	14.9	17	9.8	57	32.8	13	7.5	5	2.9	98	56.3	83	47.7	133	76.4
Georgia	147	7	4.8	24	16.3	34	23.1	23	15.6	5	3.4	11	7.5	94	63.9	79	53.7	111	75.5
Maryland	65	6	9.2	21	32.3	6	9.2	20	30.8	7	10.8	2	3.1	45	69.2	35	53.8	47	72.3
North Carolina	102	7	6.9	17	16.7	21	20.6	24	23.5	10	9.8	2	2.0	63	61.8	72	70.6	81	79.4
South Carolina	72	3	4.2	15	20.8	0	0.0	15	20.8	3	4.2	6	8.3	36	50.0	43	59.7	52	72.2
Virginia	78	6	7.7	19	24.4	9	11.5	22	28.2	4	5.1	6	7.7	56	71.8	50	64.1	64	82.1
West Virginia	64	1	1.6	12	18.8	8	12.5	9	14.1	5	7.8	1	1.6	37	57.8	33	51.6	46	71.9
CENSUS DIVISION 4, EAST NORTH CENTRAL	687	74	10.8	181	26.3	149	21.7	201	29.3	70	10.2	49	7.1	479	69.7	494	71.9	593	86.3
Illinois	174	22	12.6	53	30.5	38	21.8	61	35.1	21	12.1	15	8.6	122	70.1	123	70.7	155	89.1
Indiana	90	8	8.9	29	32.2	33	36.7	25	27.8	6	6.7	8	8.9	54	60.0	72	80.0	79	87.8
Michigan	146	12	8.2	38	26.0	17	11.6	35	24.0	10	6.8	11	7.5	106	72.6	92	63.0	125	85.6
Ohio	148	14	9.5	43	29.1	18	12.2	53	35.8	15	10.1	5	3.4	105	70.9	108	73.0	131	88.5
Wisconsin	129	18	14.0	18	14.0	43	33.3	27	20.9	18	14.0	10	7.8	92	71.3	99	76.7	103	79.8
CENSUS DIVISION 5, EAST SOUTH CENTRAL	399	16	4.0	53	13.3	71	17.8	73	18.3	13	3.3	13	3.3	185	46.4	205	51.4	287	71.9
Alabama	74	3	4.1	9	12.2	17	23.0	20	27.0	3	4.1	7	9.5	45	60.8	40	54.1	60	81.1
Kentucky	99	8	8.1	14	14.1	13	13.1	21	21.2	4	4.0	1	1.0	61	61.6	50	50.5	79	79.8
Mississippi	97	2	2.1	11	11.3	15	15.5	0	0.0	2	2.1	0	0.0	22	22.7	47	48.5	59	60.8
Tennessee	129	3	2.3	19	14.7	26	20.2	32	24.8	4	3.1	5	3.9	57	44.2	68	52.7	89	69.0
CENSUS DIVISION 6, WEST NORTH CENTRAL	686	92	13.4	119	17.3	151	22.0	118	17.2	27	3.9	83	12.1	479	69.8	436	63.6	488	71.1
Iowa	123	15	12.2	26	21.1	54	43.9	18	14.6	3	2.4	8	6.5	108	87.8	87	70.7	110	89.4
Kansas	144	18	12.5	10	6.9	25	17.4	15	10.4	0	0.0	13	9.0	80	55.6	81	56.3	79	54.9
Minnesota	120	27	22.5	33	27.5	37	30.8	17	14.2	3	2.5	21	17.5	85	70.8	93	77.5	90	75.0
Missouri	139	6	4.3	28	20.1	2	1.4	46	33.1	15	10.8	5	3.6	106	76.3	75	54.0	106	76.3
Nebraska	70	14	20.0	9	12.9	14	20.0	12	17.1	1	1.4	10	14.3	42	60.0	52	74.3	50	71.4
North Dakota	33	3	9.1	6	18.2	8	24.2	6	18.2	4	12.1	3	9.1	25	75.8	19	57.6	22	66.7
South Dakota	57	9	15.8	7	12.3	11	19.3	4	7.0	1	1.8	23	40.4	33	57.9	29	50.9	31	54.4
CENSUS DIVISION 7, WEST SOUTH CENTRAL	762	43	5.6	72	9.4	117	15.4	185	24.3	20	2.6	20	2.6	417	54.7	374	49.1	438	57.5
Arkansas	95	9	9.5	11	11.6	22	23.2	21	22.1	3	3.2	1	1.1	63	66.3	49	51.6	60	63.2
Louisiana	107	8	7.5	16	15.0	13	12.1	30	28.0	4	3.7	1	0.9	54	50.5	42	39.3	70	65.4
Oklahoma	93	18	19.4	3	3.2	8	8.6	18	19.4	2	2.2	5	5.4	56	60.2	47	50.5	51	54.8
Texas	467	8	1.7	42	9.0	74	15.8	116	24.8	11	2.4	13	2.8	244	52.2	236	50.5	257	55.0
CENSUS DIVISION 8, MOUNTAIN	337	42	12.5	58	17.2	61	18.1	85	25.2	19	5.6	22	6.5	192	57.0	214	63.5	223	66.2
Arizona	54	4	7.4	7	13.0	4	7.4	26	48.1	3	5.6	1	1.9	27	50.0	29	53.7	33	61.1
Colorado	64	6	9.4	12	18.8	18	28.1	18	28.1	5	7.8	4	6.3	39	60.9	43	67.2	49	76.6
Idaho	34	5	14.7	5	14.7	8	23.5	6	17.6	1	2.9	0	0.0	27	79.4	25	73.5	21	61.8
Montana	54	19	35.2	5	9.3	13	24.1	7	13.0	2	3.7	12	22.2	32	59.3	31	57.4	36	66.7
Nevada	28	2	7.1	5	17.9	2	7.1	10	35.7	2	7.1	0	0.0	13	46.4	16	57.1	15	53.6
New Mexico	38	2	5.3	8	21.1	4	10.5	4	10.5	3	7.9	2	5.3	19	50.0	19	50.0	20	52.6
Utah	37	3	8.1	7	18.9	3	8.1	11	29.7	3	8.1	1	2.7	18	48.6	31	83.8	27	73.0
Wyoming	28	1	3.6	9	32.1	9	32.1	3	10.7	0	0.0	2	7.1	17	60.7	20	71.4	22	78.6
CENSUS DIVISION 9, PACIFIC	480	41	8.5	88	18.3	56	11.7	156	32.5	25	5.2	13	2.7	265	55.2	324	67.5	345	71.9
Alaska	13	1	7.7	7	53.8	4	30.8	2	15.4	0	0.0	0	0.0	4	30.8	12	92.3	11	84.6
California	305	24	7.9	54	17.7	29	9.5	107	35.1	18	5.9	5	1.6	171	56.1	190	62.3	221	72.5
Hawaii	22	2	9.1	3	13.6	1	4.5	6	27.3	1	4.5	0	0.0	9	40.9	11	50.0	12	54.5
Oregon	61	6	9.8	9	14.8	10	16.4	17	27.9	3	4.9	3	4.9	43	70.5	55	90.2	49	80.3
Washington	79	8	10.1	15	19.0	12	15.2	24	30.4	3	3.8	5	6.3	38	48.1	56	70.9	52	65.8

Table 7 (Continued)

These data include only hospital-based facilities and services as reported by responding hospitals in Section C of the 2001 AHA Annual Survey, beginning on page 197. All hospitals are represented with Community Hospitals listed separately under United States. No estimates have been made for nonresponding hospitals. Definitions of facilities and services are listed in the Glossary, page 187.

CLASSIFICATION	HOSPITALS REPORTING	CARDIAC CATHETERIZATION LABORATORY		CASE MANAGEMENT		CHILDREN WELLNESS PROGRAM		CHIROPRACTIC SERVICES		COMMUNITY OUTREACH		COMPLEMENTARY MEDICINE SERVICES		CRISIS PREVENTION		CT SCANNER		DENTAL SERVICES		DIAGNOSTIC RADIOISOTOPE FACILITY		EMERGENCY DEPARTMENT	
		Number	Percent	Number	Percent	Number	Percent	Number	Percent	Number	Percent	Number	Percent	Number	Percent	Number	Percent	Number	Percent	Number	Percent	Number	Percent
UNITED STATES	4,728	1,665	35.2	3,376	71.4	870	18.4	88	1.9	2,959	62.6	746	15.8	904	19.1	3,779	79.9	1,129	23.9	2,692	56.9	4,045	85.6
COMMUNITY HOSPITALS	4,150	1,605	38.7	3,059	73.7	825	19.9	75	1.8	2,731	65.8	698	16.8	756	18.2	3,625	87.3	908	21.9	2,590	62.4	3,872	93.3
CENSUS DIVISION 1, NEW ENGLAND	218	66	30.3	173	79.4	66	30.3	7	3.2	173	79.4	57	26.1	59	27.1	169	77.5	63	28.9	139	63.8	172	78.9
Connecticut	35	16	45.7	32	91.4	14	40.0	1	2.9	33	94.3	8	22.9	17	48.6	27	77.1	18	51.4	28	80.0	28	80.0
Maine	38	6	15.8	27	71.1	8	21.1	0	0.0	28	73.7	6	15.8	3	7.9	32	84.2	5	13.2	23	60.5	34	89.5
Massachusetts	82	25	30.5	65	79.3	23	28.0	3	3.7	61	74.4	27	32.9	25	30.5	58	70.7	22	26.8	46	56.1	56	68.3
New Hampshire	30	12	40.0	25	83.3	12	40.0	2	6.7	26	86.7	9	30.0	8	26.7	27	90.0	11	36.7	18	60.0	27	90.0
Rhode Island	16	5	31.3	12	75.0	4	25.0	1	6.3	12	75.0	2	12.5	3	18.8	11	68.8	5	31.3	11	68.8	12	75.0
Vermont	17	2	11.8	12	70.6	5	29.4	0	0.0	13	76.5	5	29.4	3	17.6	14	82.4	2	11.8	13	76.5	15	88.2
CENSUS DIVISION 2, MIDDLE ATLANTIC	438	177	40.4	370	84.5	138	31.5	10	2.3	349	79.7	116	26.5	150	34.2	369	84.2	189	43.2	322	73.5	371	84.7
New Jersey	76	41	53.9	68	89.5	35	46.1	2	2.6	65	85.5	25	32.9	37	48.7	65	85.5	38	50.0	61	80.3	65	85.5
New York	177	50	28.2	148	83.6	51	28.8	3	1.7	140	79.1	44	24.9	70	39.5	148	83.6	79	44.6	122	68.9	147	83.1
Pennsylvania	185	86	46.5	154	83.2	52	28.1	5	2.7	144	77.8	47	25.4	43	23.2	156	84.3	72	38.9	139	75.1	159	85.9
CENSUS DIVISION 3, SOUTH ATLANTIC	721	318	44.1	558	77.4	132	18.3	11	1.5	491	68.1	114	15.8	139	19.3	594	82.4	176	24.4	465	64.5	603	83.6
Delaware	7	5	71.4	6	85.7	1	14.3	0	0.0	6	85.7	4	57.1	3	42.9	6	85.7	3	42.9	5	71.4	7	100.0
District of Columbia	12	10	83.3	12	100.0	3	25.0	2	16.7	11	91.7	5	41.7	7	58.3	10	83.3	6	50.0	9	75.0	10	83.3
Florida	174	100	57.5	149	85.6	26	14.9	1	0.6	111	63.8	24	13.8	23	13.2	144	82.8	29	16.7	116	66.7	147	84.5
Georgia	147	51	34.7	107	72.8	18	12.2	1	0.7	91	61.9	19	12.9	28	19.0	125	85.0	32	21.8	82	55.8	127	86.4
Maryland	65	35	53.8	51	78.5	13	20.0	2	3.1	48	73.8	17	26.2	27	41.5	47	72.3	17	26.2	43	66.2	47	72.3
North Carolina	102	39	38.2	84	82.4	16	15.7	3	2.9	69	67.6	19	18.6	16	15.7	93	91.2	38	37.3	70	68.6	90	88.2
South Carolina	72	25	34.7	38	52.8	24	33.3	0	0.0	61	84.7	3	4.2	7	9.7	55	76.4	14	19.4	45	62.5	56	77.8
Virginia	78	38	48.7	66	84.6	16	20.5	2	2.6	53	67.9	16	20.5	19	24.4	65	83.3	25	32.1	56	71.8	64	82.1
West Virginia	64	15	23.4	45	70.3	15	23.4	0	0.0	41	64.1	7	10.9	9	14.1	49	76.6	12	18.8	39	60.9	55	85.9
CENSUS DIVISION 4, EAST NORTH CENTRAL	687	283	41.2	522	76.0	144	21.0	16	2.3	474	69.0	175	25.5	180	26.2	614	89.4	182	26.5	479	69.7	625	91.0
Illinois	174	76	43.7	136	78.2	42	24.1	5	2.9	129	74.1	31	17.8	46	26.4	160	92.0	53	30.5	126	72.4	162	93.1
Indiana	90	38	42.2	71	78.9	21	23.3	2	2.2	70	77.8	21	23.3	23	25.6	81	90.0	33	36.7	66	73.3	80	88.9
Michigan	146	59	40.4	107	73.3	32	21.9	3	2.1	108	74.0	41	28.1	42	28.8	126	86.3	48	32.9	101	69.2	129	88.4
Ohio	148	75	50.7	120	81.1	33	22.3	5	3.4	118	79.7	51	34.5	38	25.7	141	95.3	38	25.7	117	79.1	139	93.9
Wisconsin	129	35	27.1	88	68.2	16	12.4	1	0.8	49	38.0	31	24.0	31	24.0	106	82.2	10	7.8	69	53.5	115	89.1
CENSUS DIVISION 5, EAST SOUTH CENTRAL	399	135	33.8	285	71.4	37	9.3	2	0.5	208	52.1	27	6.8	40	10.0	337	84.5	92	23.1	219	54.9	339	85.0
Alabama	74	30	40.5	60	81.1	5	6.8	0	0.0	44	59.5	3	4.1	6	8.1	67	90.5	8	10.8	48	64.9	68	91.9
Kentucky	99	40	40.4	75	75.8	17	17.2	1	1.0	51	51.5	13	13.1	9	9.1	87	87.9	25	25.3	53	53.5	85	85.9
Mississippi	97	25	25.8	54	55.7	4	4.1	1	1.0	58	59.8	4	4.1	7	7.2	76	78.4	36	37.1	51	52.6	81	83.5
Tennessee	129	40	31.0	96	74.4	11	8.5	0	0.0	55	42.6	7	5.4	18	14.0	107	82.9	23	17.8	67	51.9	105	81.4
CENSUS DIVISION 6, WEST NORTH CENTRAL	686	146	21.3	363	52.9	100	14.6	16	2.3	410	59.8	102	14.9	119	17.3	498	72.6	133	19.4	255	37.2	624	91.0
Iowa	123	22	17.9	80	65.0	27	22.0	3	2.4	83	67.5	23	18.7	22	17.9	103	83.7	30	24.4	47	38.2	118	95.9
Kansas	144	21	14.6	62	43.1	15	10.4	1	0.7	53	36.8	9	6.3	12	8.3	91	63.2	18	12.5	46	31.9	126	87.5
Minnesota	120	21	17.5	54	45.0	16	13.3	3	2.5	85	70.8	24	20.0	18	15.0	88	73.3	17	14.2	43	35.8	109	90.8
Missouri	139	56	40.3	100	71.9	20	14.4	5	3.6	89	64.0	28	20.1	48	34.5	115	82.7	48	34.5	75	54.0	120	86.3
Nebraska	70	13	18.6	29	41.4	8	11.4	0	0.0	46	65.7	6	8.6	10	14.3	47	67.1	11	15.7	20	28.6	65	92.9
North Dakota	33	6	18.2	14	42.4	7	21.2	3	9.1	24	72.7	8	24.2	6	18.2	22	66.7	2	6.1	11	33.3	32	97.0
South Dakota	57	7	12.3	24	42.1	7	12.3	1	1.8	30	52.6	4	7.0	3	5.3	32	56.1	7	12.3	13	22.8	54	94.7
CENSUS DIVISION 7, WEST SOUTH CENTRAL	762	241	31.6	533	69.9	92	12.1	6	0.8	352	46.2	50	6.6	73	9.6	552	72.4	140	18.4	363	47.6	616	80.8
Arkansas	95	32	33.7	66	69.5	6	6.3	1	1.1	54	56.8	10	10.5	9	9.5	77	81.1	16	16.8	50	52.6	79	83.2
Louisiana	107	39	36.4	81	75.7	21	19.6	2	1.9	45	42.1	8	7.5	11	10.3	86	80.4	20	18.7	56	52.3	87	81.3
Oklahoma	93	25	26.9	61	65.6	6	6.5	0	0.0	42	45.2	4	4.3	10	10.8	68	73.1	21	22.6	40	43.0	83	89.2
Texas	467	145	31.0	325	69.6	59	12.6	3	0.6	211	45.2	28	6.0	43	9.2	321	68.7	83	17.8	217	46.5	367	78.6
CENSUS DIVISION 8, MOUNTAIN	337	101	30.0	232	68.8	64	19.0	9	2.7	200	59.3	49	14.5	54	16.0	251	74.5	71	21.1	161	47.8	290	86.1
Arizona	54	29	53.7	48	88.9	17	31.5	0	0.0	34	63.0	11	20.4	8	14.8	40	74.1	14	25.9	28	51.9	45	83.3
Colorado	64	21	32.8	48	75.0	8	12.5	4	6.3	47	73.4	20	31.3	12	18.8	54	84.4	19	29.7	33	51.6	56	87.5
Idaho	34	6	17.6	20	58.8	8	23.5	2	5.9	22	64.7	1	2.9	3	8.8	28	82.4	7	20.6	13	38.2	31	91.2
Montana	54	9	16.7	24	44.4	12	22.2	1	1.9	30	55.6	6	11.1	5	9.3	31	57.4	5	9.3	23	42.6	51	94.4
Nevada	28	12	42.9	22	78.6	3	10.7	1	3.6	14	50.0	1	3.6	3	10.7	20	71.4	2	7.1	15	53.6	21	75.0
New Mexico	38	6	15.8	23	60.5	7	18.4	0	0.0	17	44.7	2	5.3	7	18.4	24	63.2	8	21.1	16	42.1	28	73.7
Utah	37	15	40.5	30	81.1	8	21.6	1	2.7	22	59.5	4	10.8	12	32.4	32	86.5	11	29.7	19	51.4	33	89.2
Wyoming	28	3	10.7	17	60.7	1	3.6	0	0.0	14	50.0	4	14.3	4	14.3	22	78.6	5	17.9	14	50.0	25	89.3
CENSUS DIVISION 9, PACIFIC	480	198	41.3	340	70.8	97	20.2	11	2.3	302	62.9	56	11.7	90	18.8	395	82.3	83	17.3	289	60.2	405	84.4
Alaska	13	2	15.4	9	69.2	4	30.8	0	0.0	7	53.8	2	15.4	5	38.5	8	61.5	4	30.8	4	30.8	12	92.3
California	305	141	46.2	239	78.4	66	21.6	9	3.0	198	64.9	32	10.5	60	19.7	253	83.0	59	19.3	189	62.0	247	81.0
Hawaii	22	7	31.8	13	59.1	3	13.6	0	0.0	8	36.4	2	9.1	3	13.6	13	59.1	4	18.2	13	59.1	17	77.3
Oregon	61	18	29.5	33	54.1	14	23.0	1	1.6	42	68.9	6	9.8	9	14.8	60	98.4	6	9.8	39	63.9	60	98.4
Washington	79	30	38.0	46	58.2	10	12.7	1	1.3	47	59.5	14	17.7	13	16.5	61	77.2	10	12.7	44	55.7	69	87.3

Table 7 (Continued)

These data include only hospital-based facilities and services as reported by responding hospitals in Section C of the 2001 AHA Annual Survey, beginning on page 197. All hospitals are represented with Community Hospitals listed separately under United States. No estimates have been made for nonresponding hospitals. Definitions of facilities and services are listed in the Glossary, page 187.

CLASSIFICATION	HOSPITALS REPORTING	ENABLING SERVICES		ENROLLMENT ASSISTANCE SERVICES		EXTRACORPOREAL SHOCK WAVE LITHOTRIPTER (ESWL)		FITNESS CENTER		GERIATRIC SERVICES		HEALTH FAIR		HEALTH INFORMATION CENTER		HEALTH SCREENINGS	
		Number	Percent	Number	Percent	Number	Percent	Number	Percent	Number	Percent	Number	Percent	Number	Percent	Number	Percent
UNITED STATES	4,728	720	15.2	1,269	26.8	900	19.0	1,244	26.3	2,006	42.4	3,328	70.4	2,078	44.0	3,352	70.9
COMMUNITY HOSPITALS	4,150	658	15.9	1,155	27.8	876	21.1	1,146	27.6	1,806	43.5	3,127	75.3	1,922	46.3	3,140	75.7
CENSUS DIVISION 1, NEW ENGLAND	218	50	22.9	83	38.1	72	33.0	49	22.5	121	55.5	163	74.8	131	60.1	183	83.9
Connecticut	35	8	22.9	13	37.1	18	51.4	12	34.3	25	71.4	26	74.3	25	71.4	28	80.0
Maine	38	3	7.9	10	26.3	10	26.3	9	23.7	16	42.1	25	65.8	15	39.5	31	81.6
Massachusetts	82	23	28.0	34	41.5	20	24.4	8	9.8	43	52.4	59	72.0	46	56.1	68	82.9
New Hampshire	30	9	30.0	17	56.7	12	40.0	13	43.3	16	53.3	27	90.0	21	70.0	27	90.0
Rhode Island	16	3	18.8	4	25.0	9	56.3	3	18.8	12	75.0	13	81.3	12	75.0	14	87.5
Vermont	17	4	23.5	5	29.4	3	17.6	4	23.5	9	52.9	13	76.5	12	70.6	15	88.2
CENSUS DIVISION 2, MIDDLE ATLANTIC	438	107	24.4	190	43.4	96	21.9	112	25.6	257	58.7	344	78.5	251	57.3	367	83.8
New Jersey	76	25	32.9	40	52.6	8	10.5	22	28.9	53	69.7	65	85.5	50	65.8	69	90.8
New York	177	35	19.8	75	42.4	39	22.0	35	19.8	102	57.6	135	76.3	101	57.1	142	80.2
Pennsylvania	185	47	25.4	75	40.5	49	26.5	55	29.7	102	55.1	144	77.8	100	54.1	156	84.3
CENSUS DIVISION 3, SOUTH ATLANTIC	721	128	17.8	206	28.6	189	26.2	200	27.7	290	40.2	557	77.3	334	46.3	556	77.1
Delaware	7	2	28.6	4	57.1	2	28.6	3	42.9	3	42.9	6	85.7	3	42.9	4	57.1
District of Columbia	12	5	41.7	6	50.0	2	16.7	4	33.3	8	66.7	11	91.7	8	66.7	11	91.7
Florida	174	31	17.8	47	27.0	51	29.3	56	32.2	83	47.7	126	72.4	81	46.6	130	74.7
Georgia	147	32	21.8	42	28.6	42	28.6	33	22.4	38	25.9	109	74.1	55	37.4	107	72.8
Maryland	65	15	23.1	25	38.5	15	23.1	15	23.1	30	46.2	50	76.9	45	69.2	49	75.4
North Carolina	102	22	21.6	35	34.3	21	20.6	28	27.5	39	38.2	79	77.5	49	48.0	83	81.4
South Carolina	72	0	0.0	0	0.0	14	19.4	23	31.9	33	45.8	62	86.1	23	31.9	56	77.8
Virginia	78	13	16.7	29	37.2	25	32.1	19	24.4	33	42.3	62	79.5	42	53.8	65	83.3
West Virginia	64	8	12.5	18	28.1	17	26.6	19	29.7	23	35.9	52	81.3	28	43.8	51	79.7
CENSUS DIVISION 4, EAST NORTH CENTRAL	687	56	22.7	224	32.6	128	18.6	237	34.5	396	57.6	503	73.2	415	60.4	542	78.9
Illinois	174	43	24.7	57	32.8	27	15.5	49	28.2	91	52.3	140	80.5	100	57.5	150	86.2
Indiana	90	13	14.4	29	32.2	30	33.3	31	34.4	35	38.9	78	86.7	57	63.3	81	90.0
Michigan	146	38	26.0	59	40.4	20	13.7	51	34.9	76	52.1	109	74.7	84	57.5	125	85.6
Ohio	148	45	30.4	60	40.5	28	18.9	56	37.8	83	56.1	127	85.8	88	59.5	135	91.2
Wisconsin	129	17	13.2	19	14.7	23	17.8	50	38.8	111	86.0	49	38.0	86	66.7	51	39.5
CENSUS DIVISION 5, EAST SOUTH CENTRAL	399	39	9.8	75	18.8	75	18.8	85	21.3	127	31.8	246	61.7	105	26.3	198	49.6
Alabama	74	7	9.5	18	24.3	10	13.5	17	23.0	23	31.1	55	74.3	26	35.1	49	66.2
Kentucky	99	16	16.2	25	25.3	17	17.2	18	18.2	37	37.4	73	73.7	39	39.4	66	66.7
Mississippi	97	5	5.2	9	9.3	16	16.5	25	25.8	26	26.8	32	33.0	10	10.3	0	0.0
Tennessee	129	11	8.5	23	17.8	32	24.8	25	19.4	41	31.8	86	66.7	30	23.3	83	64.3
CENSUS DIVISION 6, WEST NORTH CENTRAL	386	54	9.3	105	15.3	75	10.9	226	32.9	259	37.8	464	67.6	264	38.5	500	72.9
Iowa	123	20	16.3	34	27.6	13	10.6	47	38.2	50	40.7	89	72.4	65	52.8	113	91.9
Kansas	144	16	11.1	23	16.0	16	11.1	41	28.5	51	35.4	86	59.7	31	21.5	71	49.3
Minnesota	120	9	7.5	22	18.3	12	10.0	31	25.8	46	38.3	69	57.5	39	32.5	78	65.0
Missouri	139	1	0.7	2	1.4	22	15.8	50	36.0	62	44.6	110	79.1	79	56.8	116	83.5
Nebraska	70	10	14.3	10	14.3	7	10.0	25	35.7	14	20.0	51	72.9	20	28.6	47	67.1
North Dakota	33	4	12.1	6	18.2	3	9.1	14	42.4	18	54.5	23	69.7	15	45.5	28	84.8
South Dakota	57	4	7.0	8	14.0	2	3.5	18	31.6	18	31.6	36	63.2	15	26.3	47	82.5
CENSUS DIVISION 7, WEST SOUTH CENTRAL	762	74	9.7	179	23.5	129	16.9	164	21.5	260	34.1	497	65.2	240	31.5	478	62.7
Arkansas	95	3	3.2	17	17.9	16	16.8	19	20.0	35	36.8	74	77.9	25	26.3	69	72.6
Louisiana	107	0	9.3	35	32.7	14	13.1	27	25.2	34	31.8	67	62.6	39	36.4	71	66.4
Oklahoma	93	6	6.5	10	10.8	14	15.1	13	14.0	30	32.3	58	62.4	27	29.0	57	61.3
Texas	467	55	11.8	117	25.1	85	18.2	105	22.5	161	34.5	298	63.8	149	31.9	281	60.2
CENSUS DIVISION 8, MOUNTAIN	337	39	11.6	78	23.1	48	14.2	83	24.6	127	37.7	243	72.1	130	38.6	217	64.4
Arizona	54	8	14.8	16	29.6	8	14.8	17	31.5	23	42.6	36	66.7	26	48.1	32	59.3
Colorado	64	10	15.6	22	34.4	9	14.1	26	40.6	26	40.6	44	68.8	29	45.3	44	68.8
Idaho	34	5	14.7	9	26.5	8	23.5	4	11.8	8	23.5	27	79.4	13	38.2	23	67.6
Montana	54	2	3.7	10	18.5	6	11.1	11	20.4	28	51.9	42	77.8	15	27.8	41	75.9
Nevada	28	2	7.1	5	17.9	2	7.1	2	7.1	8	28.6	20	71.4	10	35.7	13	46.4
New Mexico	38	3	7.9	7	18.4	7	18.4	5	13.2	7	18.4	20	52.6	9	23.7	19	50.0
Utah	37	9	24.3	7	18.9	4	10.8	12	32.4	17	45.9	32	86.5	23	62.2	27	73.0
Wyoming	28	0	0.0	2	7.1	4	14.3	6	21.4	10	35.7	22	78.6	5	17.9	18	64.3
CENSUS DIVISION 9, PACIFIC	480	63	13.1	129	26.9	88	18.3	88	18.3	169	35.2	311	64.8	208	43.3	311	64.8
Alaska	13	1	7.7	7	53.8	2	15.4	2	15.4	2	15.4	11	84.6	5	38.5	8	61.5
California	305	30	9.8	71	23.3	60	19.7	52	17.0	115	37.7	196	64.3	134	43.9	193	63.3
Hawaii	22	3	13.6	3	13.6	4	18.2	2	9.1	6	27.3	7	31.8	5	22.7	10	45.5
Oregon	31	15	26.2	25	41.0	7	11.5	17	27.9	23	37.7	44	72.1	28	45.9	49	80.3
Washington	79	13	16.5	23	29.1	15	19.0	15	19.0	23	29.1	53	67.1	36	45.6	51	64.6

Table 7 (Continued)

These data include only hospital-based facilities and services as reported by responding hospitals in Section C of the 2001 AHA Annual Survey, beginning on page 197. All hospitals are represented with Community Hospitals listed separately under United States. No estimates have been made for nonresponding hospitals. Definitions of facilities and services are listed in the Glossary, page 187.

CLASSIFICATION	HOSPITALS REPORTING	HEMODIALYSIS		HIV/AIDS SERVICES		HOME HEALTH SERVICES		HOSPICE		MAGNETIC RESONANCE IMAGING (MRI)		MEALS ON WHEELS		NUTRITION PROGRAMS CENTER		OCCUPATIONAL HEALTH SERVICES	
		Number	Percent	Number	Percent	Number	Percent	Number	Percent	Number	Percent	Number	Percent	Number	Percent	Number	Percent
UNITED STATES	4,728	1,208	25.5	1,436	30.4	1,915	40.5	1,118	23.6	2,412	51.0	675	14.3	3,065	64.8	2,947	62.3
COMMUNITY HOSPITALS	4,150	1,134	27.3	1,300	31.3	1,833	44.2	1,056	25.4	2,333	56.2	660	15.9	2,801	67.5	2,750	66.3
CENSUS DIVISION 1, NEW ENGLAND	218	67	30.7	105	48.2	59	27.1	64	29.4	104	47.7	30	13.8	179	82.1	163	74.8
Connecticut	35	14	40.0	24	68.6	8	22.9	21	60.0	24	68.6	7	20.0	31	88.6	23	65.7
Maine	38	6	15.8	14	36.8	14	36.8	6	15.8	11	28.9	5	13.2	31	81.6	27	71.1
Massachusetts	82	28	34.1	37	45.1	21	25.6	18	22.0	35	42.7	10	12.2	63	76.8	60	73.2
New Hampshire	30	8	26.7	15	50.0	9	30.0	10	33.3	15	50.0	2	6.7	28	93.3	28	93.3
Rhode Island	16	9	56.3	9	56.3	6	37.5	3	18.8	9	56.3	4	25.0	12	75.0	11	68.8
Vermont	17	2	11.8	6	35.3	1	5.9	6	35.3	10	58.8	2	11.8	14	82.4	14	82.4
CENSUS DIVISION 2, MIDDLE ATLANTIC	438	183	41.8	211	48.2	156	35.6	119	27.2	242	55.3	60	13.7	334	76.3	307	70.1
New Jersey	76	45	59.2	46	60.5	26	34.2	22	28.9	41	53.9	18	23.7	63	82.9	58	76.3
New York	177	86	48.6	85	48.0	48	27.1	40	22.6	96	54.2	24	13.6	125	70.6	116	65.5
Pennsylvania	185	52	28.1	80	43.2	82	44.3	57	30.8	105	56.8	18	9.7	146	78.9	133	71.9
CENSUS DIVISION 3, SOUTH ATLANTIC	721	239	33.1	269	37.3	256	35.5	139	19.3	416	57.7	53	7.4	477	66.2	465	64.5
Delaware	7	4	57.1	5	71.4	4	57.1	0	0.0	5	71.4	0	0.0	5	71.4	5	71.4
District of Columbia	12	9	75.0	9	75.0	3	25.0	3	25.0	9	75.0	1	8.3	9	75.0	11	91.7
Florida	174	75	43.1	65	37.4	68	39.1	33	19.0	119	68.4	10	5.7	117	67.2	114	65.5
Georgia	147	43	29.3	42	28.6	32	21.8	23	15.6	76	51.7	4	2.7	89	60.5	90	61.2
Maryland	65	30	46.2	27	41.5	13	20.0	9	13.8	33	50.8	6	9.2	46	70.8	43	66.2
North Carolina	102	35	34.3	31	30.4	49	48.0	25	24.5	61	59.8	8	7.8	76	74.5	72	70.6
South Carolina	72	2	2.8	45	62.5	18	25.0	10	13.9	30	41.7	10	13.9	38	52.8	39	54.2
Virginia	78	27	34.6	30	38.5	37	47.4	26	33.3	50	64.1	11	14.1	56	71.8	53	67.9
West Virginia	64	14	21.9	15	23.4	32	50.0	10	15.6	33	51.6	3	4.7	41	64.1	38	59.4
CENSUS DIVISION 4, EAST NORTH CENTRAL	687	198	28.8	216	31.4	310	45.1	229	33.3	381	55.5	186	27.1	556	80.9	512	74.5
Illinois	174	46	26.4	70	40.2	86	49.4	68	39.1	94	54.0	46	26.4	135	77.6	122	70.1
Indiana	90	16	17.8	25	27.8	56	62.2	34	37.8	62	68.9	29	32.2	73	81.1	73	81.1
Michigan	146	42	28.8	56	38.4	68	46.6	49	33.6	68	46.6	23	15.8	121	82.9	112	76.7
Ohio	148	62	41.9	55	37.2	70	47.3	41	27.7	104	70.3	43	29.1	120	81.1	116	78.4
Wisconsin	129	32	24.8	10	7.8	30	23.3	37	28.7	53	41.1	45	34.9	107	82.9	89	69.0
CENSUS DIVISION 5, EAST SOUTH CENTRAL	399	81	20.3	98	24.6	142	35.6	66	16.5	194	48.6	15	3.8	216	54.1	195	48.9
Alabama	74	19	25.7	20	27.0	35	47.3	15	20.3	43	58.1	6	8.1	40	54.1	33	44.6
Kentucky	99	18	18.2	25	25.3	44	44.4	18	18.2	39	39.4	6	6.1	59	59.6	59	59.6
Mississippi	97	15	15.5	29	29.9	21	21.6	11	11.3	37	38.1	2	2.1	41	42.3	26	26.8
Tennessee	129	29	22.5	24	18.6	42	32.6	22	17.1	75	58.1	1	0.8	76	58.9	77	59.7
CENSUS DIVISION 6, WEST NORTH CENTRAL	686	88	12.8	173	25.2	343	50.0	229	33.4	283	41.3	203	29.6	434	63.3	448	65.3
Iowa	123	25	20.3	33	26.8	76	61.8	59	48.0	55	44.7	56	45.5	97	78.9	92	74.8
Kansas	144	11	7.6	22	15.3	63	43.8	21	14.6	44	30.6	48	33.3	68	47.2	71	49.3
Minnesota	120	24	20.0	20	16.7	74	61.7	51	42.5	50	41.7	36	30.0	72	60.0	92	76.7
Missouri	139	2	1.4	71	51.1	39	28.1	37	26.6	81	58.3	26	18.7	109	78.4	103	74.1
Nebraska	70	8	11.4	11	15.7	43	61.4	26	37.1	24	34.3	15	21.4	38	54.3	40	57.1
North Dakota	33	7	21.2	5	15.2	17	51.5	13	39.4	13	39.4	7	21.2	23	69.7	19	57.6
South Dakota	57	11	19.3	11	19.3	31	54.4	22	38.6	16	28.1	15	26.3	27	47.4	31	54.4
CENSUS DIVISION 7, WEST SOUTH CENTRAL	762	156	20.5	146	19.2	295	38.7	95	12.5	352	46.2	51	6.7	390	51.2	366	48.0
Arkansas	95	19	20.0	17	17.9	67	70.5	24	25.3	48	50.5	7	7.4	39	41.1	46	48.4
Louisiana	107	32	29.9	23	21.5	35	32.7	11	10.3	48	44.9	3	2.8	58	54.2	53	49.5
Oklahoma	93	13	14.0	18	19.4	54	58.1	14	15.1	34	36.6	16	17.2	35	37.6	37	39.8
Texas	467	92	19.7	88	18.8	139	29.8	46	9.9	222	47.5	25	5.4	258	55.2	230	49.3
CENSUS DIVISION 8, MOUNTAIN	337	69	20.5	70	20.8	154	45.7	78	23.1	175	51.9	38	11.3	198	58.8	193	57.3
Arizona	54	17	31.5	17	31.5	17	31.5	9	16.7	31	57.4	6	11.1	36	66.7	33	61.1
Colorado	64	15	23.4	16	25.0	32	50.0	12	18.8	40	62.5	10	15.6	43	67.2	45	70.3
Idaho	34	3	8.8	5	14.7	17	50.0	11	32.4	18	52.9	4	11.8	23	67.6	23	67.6
Montana	54	9	16.7	11	20.4	33	61.1	19	35.2	17	31.5	11	20.4	25	46.3	25	46.3
Nevada	28	5	17.9	4	14.3	8	28.6	2	7.1	17	60.7	1	3.6	14	50.0	17	60.7
New Mexico	38	5	13.2	5	13.2	14	36.8	5	13.2	13	34.2	3	7.9	14	36.8	10	26.3
Utah	37	9	24.3	9	24.3	16	43.2	10	27.0	23	62.2	1	2.7	27	73.0	23	62.2
Wyoming	28	6	21.4	3	10.7	17	60.7	10	35.7	16	57.1	2	7.1	16	57.1	17	60.7
CENSUS DIVISION 9, PACIFIC	480	127	26.5	148	30.8	200	41.7	99	20.6	265	55.2	39	8.1	281	58.5	298	62.1
Alaska	13	3	23.1	4	30.8	8	61.5	0	0.0	4	30.8	1	7.7	7	53.8	6	46.2
California	305	89	29.2	105	34.4	117	38.4	55	18.0	185	60.7	27	8.9	171	56.1	190	62.3
Hawaii	22	6	27.3	5	22.7	5	22.7	2	9.1	10	45.5	2	9.1	13	59.1	13	59.1
Oregon	61	12	19.7	14	23.0	44	72.1	24	39.3	34	55.7	2	3.3	42	68.9	39	63.9
Washington	79	17	21.5	20	25.3	26	32.9	18	22.8	32	40.5	7	8.9	48	60.8	50	63.3

Table 7 (Continued)

These data include only hospital-based facilities and services as reported by responding hospitals in Section C of the 2001 AHA Annual Survey, beginning on page 197. All hospitals are represented with Community Hospitals listed separately under United States. No estimates have been made for nonresponding hospitals. Definitions of facilities and services are listed in the Glossary, page 187.

CLASSIFICATION	HOSPITALS REPORTING	ONCOLOGY SERVICES		OPEN HEART SURGERY		OUTPATIENT CARE CENTER (FREESTANDING)		OUTPATIENT CARE CENTER SERVICES (HOSPITAL BASED)		OUTPATIENT SURGERY		PAIN MANAGEMENT PROGRAM		PALLIATIVE CARE PROGRAM		PATIENT EDUCATION CENTER		PATIENT REPRESENTATIVE SERVICES	
		Number	Percent	Number	Percent	Number	Percent	Number	Percent	Number	Percent	Number	Percent	Number	Percent	Number	Percent	Number	Percent
UNITED STATES	4,728	2,556	54.1	971	20.5	1,217	25.7	3,320	70.2	3,985	84.3	2,102	44.5	806	17.0	2,587	54.7	2,899	61.3
COMMUNITY HOSPITALS	4,150	2,456	59.2	936	22.6	1,084	26.1	3,085	74.3	3,822	92.1	1,943	46.8	717	17.3	2,351	56.7	2,623	63.2
CENSUS DIVISION 1, NEW ENGLAND	218	169	77.5	26	11.9	73	33.5	169	77.5	177	81.2	135	61.9	63	28.9	138	63.3	148	67.9
Connecticut	35	28	80.0	7	20.0	17	48.6	28	80.0	28	80.0	25	71.4	12	34.3	25	71.4	25	71.4
Maine	38	30	78.9	2	5.3	11	28.9	29	76.3	34	89.5	20	52.6	9	23.7	20	52.6	19	50.0
Massachusetts	82	61	74.4	9	11.0	25	30.5	62	75.6	61	74.4	50	61.0	19	23.2	48	58.5	59	72.0
New Hampshire	30	25	83.3	5	16.7	10	33.3	24	80.0	27	90.0	21	70.0	11	36.7	21	70.0	22	73.3
Rhode Island	16	12	75.0	2	12.5	6	37.5	12	75.0	12	75.0	9	56.3	3	18.8	10	62.5	10	62.5
Vermont	17	13	76.5	1	5.9	4	23.5	14	82.4	15	88.2	10	58.8	9	52.9	14	82.4	13	76.5
CENSUS DIVISION 2, MIDDLE ATLANTIC	438	312	71.2	90	20.5	192	43.8	341	77.9	377	86.1	290	66.2	119	27.2	295	67.4	327	74.7
New Jersey	76	64	84.2	13	17.1	30	39.5	58	76.3	66	86.8	58	76.3	22	28.9	61	80.3	66	86.8
New York	177	116	65.5	27	15.3	100	56.5	136	76.8	151	85.3	111	62.7	46	26.0	118	66.7	134	75.7
Pennsylvania	185	132	71.4	50	27.0	62	33.5	147	79.5	160	86.5	121	65.4	51	27.6	116	62.7	127	68.6
CENSUS DIVISION 3, SOUTH ATLANTIC	721	386	53.5	142	19.7	226	31.3	517	71.7	612	84.9	374	51.9	129	17.9	449	62.3	472	65.5
Delaware	7	5	71.4	2	28.6	4	57.1	4	57.1	7	100.0	5	71.4	2	28.6	4	57.1	6	85.7
District of Columbia	12	10	83.3	7	58.3	7	58.3	12	100.0	10	83.3	10	83.3	7	58.3	11	91.7	10	83.3
Florida	174	99	56.9	51	29.3	63	36.2	125	71.8	150	86.2	100	57.5	37	21.3	96	55.2	104	59.8
Georgia	147	63	42.9	18	12.2	45	30.6	102	69.4	127	86.4	69	46.9	19	12.9	85	57.8	97	66.0
Maryland	65	45	69.2	10	15.4	21	32.3	42	64.6	49	75.4	41	63.1	14	21.5	37	56.9	44	67.7
North Carolina	102	63	61.8	20	19.6	28	27.5	73	71.6	93	91.2	49	48.0	22	21.6	62	60.8	69	67.6
South Carolina	72	21	29.2	13	18.1	21	29.2	57	79.2	58	80.6	33	45.8	0	0.0	68	94.4	43	59.7
Virginia	78	48	61.5	16	20.5	24	30.8	56	71.8	67	85.9	46	59.0	15	19.2	52	66.7	64	82.1
West Virginia	64	32	50.0	5	7.8	13	20.3	46	71.9	51	79.7	21	32.8	13	20.3	34	53.1	35	54.7
CENSUS DIVISION 4, EAST NORTH CENTRAL	687	485	70.6	177	25.8	238	34.6	567	82.5	627	91.3	403	58.7	138	20.1	479	69.7	491	71.5
Illinois	174	126	72.4	53	30.5	51	29.3	141	81.0	160	92.0	104	59.8	40	23.0	117	67.2	121	69.5
Indiana	90	67	74.4	22	24.4	33	36.7	72	80.0	81	90.0	53	58.9	22	24.4	52	57.8	58	64.4
Michigan	146	98	67.1	29	19.9	53	36.3	109	74.7	130	89.0	84	57.5	37	25.3	95	65.1	103	70.5
Ohio	148	114	77.0	49	33.1	56	37.8	121	81.8	142	95.9	88	59.5	39	26.4	94	63.5	117	79.1
Wisconsin	129	80	62.0	24	18.6	45	34.9	124	96.1	114	88.4	74	57.4	0	0.0	121	93.8	92	71.3
CENSUS DIVISION 5, EAST SOUTH CENTRAL	399	175	43.9	75	18.8	48	12.0	214	53.6	329	82.5	129	32.3	41	10.3	192	48.1	249	62.4
Alabama	74	43	58.1	19	25.7	9	12.2	53	71.6	67	90.5	35	47.3	11	14.9	38	51.4	43	58.1
Kentucky	99	48	48.5	18	18.2	20	20.2	67	67.7	85	85.9	39	39.4	14	14.1	47	47.5	59	59.6
Mississippi	97	32	33.0	16	16.5	0	0.0	27	27.8	71	73.2	13	13.4	0	0.0	52	53.6	63	64.9
Tennessee	129	52	40.3	22	17.1	19	14.7	67	51.9	106	82.2	42	32.6	16	12.4	55	42.6	84	65.1
CENSUS DIVISION 6, WEST NORTH CENTRAL	686	337	49.1	96	14.0	92	13.4	507	73.9	604	88.0	229	33.4	95	13.8	339	49.4	346	50.4
Iowa	123	72	58.5	13	10.6	13	10.6	103	83.7	116	94.3	41	33.3	22	17.9	73	59.3	58	47.2
Kansas	144	55	38.2	14	9.7	14	9.7	92	63.9	116	80.6	36	25.0	26	18.1	48	33.3	61	42.4
Minnesota	120	63	52.5	16	13.3	12	10.0	92	76.7	113	94.2	35	29.2	26	21.7	62	51.7	60	50.0
Missouri	139	77	55.4	35	25.2	39	28.1	114	82.0	118	84.9	69	49.6	1	0.7	84	60.4	108	77.7
Nebraska	70	37	52.9	8	11.4	8	11.4	49	70.0	65	92.9	19	27.1	4	5.7	28	40.0	26	37.1
North Dakota	33	15	45.5	6	18.2	2	6.1	20	60.6	30	90.9	11	33.3	9	27.3	17	51.5	18	54.5
South Dakota	57	18	31.6	4	7.0	4	7.0	37	64.9	46	80.7	18	31.6	7	12.3	27	47.4	15	26.3
CENSUS DIVISION 7, WEST SOUTH CENTRAL	762	283	37.1	170	22.3	146	19.2	464	60.9	577	75.7	231	30.3	73	9.6	316	41.5	395	51.8
Arkansas	95	37	38.9	20	21.1	17	17.9	64	67.4	77	81.1	25	26.3	9	9.5	37	38.9	43	45.3
Louisiana	107	45	42.1	29	27.1	25	23.4	66	61.7	84	78.5	29	27.1	14	13.1	43	40.2	62	57.9
Oklahoma	93	32	34.4	14	15.1	11	11.8	43	46.2	76	81.7	32	34.4	12	12.9	31	33.3	37	39.8
Texas	467	169	36.2	107	22.9	93	19.9	291	62.3	340	72.8	145	31.0	38	8.1	205	43.9	253	54.2
CENSUS DIVISION 8, MOUNTAIN	337	141	41.8	57	16.9	77	22.8	215	63.8	266	78.9	126	37.4	56	16.6	150	44.5	191	56.7
Arizona	54	29	53.7	16	29.6	20	37.0	33	61.1	43	79.6	23	42.6	10	18.5	27	50.0	35	64.8
Colorado	64	36	56.3	13	20.3	22	34.4	49	75.6	54	84.4	33	51.6	15	23.4	34	53.1	51	79.7
Idaho	34	14	41.2	3	8.8	6	17.6	20	58.8	28	82.4	12	35.3	5	14.7	14	41.2	15	44.1
Montana	54	17	31.5	4	7.4	2	3.7	31	57.4	39	72.2	16	29.6	10	18.5	17	31.5	21	38.9
Nevada	28	12	42.9	7	25.0	9	32.1	18	64.3	17	60.7	9	32.1	2	7.1	9	32.1	13	46.4
New Mexico	38	10	26.3	4	10.5	4	10.5	20	52.6	27	71.1	9	23.7	5	13.2	11	28.9	19	50.0
Utah	37	13	35.1	8	21.6	13	35.1	23	62.2	34	91.9	18	48.6	6	16.2	25	67.6	24	64.9
Wyoming	28	10	35.7	2	7.1	1	3.6	21	75.0	24	85.7	6	21.4	3	10.7	13	46.4	13	46.4
CENSUS DIVISION 9, PACIFIC	480	268	55.8	138	28.8	125	26.0	326	67.9	416	86.7	185	38.5	92	19.2	229	47.7	280	58.3
Alaska	13	5	46.2	2	15.4	3	23.1	11	84.6	12	92.3	4	30.8	3	23.1	5	38.5	7	53.8
California	305	173	58.4	102	33.4	87	28.5	210	68.9	266	87.2	114	37.4	51	16.7	141	46.2	182	59.7
Hawaii	22	11	50.0	6	27.3	4	18.2	11	50.0	13	59.1	9	40.9	4	18.2	6	27.3	9	40.9
Oregon	61	30	49.2	11	18.0	14	23.0	45	73.8	59	96.7	26	42.6	15	24.6	35	57.4	34	55.7
Washington	79	43	54.4	17	21.5	17	21.5	49	62.0	66	83.5	32	40.5	19	24.1	42	53.2	48	60.8

Table 7 (Continued)

These data include only hospital-based facilities and services as reported by responding hospitals in Section C of the 2001 AHA Annual Survey, beginning on page 197. All hospitals are represented with Community Hospitals listed separately under United States. No estimates have been made for nonresponding hospitals. Definitions of facilities and services are listed in the Glossary, page 187.

CLASSIFICATION	HOSPITALS REPORTING	PHYSICAL REHABILITATION OUTPATIENT SERVICES		POSITRON EMISSION TOMOGRAPHY (PET)		PRIMARY CARE DEPARTMENT		PSYCHIATRIC CHILD/ADOLESCENT SERVICES		PSYCHIATRIC CONSULTATION/ LIAISON SERVICES		PSYCHIATRIC EDUCATION SERVICES		PSYCHIATRIC EMERGENCY SERVICES		PSYCHIATRIC GERIATRIC SERVICES	
		Number	Percent	Number	Percent	Number	Percent	Number	Percent	Number	Percent	Number	Percent	Number	Percent	Number	Percent
UNITED STATES	4,728	3,649	77.2	448	9.5	1,661	35.1	909	19.2	1,526	32.3	1,199	25.4	1,624	34.3	1,492	31.6
COMMUNITY HOSPITALS	4,150	3,452	83.2	440	10.6	1,500	36.1	684	16.5	1,246	30.0	926	22.3	1,376	33.2	1,218	29.3
CENSUS DIVISION 1, NEW ENGLAND	218	178	81.7	24	11.0	103	47.2	71	32.6	115	52.8	86	39.4	109	50.0	107	49.1
Connecticut	35	25	71.4	13	37.1	19	54.3	20	57.1	26	74.3	23	65.7	26	74.3	26	74.3
Maine	38	33	86.8	1	2.6	11	28.9	8	21.1	12	31.6	7	18.4	12	31.6	11	28.9
Massachusetts	82	65	79.3	6	7.3	36	43.9	28	34.1	46	56.1	35	42.7	37	45.1	37	45.1
New Hampshire	30	29	96.7	3	10.0	16	53.3	8	26.7	12	40.0	8	26.7	14	46.7	14	46.7
Rhode Island	16	11	68.8	0	0.0	10	62.5	2	12.5	10	62.5	6	37.5	12	75.0	11	68.8
Vermont	17	15	88.2	1	5.9	11	64.7	5	29.4	9	52.9	7	41.2	8	47.1	8	47.1
CENSUS DIVISION 2, MIDDLE ATLANTIC	438	364	83.1	63	14.4	235	53.7	138	31.5	230	52.5	177	40.4	222	50.7	203	46.3
New Jersey	76	68	89.5	10	13.2	46	60.5	28	36.8	44	57.9	34	44.7	44	57.9	35	46.1
New York	177	144	81.4	27	15.3	118	66.7	58	32.8	98	55.4	73	41.2	95	53.7	78	44.1
Pennsylvania	185	152	82.2	26	14.1	71	38.4	52	28.1	88	47.6	70	37.8	83	44.9	90	48.6
CENSUS DIVISION 3, SOUTH ATLANTIC	721	570	79.1	110	15.3	236	32.7	146	20.2	245	34.0	204	28.3	282	39.1	232	32.2
Delaware	7	5	71.4	0	0.0	5	71.4	1	14.3	2	28.6	1	14.3	4	57.1	3	42.9
District of Columbia	12	12	100.0	3	25.0	9	75.0	5	41.7	10	83.3	7	58.3	10	83.3	8	66.7
Florida	174	143	82.2	42	24.1	61	35.1	22	12.6	44	25.3	42	24.1	63	36.2	48	27.6
Georgia	147	112	76.2	20	13.6	44	29.9	28	19.0	39	26.5	34	23.1	44	29.9	36	24.5
Maryland	65	46	70.8	11	16.9	23	35.4	28	43.1	42	64.6	31	47.7	44	67.7	33	50.8
North Carolina	102	93	91.2	9	8.8	31	30.4	21	20.6	35	34.3	32	31.4	44	43.1	41	40.2
South Carolina	72	47	65.3	2	2.8	17	23.6	16	22.2	23	31.9	20	27.8	24	33.3	19	26.4
Virginia	78	62	79.5	9	11.5	22	28.2	16	20.5	32	41.0	21	26.9	32	41.0	26	33.3
West Virginia	64	50	78.1	14	21.9	24	37.5	9	14.1	18	28.1	16	25.0	17	26.6	18	28.1
CENSUS DIVISION 4, EAST NORTH CENTRAL	687	605	88.1	66	9.6	315	45.9	172	25.0	298	43.4	244	35.5	307	44.7	267	38.9
Illinois	174	157	90.2	18	10.3	74	42.5	43	24.7	77	44.3	61	35.1	81	46.6	69	39.7
Indiana	90	80	88.9	11	12.2	41	45.6	23	25.6	35	38.9	30	33.3	35	38.9	33	36.7
Michigan	146	125	85.6	4	2.7	88	60.3	24	16.4	66	45.2	52	35.6	68	46.6	48	32.9
Ohio	148	138	93.2	27	18.2	72	48.6	41	27.7	70	47.3	62	41.9	71	48.0	67	45.3
Wisconsin	129	105	81.4	6	4.7	40	31.0	41	31.8	50	38.8	39	30.2	52	40.3	50	38.8
CENSUS DIVISION 5, EAST SOUTH CENTRAL	399	285	71.4	25	6.3	94	23.6	46	11.5	101	25.3	82	20.6	102	25.6	128	32.1
Alabama	74	57	77.0	5	6.8	20	27.0	9	12.2	20	27.0	17	23.0	23	31.1	22	29.7
Kentucky	99	75	75.8	8	8.1	27	27.3	11	11.1	26	26.3	21	21.2	29	29.3	26	26.3
Mississippi	97	52	53.6	2	2.1	16	16.5	9	9.3	20	20.6	17	17.5	18	18.6	36	37.1
Tennessee	129	101	78.3	10	7.8	31	24.0	17	13.2	35	27.1	27	20.9	32	24.8	44	34.1
CENSUS DIVISION 6, WEST NORTH CENTRAL	686	543	79.2	41	6.0	234	34.1	120	17.5	175	25.5	135	19.7	188	27.4	165	24.1
Iowa	123	98	79.7	9	7.3	52	42.3	31	25.2	35	28.5	32	26.0	46	37.4	28	22.8
Kansas	144	114	79.2	9	6.3	36	25.0	14	9.7	18	12.5	15	10.4	20	13.9	32	22.2
Minnesota	120	103	85.8	7	5.8	37	30.8	28	23.3	39	32.5	26	21.7	35	29.2	33	27.5
Missouri	139	113	81.3	6	4.3	58	41.7	27	19.4	59	42.4	44	31.7	53	38.1	47	33.8
Nebraska	70	44	62.9	4	5.7	15	21.4	9	12.9	12	17.1	8	11.4	15	21.4	10	14.3
North Dakota	33	28	84.8	2	6.1	17	51.5	6	18.2	6	18.2	5	15.2	9	27.3	7	21.2
South Dakota	57	43	75.4	4	7.0	19	33.3	5	8.8	6	10.5	5	8.8	10	17.5	8	14.0
CENSUS DIVISION 7, WEST SOUTH CENTRAL	762	520	68.2	48	6.3	180	23.6	83	10.9	142	18.6	112	14.7	163	21.4	194	25.5
Arkansas	95	70	73.7	2	2.1	18	18.9	11	11.6	19	20.0	15	15.8	23	24.2	32	33.7
Louisiana	107	64	59.8	5	4.7	35	32.7	9	8.4	27	25.2	14	13.1	31	29.0	40	37.4
Oklahoma	93	60	64.5	8	8.6	25	26.9	13	14.0	17	18.3	15	16.1	24	25.8	28	30.1
Texas	467	326	69.8	33	7.1	102	21.8	50	10.7	79	16.9	68	14.6	85	18.2	94	20.1
CENSUS DIVISION 8, MOUNTAIN	337	247	73.3	23	6.8	119	35.3	66	19.6	92	27.3	67	19.9	106	31.5	79	23.4
Arizona	54	43	79.6	3	5.6	18	33.3	9	16.7	16	29.6	12	22.2	18	33.3	14	25.9
Colorado	64	55	85.9	6	9.4	33	51.6	13	20.3	20	31.3	15	23.4	24	37.5	16	25.0
Idaho	34	24	70.6	2	5.9	8	23.5	5	14.7	7	20.6	5	14.7	8	23.5	5	14.7
Montana	54	40	74.1	1	1.9	24	44.4	9	16.7	11	20.4	9	16.7	16	29.6	10	18.5
Nevada	28	18	64.3	3	10.7	5	17.9	3	10.7	5	17.9	4	14.3	5	17.9	6	21.4
New Mexico	38	22	57.9	1	2.6	9	23.7	12	31.6	13	34.2	6	15.8	12	31.6	10	26.3
Utah	37	23	62.2	4	10.8	14	37.8	8	21.6	12	32.4	8	21.6	14	37.8	10	27.0
Wyoming	28	22	78.6	3	10.7	8	28.6	7	25.0	8	28.6	8	28.6	9	32.1	8	28.6
CENSUS DIVISION 9, PACIFIC	480	337	70.2	48	10.0	145	30.2	67	14.0	128	26.7	92	19.2	145	30.2	117	24.4
Alaska	13	8	61.5	0	0.0	4	30.8	2	15.4	5	38.5	2	15.4	6	46.2	2	15.4
California	305	210	68.9	34	11.1	79	25.9	44	14.4	79	25.9	57	18.7	84	27.5	81	26.6
Hawaii	22	14	63.6	1	4.5	4	18.2	3	13.6	5	22.7	4	18.2	5	22.7	4	18.2
Oregon	61	51	83.6	2	3.3	22	36.1	6	9.8	14	23.0	11	18.0	23	37.7	10	16.4
Washington	79	54	68.4	11	13.9	36	45.6	12	15.2	25	31.6	18	22.8	27	34.2	20	25.3

Table 7 (Continued)

These data include only hospital-based facilities and services as reported by responding hospitals in Section C of the 2001 AHA Annual Survey, beginning on page 197. All hospitals are represented with Community Hospitals listed separately under United States. No estimates have been made for nonresponding hospitals. Definitions of facilities and services are listed in the Glossary, page 187.

CLASSIFICATION	HOSPITALS REPORTING	PSYCHIATRIC OUTPATIENT SERVICES		PSYCHIATRIC PARTIAL HOSPITILIZATION PROGRAM		RADIATION THERAPY		REPRODUCTIVE HEALTH		RETIREMENT HOUSING		SLEEP CENTER		SINGLE PHOTON EMISSION COMPUTED TOMOGRAPHY (SPECT)		SOCIAL WORK SERVICES		SPORTS MEDICINE	
		Number	Percent	Number	Percent	Number	Percent	Number	Percent	Number	Percent	Number	Percent	Number	Percent	Number	Percent	Number	Percent
UNITED STATES	4,728	1,344	28.4	1,007	21.3	1,191	25.2	795	16.8	182	3.8	1,542	32.6	1,506	31.9	4,045	85.6	1,623	34.3
COMMUNITY HOSPITALS	4,150	1,067	25.7	809	19.5	1,150	27.7	739	17.8	179	4.3	1,481	35.7	1,457	35.1	3,584	86.4	1,597	38.5
CENSUS DIVISION 1, NEW ENGLAND	218	113	51.8	82	37.6	66	30.3	66	30.3	10	4.6	101	46.3	102	46.8	204	93.6	85	39.0
Connecticut	35	25	71.4	21	60.0	20	57.1	14	40.0	3	8.6	18	51.4	21	60.0	35	100.0	15	42.9
Maine	38	13	34.2	9	23.7	6	15.8	6	15.8	2	5.3	13	34.2	16	42.1	36	94.7	9	23.7
Massachusetts	82	45	54.9	33	40.2	28	34.1	27	32.9	1	1.2	39	47.6	36	43.9	71	86.6	34	41.5
New Hampshire	30	11	36.7	7	23.3	6	20.0	11	36.7	2	6.7	15	50.0	14	46.7	29	96.7	14	46.7
Rhode Island	16	7	43.8	6	37.5	3	18.8	3	18.8	1	6.3	11	68.8	8	50.0	16	100.0	5	31.3
Vermont	17	12	70.6	6	35.3	3	17.6	5	29.4	1	5.9	5	29.4	7	41.2	17	100.0	8	47.1
CENSUS DIVISION 2, MIDDLE ATLANTIC	438	180	41.1	123	28.1	166	37.9	133	30.4	13	3.0	186	42.5	193	44.1	421	96.1	176	40.2
New Jersey	76	35	46.1	32	42.1	33	43.4	26	34.2	2	2.6	40	52.6	41	53.9	75	98.7	27	35.5
New York	177	78	44.1	42	23.7	64	36.2	64	36.2	4	2.3	58	32.8	66	37.3	169	95.5	68	38.4
Pennsylvania	185	67	36.2	49	26.5	69	37.3	43	23.2	7	3.8	88	47.6	86	46.5	177	95.7	81	43.8
CENSUS DIVISION 3, SOUTH ATLANTIC	721	210	29.1	169	23.4	223	30.9	111	15.4	15	2.1	272	37.7	276	38.3	619	85.9	242	33.6
Delaware	7	4	57.1	2	28.6	1	14.3	1	14.3	0	0.0	4	57.1	5	71.4	6	85.7	3	42.9
District of Columbia	12	9	75.0	6	50.0	8	66.7	6	50.0	0	0.0	7	58.3	7	58.3	12	100.0	8	66.7
Florida	174	41	23.6	37	21.3	62	35.6	31	17.8	1	0.6	66	37.9	78	44.8	134	77.0	60	34.5
Georgia	147	37	25.2	28	19.0	33	22.4	17	11.6	6	4.1	63	42.9	33	22.4	120	81.6	45	30.6
Maryland	65	37	56.9	27	41.5	20	30.8	18	27.7	0	0.0	35	53.8	27	41.5	62	95.4	18	27.7
North Carolina	102	31	30.4	19	18.6	37	36.3	13	12.7	3	2.9	53	52.0	44	43.1	93	91.2	28	27.5
South Carolina	72	14	19.4	15	20.8	20	27.8	8	11.1	4	5.6	0	0.0	16	22.2	63	87.5	24	33.3
Virginia	78	24	30.8	28	35.9	29	37.2	11	14.1	0	0.0	26	33.3	40	51.3	69	88.5	29	37.2
West Virginia	64	13	20.3	7	10.9	13	20.3	6	9.4	1	1.6	18	28.1	26	40.6	60	93.8	27	42.2
CENSUS DIVISION 4, EAST NORTH CENTRAL	687	274	39.9	201	29.3	221	32.2	140	20.4	35	5.1	307	44.7	310	45.1	642	93.4	366	53.3
Illinois	174	71	40.8	64	36.8	61	35.1	37	21.3	9	5.2	86	49.4	71	40.8	159	91.4	83	47.7
Indiana	90	32	35.6	22	24.4	30	33.3	19	21.1	1	1.1	44	48.9	36	40.0	82	91.1	44	48.9
Michigan	146	55	37.7	32	21.9	43	29.5	40	27.4	5	3.4	69	47.3	69	47.3	137	93.8	74	50.7
Ohio	148	70	47.3	55	37.2	60	40.5	28	18.9	4	2.7	80	54.1	85	57.4	142	95.9	83	56.1
Wisconsin	129	46	35.7	28	21.7	27	20.9	16	12.4	16	12.4	28	21.7	49	38.0	122	94.6	82	63.6
CENSUS DIVISION 5, EAST SOUTH CENTRAL	399	78	19.5	57	14.3	84	21.1	39	9.8	9	2.3	108	27.1	104	26.1	343	86.0	125	31.3
Alabama	74	15	20.3	10	13.5	23	31.1	9	12.2	3	4.1	25	33.8	14	18.9	62	83.8	27	36.5
Kentucky	99	22	22.2	15	15.2	24	24.2	7	7.1	2	2.0	29	29.3	26	26.3	82	82.8	30	30.3
Mississippi	97	16	16.5	10	10.3	1	1.0	5	5.2	3	3.1	13	13.4	31	32.0	92	94.8	21	21.6
Tennessee	129	25	19.4	22	17.1	36	27.9	18	14.0	1	0.8	41	31.8	33	25.6	107	82.9	47	36.4
CENSUS DIVISION 6, WEST NORTH CENTRAL	686	169	24.6	106	15.5	108	15.7	91	13.3	77	11.2	160	23.3	146	21.3	552	80.5	241	35.1
Iowa	123	41	33.3	26	21.1	20	16.3	18	14.6	16	13.0	46	37.4	26	21.1	101	82.1	57	46.3
Kansas	144	15	10.4	10	6.9	14	9.7	13	9.0	13	9.0	43	29.9	22	15.3	98	68.1	29	20.1
Minnesota	120	39	32.5	20	16.7	16	13.3	16	13.3	17	14.2	32	26.7	14	11.7	105	87.5	36	30.0
Missouri	139	43	30.9	28	20.1	31	22.3	24	17.3	2	1.4	3	2.2	54	38.8	128	92.1	63	45.3
Nebraska	70	14	20.0	10	14.3	13	18.6	6	8.6	6	8.6	17	24.3	16	22.9	52	74.3	27	38.6
North Dakota	33	9	27.3	6	18.2	7	21.2	6	18.2	12	36.4	8	24.2	8	24.2	30	90.9	13	39.4
South Dakota	57	8	14.0	6	10.5	7	12.3	8	14.0	11	19.3	11	19.3	6	10.5	38	66.7	16	28.1
CENSUS DIVISION 7, WEST SOUTH CENTRAL	762	122	16.0	111	14.6	120	15.7	82	10.8	9	1.2	210	27.6	167	21.9	599	78.6	191	25.1
Arkansas	95	15	15.8	9	9.5	9	9.5	10	10.5	2	2.1	30	31.6	18	18.9	74	77.9	23	24.2
Louisiana	107	23	21.5	23	21.5	20	18.7	17	15.9	2	1.9	38	35.5	26	24.3	88	82.2	22	20.6
Oklahoma	93	18	19.4	9	9.7	19	20.4	6	6.5	2	2.2	28	30.1	23	24.7	62	66.7	26	28.0
Texas	467	66	14.1	70	15.0	72	15.4	49	10.5	3	0.6	114	24.4	100	21.4	375	80.3	120	25.7
CENSUS DIVISION 8, MOUNTAIN	337	87	25.8	60	17.8	57	16.9	55	16.3	4	1.2	92	27.3	74	22.0	270	80.1	90	26.7
Arizona	54	19	35.2	8	14.8	13	24.1	5	9.3	0	0.0	15	27.8	14	25.9	47	87.0	6	11.1
Colorado	64	18	28.1	15	23.4	12	18.8	12	18.8	2	3.1	23	35.9	19	29.7	49	76.6	27	42.2
Idaho	34	5	14.7	2	5.9	7	20.6	2	5.9	0	0.0	9	26.5	5	14.7	29	85.3	11	32.4
Montana	54	10	18.5	9	16.7	5	9.3	9	16.7	2	3.7	10	18.5	11	20.4	43	79.6	18	33.3
Nevada	28	5	17.9	5	17.9	4	14.3	2	7.1	0	0.0	5	17.9	6	21.4	22	78.6	3	10.7
New Mexico	38	13	34.2	7	18.4	5	13.2	8	21.1	0	0.0	6	15.8	6	15.8	29	76.3	7	18.4
Utah	37	8	21.6	11	29.7	8	21.6	12	32.4	0	0.0	16	43.2	7	18.9	29	78.4	12	32.4
Wyoming	28	9	32.1	3	10.7	3	10.7	5	17.9	0	0.0	8	28.6	6	21.4	22	78.6	6	21.4
CENSUS DIVISION 9, PACIFIC	480	111	23.1	98	20.4	146	30.4	78	16.3	10	2.1	106	22.1	134	27.9	395	82.3	107	22.3
Alaska	13	5	38.5	3	23.1	2	15.4	2	15.4	0	0.0	4	30.8	2	15.4	11	84.6	2	15.4
California	305	76	24.9	71	23.3	102	33.4	52	17.0	5	1.6	53	17.4	90	29.5	259	84.9	60	19.7
Hawaii	22	4	18.2	4	18.2	5	22.7	5	22.7	0	0.0	4	18.2	4	18.2	19	86.4	6	27.3
Oregon	61	10	16.4	5	8.2	15	24.6	7	11.5	4	6.6	18	29.5	24	39.3	47	77.0	15	24.6
Washington	79	16	20.3	15	19.0	22	27.8	12	5.2	1	1.3	27	34.2	14	17.7	59	74.7	24	30.4

Table 7 (Continued)

These data include only hospital-based facilities and services as reported by responding hospitals in Section C of the 2001 AHA Annual Survey, beginning on page 197. All hospitals are represented with Community Hospitals listed separately under United States. No estimates have been made for nonresponding hospitals. Definitions of facilities and services are listed in the Glossary, page 187.

CLASSIFICATION	HOSPITALS REPORTING	SUPPORT GROUPS		TEEN OUTREACH SERVICES		TOBACCO TREATMENT		TRANSPLANT SERVICES		TRANSPORTATION TO HEALTH FACILITIES		TRAUMA CENTER (CERTIFIED)		ULTRASOUND		URGENT CARE CENTER		VOLUNTEER SERVICES DEPARTMENT		WOMEN'S HEALTH SERVICES	
		Number	Percent	Number	Percent	Number	Percent	Number	Percent	Number	Percent	Number	Percent	Number	Percent	Number	Percent	Number	Percent	Number	Percent
UNITED STATES	4,728	2,913	61.6	666	14.1	1,401	29.6	402	8.5	1,337	28.3	1,377	29.1	3,819	80.8	1,186	25.1	3,554	75.2	2,031	43.0
COMMUNITY HOSPITALS	4,150	2,648	63.8	633	15.3	1,260	30.4	386	9.3	1,143	27.5	1,353	32.6	3,642	87.8	1,098	26.5	3,252	78.4	1,895	45.7
CENSUS DIVISION 1, NEW ENGLAND	218	185	84.9	59	27.1	130	59.6	19	8.7	66	30.3	62	28.4	175	80.3	98	45.0	199	91.3	131	60.1
Connecticut	35	35	100.0	16	45.7	22	62.9	4	11.4	9	25.7	16	45.7	29	82.9	20	57.1	33	94.3	24	68.6
Maine	38	30	78.9	5	13.2	26	68.4	1	2.6	6	15.8	8	21.1	31	81.6	15	39.5	32	84.2	19	50.0
Massachusetts	82	63	76.8	28	34.1	39	47.6	9	11.0	26	31.7	18	22.0	61	74.4	34	41.5	74	90.2	46	56.1
New Hampshire	30	27	90.0	6	20.0	22	73.3	2	6.7	11	36.7	15	50.0	27	90.0	13	43.3	29	96.7	24	80.0
Rhode Island	16	14	87.5	4	25.0	8	50.0	2	12.5	7	43.8	1	6.3	13	81.3	7	43.8	15	93.8	10	62.5
Vermont	17	16	94.1	0	0.0	13	76.5	1	5.9	7	41.2	4	23.5	14	82.4	9	52.9	16	94.1	8	47.1
CENSUS DIVISION 2, MIDDLE ATLANTIC	438	337	76.9	119	27.2	193	44.1	51	11.6	162	37.0	97	22.1	377	86.1	105	24.0	393	89.7	255	58.2
New Jersey	76	67	88.2	33	43.4	38	50.0	8	10.5	47	61.8	16	21.1	66	86.8	22	28.9	72	94.7	49	64.5
New York	177	132	74.6	45	25.4	71	40.1	21	11.9	57	32.2	46	26.0	151	85.3	49	27.7	156	88.1	107	60.5
Pennsylvania	185	138	74.6	41	22.2	84	45.4	22	11.9	58	31.4	35	18.9	160	86.5	34	18.4	165	89.2	99	53.5
CENSUS DIVISION 3, SOUTH ATLANTIC	721	474	65.7	96	13.3	209	29.0	108	15.0	215	29.8	172	23.9	604	83.8	169	23.4	605	83.9	356	49.4
Delaware	7	6	85.7	1	14.3	3	42.9	3	42.9	1	14.3	6	85.7	6	85.7	0	0.0	6	85.7	5	71.4
District of Columbia	12	12	100.0	3	25.0	5	41.7	6	50.0	8	66.7	6	50.0	11	91.7	5	41.7	12	100.0	10	83.3
Florida	174	117	67.2	15	8.6	45	25.9	16	9.2	63	36.2	35	20.1	149	85.6	44	25.3	146	83.9	85	48.9
Georgia	147	82	55.8	22	15.0	45	30.6	11	7.5	35	23.8	26	17.7	127	86.4	35	23.8	117	79.6	66	44.9
Maryland	65	50	76.9	14	21.5	29	44.6	4	6.2	22	33.8	15	23.1	49	75.4	15	23.1	59	90.8	34	52.3
North Carolina	102	72	70.6	15	14.7	34	33.3	6	5.9	29	28.4	20	19.6	91	89.2	31	30.4	93	91.2	42	41.2
South Carolina	72	43	59.7	11	15.3	0	0.0	51	70.8	25	34.7	25	34.7	55	76.4	10	13.9	54	75.0	45	62.5
Virginia	78	56	71.8	10	12.8	23	29.5	7	9.0	16	20.5	18	23.1	67	85.9	16	20.5	67	85.9	39	50.0
West Virginia	64	36	56.3	5	7.8	25	39.1	4	6.3	16	25.0	21	32.8	49	76.6	13	20.3	51	79.7	30	46.9
CENSUS DIVISION 4, EAST NORTH CENTRAL	687	504	73.4	119	17.3	294	42.8	55	8.0	226	32.9	241	35.1	602	87.6	287	41.8	569	82.8	358	52.1
Illinois	174	139	79.9	33	19.0	76	43.7	16	9.2	74	42.5	68	39.1	157	90.2	49	28.2	154	88.5	95	54.6
Indiana	90	73	81.1	16	17.8	48	53.3	5	5.6	21	23.3	19	21.1	80	88.9	35	38.9	82	91.1	52	57.8
Michigan	146	119	81.5	26	17.8	67	45.9	13	8.9	52	35.6	54	37.0	130	89.0	75	51.4	129	88.4	74	50.7
Ohio	148	117	79.1	35	23.6	68	45.9	17	11.5	53	35.8	44	29.7	139	93.9	55	37.2	140	94.6	83	56.1
Wisconsin	129	56	43.4	9	7.0	35	27.1	4	3.1	26	20.2	56	43.4	96	74.4	73	56.6	64	49.6	54	41.9
CENSUS DIVISION 5, EAST SOUTH CENTRAL	399	206	51.6	36	9.0	99	24.8	23	5.8	90	22.6	113	28.3	339	85.0	44	11.0	233	58.4	148	37.1
Alabama	74	43	58.1	11	14.9	22	29.7	4	5.4	19	25.7	26	35.1	68	91.9	9	12.2	61	82.4	32	43.2
Kentucky	99	56	56.6	10	10.1	37	37.4	4	4.0	17	17.2	23	23.2	85	85.9	16	16.2	76	76.8	40	40.4
Mississippi	97	39	40.2	7	7.2	9	9.3	1	1.0	24	24.7	46	47.4	79	81.4	7	7.2	0	0.0	29	29.9
Tennessee	129	68	52.7	8	6.2	31	24.0	14	10.9	30	23.3	18	14.0	107	82.9	12	9.3	96	74.4	47	36.4
CENSUS DIVISION 6, WEST NORTH CENTRAL	686	401	58.5	72	10.5	152	22.2	33	4.8	195	28.4	187	27.3	502	73.2	138	20.1	466	67.9	189	27.6
Iowa	123	88	71.5	21	17.1	44	35.8	8	6.5	37	30.1	76	61.8	105	85.4	26	21.1	94	76.4	35	28.5
Kansas	144	58	40.3	8	5.6	22	15.3	4	2.8	35	24.3	13	9.0	81	56.3	13	9.0	82	56.9	28	19.4
Minnesota	120	85	70.8	11	9.2	43	35.8	4	3.3	29	24.2	28	23.3	91	75.8	36	30.0	86	71.7	31	25.8
Missouri	139	97	69.8	20	14.4	1	0.7	9	6.5	54	38.8	34	24.5	112	80.6	39	28.1	117	84.2	57	41.0
Nebraska	70	31	44.3	6	8.6	18	25.7	4	5.7	17	24.3	13	18.6	50	71.4	9	12.9	35	50.0	16	22.9
North Dakota	33	20	60.6	5	15.2	8	24.2	2	6.1	9	27.3	16	48.5	20	60.6	6	18.2	25	75.8	13	39.4
South Dakota	57	22	38.6	1	1.8	16	28.1	2	3.5	14	24.6	7	12.3	43	75.4	9	15.8	27	47.4	9	15.8
CENSUS DIVISION 7, WEST SOUTH CENTRAL	762	351	46.1	40	5.2	107	14.0	45	5.9	161	21.1	259	34.0	546	71.7	110	14.4	480	63.0	256	33.6
Arkansas	95	52	54.7	8	8.4	19	20.0	4	4.2	24	25.3	13	13.7	76	80.0	10	10.5	60	63.2	31	32.6
Louisiana	107	44	41.1	5	4.7	18	16.8	7	6.5	23	21.5	19	17.8	88	82.2	25	23.4	70	65.4	42	39.3
Oklahoma	93	33	35.5	2	2.2	15	16.1	0	0.0	16	17.2	28	30.1	64	68.8	17	18.3	59	63.4	27	29.0
Texas	467	222	47.5	25	5.4	55	11.8	34	7.3	98	21.0	199	42.6	318	68.1	58	12.4	291	62.3	156	33.4
CENSUS DIVISION 8, MOUNTAIN	337	175	51.9	55	16.3	100	29.7	22	6.5	86	25.5	103	30.6	271	80.4	91	27.0	232	68.8	131	38.9
Arizona	54	37	68.5	9	16.7	17	31.5	5	9.3	12	22.2	8	14.8	47	87.0	17	31.5	42	77.8	23	42.6
Colorado	64	38	59.4	12	18.8	25	39.1	4	6.3	20	31.3	45	70.3	53	82.8	16	25.0	48	75.0	29	45.3
Idaho	34	15	44.1	8	23.5	11	32.4	4	11.8	10	29.4	8	23.5	28	82.4	7	20.6	24	70.6	12	35.3
Montana	54	20	37.0	8	14.8	17	31.5	1	1.9	16	29.6	9	16.7	38	70.4	11	20.4	33	61.1	14	25.9
Nevada	28	10	35.7	1	3.6	4	14.3	3	10.7	8	28.6	4	14.3	19	67.9	9	32.1	19	67.9	10	35.7
New Mexico	38	13	34.2	8	21.1	9	23.7	1	2.6	7	18.4	3	7.9	27	71.1	12	31.6	15	39.5	10	26.3
Utah	37	24	64.9	7	18.9	9	24.3	4	10.8	6	16.2	12	32.4	33	89.2	14	37.8	33	89.2	23	62.2
Wyoming	28	18	64.3	2	7.1	8	28.6	0	0.0	7	25.0	14	50.0	26	92.9	5	17.9	18	64.3	10	35.7
CENSUS DIVISION 9, PACIFIC	480	280	58.3	70	14.6	117	24.4	46	9.6	136	28.3	143	29.8	403	84.0	144	30.0	377	78.5	207	43.1
Alaska	13	7	53.8	5	38.5	4	30.8	0	0.0	2	15.4	0	0.0	13	100.0	2	15.4	6	46.2	5	38.5
California	305	172	56.4	52	17.0	55	18.0	33	10.8	106	34.8	51	16.7	255	83.6	98	32.1	248	81.3	136	44.6
Hawaii	22	11	50.0	2	9.1	4	18.2	2	9.1	3	13.6	3	13.6	14	63.6	4	18.2	16	72.7	6	27.3
Oregon	61	45	73.8	6	9.8	28	45.9	6	9.8	13	21.3	40	65.6	60	98.4	15	24.6	50	82.0	28	45.9
Washington	79	45	57.0	5	6.3	26	32.9	5	6.3	12	15.2	49	62.0	61	77.2	25	31.6	57	72.2	32	40.5

Table 8

MSAs

Metropolitan Statistical Areas

According to the U.S. Office of Management and Budget, an MSA is a geographical designation that represents an integrated social and economic unit with a large population nucleus. Under these standards, an area qualifies for recognition as an MSA if there is a city within the area of at least 50,000 population or an urban area of at least 50,000 with a total metropolitan population of at least 100,000. MSAs are defined as entire counties. In addition to the county containing the main city, an MSA also includes additional counties having strong economic and social ties to the central county. Such counties must have a specified level of commuting to the central counties and must meet certain standards regarding metropolitan character, such as population density.

When an MSA encompasses two or more central cities, up to three cities may be specified in the MSA title. They will be listed in order of population size. When a single central city exists, the MSA is named for that particular city. The official MSA title will also include a list of each of the states it covers.

This publication includes the most current MSAs as defined by the Office of Management and Budget.

TABLE 8

U.S. CENSUS DIVISION 1, NEW ENGLAND

U.S. Community Hospitals
(Nonfederal, short-term general and other special hospitals)

2001 Utilization, Personnel and Finances

										NEWBORNS		OUTPATIENT VISITS	
CLASSIFICATION	Hospitals	Beds	Admissions	Inpatient Days	Adjusted Patient Days	Average Daily Census	Adjusted Average Daily Census	Average Stay (days)	Surgical Operations	Bassinets	Births	Emergency	Total
UNITED STATES	4,907	824,676	33,765,589	193,754,932	314,740,801	531,715	863,683	5.7	26,432,095	60,351	3,868,995	105,865,778	536,588,378
Nonmetropolitan	2,166	174,945	5,372,241	35,717,503	71,393,393	97,918	195,777	6.6	4,479,968	13,831	533,148	22,155,102	110,466,485
Metropolitan	2,741	649,731	28,393,348	158,037,429	243,347,408	433,797	667,906	5.6	21,952,127	46,520	3,335,847	83,710,676	426,121,893
CENSUS DIVISION 1, NEW ENGLAND	205	35,385	1,567,000	9,144,828	16,403,419	25,057	44,951	5.8	1,432,306	2,715	169,198	5,973,441	35,152,531
Nonmetropolitan	77	6,784	265,728	1,573,750	3,325,360	4,312	9,119	5.9	262,198	703	28,629	1,322,154	7,186,564
Metropolitan	128	28,601	1,301,272	7,571,078	13,078,059	20,745	35,832	5.8	1,170,108	2,012	140,569	4,651,287	27,965,967
Connecticut	35	8,041	360,007	2,184,918	3,355,992	5,985	9,195	6.1	295,397	588	42,694	1,328,651	6,489,426
Nonmetropolitan	6	479	26,264	113,259	233,924	309	641	4.3	23,017	61	2,855	133,181	819,057
Metropolitan	29	7,562	333,743	2,071,659	3,122,068	5,676	8,554	6.2	272,380	527	39,839	1,195,470	5,670,369
Bridgeport	4	843	44,642	235,395	353,096	645	968	5.3	32,147	79	5,389	158,964	504,071
Danbury	2	340	18,463	80,175	143,202	220	392	4.3	16,567	36	2,719	79,515	260,039
Hartford	10	2,770	116,123	761,939	1,164,053	2,087	3,189	6.6	108,249	150	12,719	392,309	2,503,906
New Haven-Meriden	6	1,973	71,591	584,620	771,707	1,602	2,114	8.2	48,818	80	7,055	219,644	1,003,857
New London-Norwich	2	439	23,963	117,149	204,359	321	560	4.9	23,336	46	2,636	124,479	347,763
Stamford-Norwalk	3	765	35,585	184,039	294,598	504	807	5.2	26,985	81	6,625	111,887	673,906
Waterbury	2	432	23,376	108,342	191,053	297	524	4.6	16,278	55	2,696	108,672	376,827
Maine	37	3,844	148,612	898,059	1,621,795	2,464	4,452	6.0	159,828	329	13,320	700,510	3,512,598
Nonmetropolitan	29	2,182	70,637	462,914	961,154	1,271	2,641	6.6	92,458	217	6,470	428,767	2,284,433
Metropolitan	8	1,662	77,975	435,145	660,641	1,193	1,811	5.6	67,370	112	6,850	271,743	1,228,165
Bangor	2	454	20,642	106,432	163,107	293	448	5.2	21,846	26	1,696	68,295	415,244
Lewiston-Auburn	2	325	13,937	78,158	132,896	214	364	5.6	11,219	38	1,264	64,239	340,066
Portland	3	804	39,374	230,508	324,451	631	889	5.9	30,779	41	3,507	115,222	388,902
Portsmouth-Rochester	1	79	4,022	20,047	40,187	55	110	5.0	3,526	7	383	23,987	83,953
Massachusetts	80	16,504	766,708	4,382,048	8,075,056	12,007	22,126	5.7	680,456	1,186	79,908	2,717,815	18,778,137
Nonmetropolitan	11	1,367	72,579	348,701	658,504	956	1,805	4.8	56,325	176	9,718	322,959	1,466,086
Metropolitan	69	15,137	694,129	4,033,347	7,416,552	11,051	20,321	5.8	624,131	1,010	70,190	2,394,856	17,312,051
Barnstable-Yarmouth	1	228	15,658	65,217	128,283	179	351	4.2	10,758	10	1,032	76,743	365,308
Boston	38	8,614	401,377	2,411,996	4,402,651	6,609	12,063	6.0	370,295	540	40,326	1,135,711	10,832,085
Brockton	2	447	23,790	109,736	212,560	301	582	4.6	21,723	40	2,372	117,369	372,929
Fitchburg-Leominster	2	285	13,139	65,710	130,013	180	356	5.0	10,004	34	1,997	69,158	409,759
Lawrence	5	638	24,989	139,072	285,383	381	782	5.6	19,793	70	3,200	126,230	436,794
Lowell	2	381	17,864	73,898	197,231	202	541	4.1	20,636	39	2,841	92,148	496,546
Pittsfield	1	398	12,606	77,965	142,281	214	390	6.2	10,045	20	754	56,625	77,539
Providence-Fall River-Warwick	3	1,037	47,953	280,444	546,128	768	1,496	5.8	52,296	95	4,991	283,722	1,348,930
Springfield	9	1,710	70,331	462,760	770,926	1,267	2,113	6.6	59,274	96	7,644	268,012	1,617,380
Worcester	6	1,399	66,422	346,549	601,096	950	1,647	5.2	49,307	66	5,033	169,138	1,354,781
New Hampshire	28	2,853	116,071	637,239	1,328,669	1,743	3,640	5.5	109,169	302	13,919	537,367	2,929,626
Nonmetropolitan	18	1,477	58,633	349,688	771,385	956	2,113	6.0	52,721	157	5,502	242,192	1,693,017
Metropolitan	10	1,376	57,438	287,551	557,284	787	1,527	5.0	56,448	145	8,417	295,175	1,236,609
Lawrence	2	159	4,297	34,463	70,639	94	193	8.0	5,619	10	595	26,367	244,357
Manchester	2	461	19,646	102,685	162,102	281	444	5.2	14,740	20	2,719	72,744	264,646
Nashua	2	308	13,863	63,849	147,077	175	403	4.6	10,070	65	2,223	77,855	351,971
Portsmouth-Rochester	4	448	19,632	86,554	177,466	237	487	4.4	26,019	50	2,880	118,209	375,635
Rhode Island	11	2,449	120,901	638,571	1,161,324	1,751	3,180	5.3	134,966	176	13,375	451,325	2,151,240
Nonmetropolitan	1	148	6,309	32,632	75,292	89	206	5.2	7,237	9	708	28,641	100,369
Metropolitan	10	2,301	114,592	605,939	1,086,032	1,662	2,974	5.3	127,729	167	12,667	422,684	2,050,871
New London-Norwich	1	125	4,636	18,483	45,274	51	124	4.0	14,008	18	480	20,413	409,368
Providence-Fall River-Warwick	9	2,176	109,956	587,456	1,040,758	1,611	2,850	5.3	113,721	149	12,187	402,271	1,641,503
Vermont	14	1,694	54,701	403,993	860,583	1,107	2,358	7.4	52,490	134	5,982	237,773	1,291,504
Nonmetropolitan	12	1,131	31,306	266,556	625,101	731	1,713	8.5	30,440	83	3,376	166,414	823,602
Metropolitan	2	563	23,395	137,437	235,482	376	645	5.9	22,050	51	2,606	71,359	467,902
Burlington	2	563	23,395	137,437	235,482	376	645	5.9	22,050	51	2,606	71,359	467,902

TABLE 8

U.S. CENSUS DIVISION 1, NEW ENGLAND

U.S. Community Hospitals
(Nonfederal, short-term general and other special hospitals)

2001 Utilization, Personnel and Finances

FULL-TIME EQUIVALENT PERSONNEL					FULL-TIME EQUIV. TRAINEES			EXPENSES							
								LABOR				TOTAL			
Physicians and Dentists	Registered Nurses	Licensed Practical Nurses	Other Salaried Personnel	Total Personnel	Medical and Dental Residents	Other Trainees	Total Trainees	Payroll (in thousands)	Employee Benefits (in thousands)	Total (in thousands)	Percent of Total	Amount (in thousands)	Adjusted per Admission	Adjusted per Inpatient Day
70,153	956,577	126,143	2,828,126	3,980,999	77,440	5,751	83,191	$161,734,716	$34,640,089	$196,374,807	51.3	$383,082,895	$6,976.34	$1,217.14
8,081	142,404	36,781	476,073	663,339	1,719	697	2,416	22,294,816	5,051,240	27,346,046	53.3	51,353,805	4,803.37	719.31
62,072	814,173	89,362	2,352,053	3,317,660	75,721	5,054	80,775	139,439,900	29,588,849	169,028,761	51.0	331,729,090	7,501.70	1,363.19
8,822	50,609	3,491	169,099	232,021	6,902	421	7,323	9,864,081	1,986,605	11,850,684	52.3	22,650,946	7,771.89	1,380.87
708	8,504	817	29,152	39,181	418	4	422	1,557,051	331,147	1,888,196	54.8	3,448,388	6,152.43	1,037.00
8,114	42,105	2,674	139,947	192,840	6,484	417	6,901	8,307,030	1,655,458	9,962,488	51.9	19,202,558	8,157.49	1,468.30
794	10,252	522	34,176	45,744	1,194	195	1,389	2,222,203	456,462	2,678,665	56.8	4,718,315	7,977.42	1,405.94
60	702	24	3,001	3,787	0	0	0	148,210	33,212	181,423	57.4	315,803	5,782.55	1,350.02
734	9,550	498	31,175	41,957	1,194	195	1,389	2,073,994	423,250	2,497,242	56.7	4,402,513	8,200.70	1,410.13
89	1,144	86	3,188	4,507	156	4	160	219,274	45,438	264,712	53.0	499,421	7,338.60	1,414.41
9	498	21	1,735	2,263	57	0	57	120,932	28,377	149,309	55.6	268,674	8,162.41	1,876.19
250	3,532	160	12,821	16,763	107	83	190	771,449	139,662	911,110	58.2	1,564,522	8,051.22	1,344.03
115	2,305	147	6,101	8,668	634	85	719	453,985	104,766	558,750	55.5	1,006,994	9,972.61	1,304.89
47	548	53	2,046	2,694	0	5	5	138,681	31,623	170,304	58.7	290,052	6,924.14	1,419.33
146	896	16	3,238	4,296	129	12	141	232,886	44,693	277,578	55.7	497,992	8,656.07	1,690.41
78	627	15	2,046	2,766	111	6	117	136,787	28,691	165,479	60.2	274,858	6,678.11	1,438.65
477	5,076	362	15,269	21,184	236	0	236	836,169	174,737	1,010,903	53.3	1,895,303	7,046.73	1,168.65
171	2,421	228	8,121	10,941	0	0	0	392,132	80,257	472,388	54.6	865,514	5,789.43	900.49
306	2,655	134	7,148	10,243	236	0	236	444,037	94,479	538,515	52.3	1,029,788	8,620.15	1,558.77
90	930	43	1,872	2,935	27	0	27	126,311	27,050	153,360	51.0	300,598	9,481.10	1,842.95
50	401	24	1,122	1,597	21	0	21	69,122	12,909	82,030	48.6	168,847	7,133.38	1,270.52
148	1,148	62	3,771	5,129	188	0	188	223,469	48,884	272,353	54.2	502,943	8,977.12	1,550.14
18	176	5	383	582	0	0	0	25,135	5,637	30,772	53.6	57,400	7,118.99	1,428.33
6,418	26,504	1,765	88,851	123,538	4,213	186	4,399	5,028,545	947,892	5,976,438	49.6	12,055,797	8,170.36	1,492.97
174	2,275	205	6,597	9,251	104	4	108	412,125	85,837	497,960	55.0	905,774	6,457.78	1,375.50
6,244	24,229	1,560	82,254	114,287	4,109	182	4,291	4,616,420	862,055	5,478,478	49.1	11,150,023	8,350.25	1,503.40
20	333	15	1,100	1,468	0	0	0	77,684	20,152	97,836	50.9	192,173	6,239.38	1,498.04
5,653	15,484	833	55,945	77,915	3,189	181	3,370	3,057,779	552,407	3,610,189	47.3	7,640,026	9,936.45	1,735.32
29	565	4	1,596	2,194	0	0	0	118,205	15,156	133,362	61.4	217,248	4,714.58	1,022.05
12	294	35	990	1,331	3	0	3	60,042	11,331	71,372	53.7	132,970	5,177.16	1,022.74
62	696	54	2,113	2,925	4	0	4	132,367	24,655	157,022	58.6	268,161	5,132.36	939.65
12	369	52	1,522	1,955	0	0	0	85,468	13,684	99,151	53.9	183,882	3,856.42	932.32
85	494	60	1,046	1,685	88	0	88	77,502	16,559	94,062	58.7	160,106	6,959.61	1,125.28
41	1,203	114	4,157	5,515	0	0	0	246,999	58,358	305,358	60.7	502,875	5,317.82	920.80
297	1,905	113	6,369	8,684	250	0	250	382,366	70,404	452,769	52.4	864,346	6,632.95	1,121.18
33	2,886	280	7,416	10,615	575	1	576	378,008	79,350	457,357	46.3	988,237	8,517.23	1,644.06
211	4,173	240	13,428	18,052	314	0	314	713,270	166,334	879,605	54.4	1,617,994	6,732.83	1,217.76
172	2,247	167	7,384	9,970	314	0	314	394,465	84,902	479,367	54.1	885,710	6,983.61	1,148.21
39	1,926	73	6,044	8,082	0	0	0	318,806	81,432	400,238	54.7	732,284	6,452.58	1,314.02
0	152	5	736	893	0	0	0	34,099	6,368	40,467	55.8	72,489	7,467.66	1,026.18
8	709	20	2,081	2,818	0	0	0	105,451	36,406	141,856	56.2	252,443	8,069.64	1,557.31
16	426	30	1,004	1,770	0	0	0	79,102	15,340	94,442	58.0	161,233	5,037.10	1,096.25
15	639	18	1,923	2,595	0	0	0	100,154	23,319	123,473	50.2	246,120	6,078.84	1,386.86
441	3,066	294	10,609	14,410	693	0	693	723,131	158,712	881,845	55.4	1,592,004	7,175.02	1,071.14
0	140	10	441	591	0	0	0	28,902	3,732	32,634	47.2	69,196	4,753.45	919.03
441	2,926	284	10,168	13,819	693	0	693	694,231	154,980	849,211	55.8	1,523,138	7,345.34	1,402.48
12	56	7	392	467	0	0	0	25,930	6,683	32,613	58.0	56,270	4,955.09	1,242.88
429	2,870	277	9,776	13,352	693	0	693	668,301	148,297	816,598	55.7	1,466,868	7,483.83	1,409.42
481	1,538	308	6,766	9,093	252	40	292	340,760	82,468	423,228	54.9	771,202	6,633.20	896.14
131	719	183	3,608	4,641	0	0	0	181,217	43,206	224,424	55.2	406,390	5,137.75	660.12
350	819	125	3,158	4,452	252	40	292	159,543	39,262	198,804	54.5	364,812	8,784.52	1,549.22
350	819	125	3,158	4,452	252	40	292	159,543	39,262	198,804	54.5	364,812	8,784.52	1,549.22

MSAs

TABLE 8

U.S. CENSUS DIVISION 2, MIDDLE ATLANTIC

U.S. Community Hospitals
(Nonfederal, short-term general and other special hospitals)

2001 Utilization, Personnel and Finances

CLASSIFICATION	Hospitals	Beds	Admissions	Inpatient Days	Adjusted Patient Days	Average Daily Census	Adjusted Average Daily Census	Average Stay (days)	Surgical Operations	NEWBORNS		OUTPATIENT VISITS	
										Bassinets	Births	Emergency	Total
UNITED STATES	4,908	825,966	33,813,589	194,106,316	315,240,946	532,678	865,053	5.7	26,464,309	60,448	3,873,395	105,957,778	538,480,378
Nonmetropolitan	2,166	174,945	5,372,241	35,717,503	71,393,393	97,918	195,777	6.6	4,479,968	13,831	533,148	22,155,102	110,466,485
Metropolitan	2,742	651,021	28,441,348	158,388,813	243,847,553	434,760	669,276	5.6	21,984,341	46,617	3,340,247	83,802,676	428,013,893
CENSUS DIVISION 2, MIDDLE ATLANTIC	495	134,007	5,303,235	35,582,339	54,081,906	97,706	148,480	6.7	4,219,552	8,032	502,368	15,262,789	96,153,757
Nonmetropolitan	80	10,643	336,417	2,440,090	4,931,284	6,728	13,600	7.3	347,042	791	27,953	1,323,356	9,057,663
Metropolitan	415	123,364	4,966,818	33,142,249	49,150,622	90,978	134,880	6.7	3,872,510	7,241	474,415	13,939,433	87,096,094
New Jersey	78	24,580	1,083,798	6,165,019	8,314,926	17,008	22,917	5.7	693,414	1,735	109,870	2,936,620	18,444,560
Metropolitan	78	24,580	1,083,798	6,165,019	8,314,926	17,008	22,917	5.7	693,414	1,735	109,870	2,936,620	18,444,560
Atlantic-Cape May	5	969	46,189	260,064	392,079	713	1,073	5.6	26,129	69	3,831	158,196	870,724
Bergen-Passaic	10	3,640	200,308	910,112	1,227,852	2,493	3,365	4.5	105,762	255	17,717	354,229	4,046,107
Jersey City	8	1,993	61,659	350,682	452,567	1,077	1,380	5.7	40,368	140	6,411	196,260	968,904
Middlesex-Somerset-Hunterdon	8	2,454	118,416	704,106	908,376	1,930	2,489	5.9	63,769	258	16,174	327,313	1,627,855
Monmouth-Ocean	8	3,321	135,221	883,045	1,185,306	2,421	3,247	6.5	99,566	213	12,611	374,233	3,563,506
Newark	21	7,508	306,425	1,960,794	2,618,474	5,371	7,172	6.4	203,154	451	30,620	847,073	4,141,796
Philadelphia	11	2,758	141,021	693,903	929,874	1,900	2,547	4.9	97,273	217	14,331	428,714	1,580,005
Trenton	6	1,380	54,955	297,126	446,979	815	1,224	5.4	39,640	103	6,224	167,509	1,396,848
Vineland-Millville-Bridgeton	1	557	19,604	105,187	153,419	288	420	5.4	17,753	29	1,951	83,093	248,815
New York	212	67,296	2,410,906	19,021,960	28,716,483	52,120	78,675	7.9	1,947,693	3,734	249,035	7,452,574	45,645,773
Nonmetropolitan	36	4,921	127,261	1,191,176	2,368,185	3,264	6,490	9.4	119,766	353	11,547	550,004	4,173,796
Metropolitan	176	62,375	2,283,645	17,830,784	26,348,298	48,856	72,185	7.8	1,827,927	3,381	237,488	6,902,570	41,471,977
Albany-Schenectady-Troy	13	2,819	103,099	729,795	1,197,138	1,999	3,281	7.1	94,940	156	8,791	374,985	2,087,292
Binghamton	2	625	28,334	166,428	362,193	456	992	5.9	33,120	65	2,789	86,362	1,232,757
Buffalo-Niagara Falls	14	5,569	161,733	1,417,536	2,133,251	3,883	5,843	8.8	155,539	295	14,198	497,278	2,825,187
Dutchess County	3	647	27,337	175,520	272,186	481	745	6.4	15,019	46	3,025	87,367	604,127
Elmira	2	505	13,980	136,744	236,337	374	647	9.8	10,204	20	1,472	50,763	340,988
Glens Falls	2	499	13,490	111,273	172,526	305	472	8.2	12,267	23	1,484	69,306	465,573
Jamestown	4	590	15,834	134,149	228,956	369	627	8.5	22,412	68	1,380	80,102	433,329
Nassau-Suffolk	26	10,076	378,313	3,181,821	4,397,236	8,716	12,048	8.4	336,943	579	42,144	949,943	4,815,579
New York	78	33,661	1,281,254	9,865,102	14,047,549	27,031	38,490	7.7	908,329	1,571	134,061	3,870,034	21,996,266
Newburgh	5	854	35,207	189,833	325,065	519	890	5.4	32,540	74	4,042	94,241	623,643
Rochester	13	3,155	103,897	785,685	1,448,392	2,154	3,968	7.6	101,288	248	11,333	391,305	3,796,250
Syracuse	9	2,185	84,933	591,463	937,652	1,621	2,567	7.0	80,249	164	9,713	238,888	1,399,721
Utica-Rome	5	1,190	36,234	345,435	589,817	948	1,615	9.5	25,077	72	3,056	111,996	851,265
Pennsylvania	205	42,131	1,808,531	10,395,360	17,050,497	28,578	46,888	5.7	1,578,445	2,563	143,463	4,873,595	32,063,424
Nonmetropolitan	44	5,722	209,156	1,248,914	2,563,099	3,464	7,110	6.0	227,276	438	16,406	773,352	4,883,867
Metropolitan	161	36,409	1,599,375	9,146,446	14,487,398	25,114	39,778	5.7	1,351,169	2,125	127,057	4,100,243	27,179,557
Allentown-Bethlehem-Easton	8	2,019	97,863	528,046	811,784	1,447	2,225	5.4	81,492	118	8,140	288,963	1,567,102
Altoona	5	485	23,823	126,391	240,355	346	658	5.3	30,868	29	2,040	68,597	650,387
Erie	7	1,168	40,562	214,464	317,983	588	871	5.3	24,141	71	3,928	130,464	443,474
Harrisburg-Lebanon-Carlisle	7	1,784	82,056	491,383	726,337	1,405	2,075	6.0	74,411	92	7,419	173,026	1,479,290
Johnstown	6	863	35,551	189,576	356,407	520	976	5.3	52,586	44	2,100	102,348	800,900
Lancaster	5	1,076	45,877	224,102	379,888	614	1,041	4.9	46,635	100	5,058	114,547	1,358,226
Philadelphia	54	13,796	639,877	3,679,870	5,460,332	10,083	14,961	5.8	475,847	910	53,439	1,576,812	10,094,212
Pittsburgh	40	9,576	409,347	2,331,366	3,773,415	6,385	10,336	5.7	352,303	415	25,694	969,920	5,733,044
Reading	3	956	41,164	249,643	424,735	683	1,164	6.1	36,163	62	4,047	115,231	983,144
Scranton--Wilkes-Barre--Hazleton	15	2,621	94,610	621,266	1,044,738	1,702	2,863	6.6	71,124	161	6,935	262,571	1,805,404
Sharon	3	561	23,990	129,411	262,518	354	720	5.4	19,444	43	1,560	81,345	587,782
State College	2	296	10,488	57,589	93,350	157	256	5.5	12,135	5	1,302	34,781	200,074
Williamsport	2	473	14,968	108,205	247,106	296	677	7.2	30,691	22	1,315	68,997	549,892
York	4	735	39,199	195,134	348,450	534	955	5.0	43,329	53	4,080	112,641	926,626

MSAs

U.S. CENSUS DIVISION 2, MIDDLE ATLANTIC

U.S. Community Hospitals
(Nonfederal, short-term general and other special hospitals)

2001 Utilization, Personnel and Finances

FULL-TIME EQUIVALENT PERSONNEL					FULL-TIME EQUIV. TRAINEES			EXPENSES						
								LABOR				TOTAL		
Physicians and Dentists	Registered Nurses	Licensed Practical Nurses	Other Salaried Personnel	Total Personnel	Medical and Dental Residents	Other Trainees	Total Trainees	Payroll (in thousands)	Employee Benefits (in thousands)	Total (in thousands)	Percent of Total	Amount (in thousands)	Adjusted per Admission	Adjusted per Inpatient Day
70,324	958,026	126,252	2,832,672	3,987,274	77,731	5,760	83,491	$162,010,407	$34,697,237	$196,707,646	51.3	$383,734,757	$6,979.53	$1,217.27
8,081	142,404	36,781	476,073	663,339	1,719	697	2,416	22,294,816	5,051,240	27,346,046	53.3	51,353,805	4,803.37	719.31
62,243	815,622	89,471	2,356,599	3,323,935	76,012	5,063	81,075	139,715,591	29,645,998	169,361,600	51.0	332,380,952	7,504.85	1,363.07
16,375	153,381	17,128	466,915	653,799	23,211	474	23,685	28,849,218	6,231,618	35,080,835	53.4	65,738,327	8,094.26	1,215.53
1,101	8,862	2,368	30,768	43,099	368	8	376	1,517,433	320,628	1,838,060	53.8	3,419,578	4,966.74	693.45
15,274	144,519	14,760	436,147	610,700	22,843	466	23,309	27,331,785	5,910,990	33,242,775	53.3	62,318,749	8,383.95	1,267.91
2,577	28,835	2,333	83,105	116,850	2,471	88	2,559	5,331,489	1,123,566	6,455,052	55.1	11,716,951	7,972.04	1,409.15
2,577	28,835	2,333	83,105	116,850	2,471	88	2,559	5,331,489	1,123,566	6,455,052	55.1	11,716,951	7,972.04	1,409.15
46	1,499	119	3,925	5,589	31	3	34	212,512	58,231	270,743	57.1	473,900	6,915.92	1,208.68
292	4,649	142	13,201	18,284	339	4	343	901,041	169,692	1,070,732	55.3	1,935,549	7,189.58	1,576.37
99	1,438	225	4,541	6,303	93	0	93	262,450	57,555	320,005	53.9	593,714	7,408.19	1,311.88
282	3,320	243	9,854	13,699	155	0	155	665,376	124,354	789,730	57.8	1,366,131	8,844.34	1,503.93
287	3,676	349	11,923	16,235	397	9	406	675,990	147,126	823,116	52.8	1,560,002	8,657.39	1,316.12
1,304	8,211	570	22,488	32,573	1,247	62	1,309	1,629,890	353,151	1,983,040	55.7	3,560,994	8,520.57	1,359.95
155	3,984	340	10,534	15,013	147	10	157	617,483	134,185	751,668	52.0	1,444,745	7,656.55	1,553.70
112	1,560	179	5,065	6,916	62	0	62	280,028	52,350	332,377	55.5	598,692	7,301.03	1,339.42
0	498	166	1,574	2,238	0	0	0	86,719	26,922	113,641	62.0	183,224	6,408.00	1,194.27
9,470	73,234	8,580	235,138	326,422	14,371	309	14,680	15,394,344	3,493,894	18,888,238	55.0	34,352,757	9,364.16	1,196.27
475	3,418	999	13,399	18,291	78	4	82	671,687	137,727	809,412	57.2	1,414,346	5,495.85	597.23
8,995	69,816	7,581	221,739	308,131	14,293	305	14,598	14,722,657	3,356,167	18,078,826	54.9	32,938,411	9,656.00	1,250.12
155	3,064	384	9,273	12,876	491	7	498	484,839	94,672	579,512	50.0	1,160,056	6,923.97	969.02
79	714	78	2,914	3,785	74	0	74	147,087	34,115	181,202	50.9	356,073	5,661.66	983.10
306	4,426	630	14,121	19,483	180	5	185	825,357	182,078	1,007,435	53.8	1,871,711	7,403.83	877.40
25	734	32	2,196	2,987	6	0	6	130,639	28,980	159,619	54.0	295,767	7,046.77	1,086.64
47	522	74	1,568	2,211	9	0	9	81,819	16,801	98,620	59.3	166,259	6,683.52	703.48
29	476	54	1,390	1,949	47	6	53	64,981	14,064	79,044	50.7	155,989	7,710.79	904.15
25	503	76	1,467	2,071	15	0	15	64,716	13,277	77,993	56.2	138,836	4,592.20	606.39
1,448	11,605	958	31,515	45,526	1,697	6	1,703	2,353,278	558,341	2,911,618	57.8	5,034,841	9,545.74	1,145.00
5,928	39,193	3,539	129,308	177,968	10,679	269	10,948	9,140,616	2,086,757	11,227,375	54.5	20,587,644	11,153.11	1,465.57
39	868	91	2,531	3,529	11	1	12	151,640	32,286	183,927	58.5	314,212	5,213.74	966.61
748	4,037	756	13,768	19,309	686	5	691	652,558	148,216	800,773	55.3	1,447,941	7,968.72	999.69
105	2,565	656	7,952	11,278	368	6	374	451,169	109,856	561,025	53.7	1,011,007	7,007.00	1,114.38
61	1,100	253	3,736	5,159	30	0	30	173,959	36,725	210,683	57.9	364,184	5,922.75	617.45
4,328	51,312	6,215	148,672	210,527	6,369	77	6,446	8,123,385	1,614,158	9,737,545	49.5	19,668,619	6,592.89	1,153.55
626	5,444	1,369	17,369	24,808	290	4	294	845,745	182,901	1,028,648	51.3	2,005,232	4,650.92	782.35
3,702	45,868	4,846	131,303	185,719	6,079	73	6,152	7,277,639	1,431,257	8,708,897	49.3	17,663,387	6,920.96	1,219.22
201	2,560	242	7,685	10,688	239	0	239	412,887	86,714	499,601	50.3	993,896	6,694.30	1,224.34
26	677	132	1,838	2,673	17	0	17	105,773	21,029	126,802	51.8	244,781	5,160.24	1,018.42
92	1,403	94	3,092	4,681	94	1	95	150,231	31,225	181,456	48.1	377,408	6,261.75	1,186.88
516	2,324	349	8,372	11,561	482	9	491	428,938	80,022	508,962	51.3	991,744	8,129.65	1,365.40
53	1,008	183	3,180	4,424	65	0	65	136,039	26,545	162,583	47.0	345,639	5,130.83	969.79
94	1,051	230	4,000	5,375	61	1	62	221,908	37,768	259,675	51.6	503,107	6,430.47	1,324.36
1,908	18,868	1,393	50,290	72,459	3,234	22	3,256	3,170,201	621,292	3,791,491	49.6	7,636,596	7,957.76	1,308.66
585	11,829	875	31,301	47,590	1,566	27	1,593	1,718,441	321,982	2,040,422	46.5	4,387,146	6,648.46	1,162.65
60	987	186	3,329	4,562	78	0	78	173,172	41,579	214,751	54.7	392,555	5,517.75	924.23
52	2,660	643	7,160	10,515	55	0	55	365,650	82,723	448,374	50.1	894,275	5,434.60	855.98
41	677	104	2,031	2,853	14	0	14	94,012	16,110	110,123	52.0	211,956	4,345.94	807.40
1	229	55	660	945	0	0	0	37,212	9,015	46,228	56.5	81,782	4,660.73	876.08
6	544	77	1,666	2,293	20	0	20	68,469	14,572	83,041	46.8	177,206	1,020.70	717.49
67	1,061	200	3,899	5,100	154	13	167	194,706	40,682	235,388	55.4	425,207	6,003.29	1,220.28

MSAs

U.S. CENSUS DIVISION 3, SOUTH ATLANTIC

U.S. Community Hospitals
(Nonfederal, short-term general and other special hospitals)

2001 Utilization, Personnel and Finances

CLASSIFICATION	Hospitals	Beds	Admissions	Inpatient Days	Adjusted Patient Days	Average Daily Census	Adjusted Average Daily Census	Average Stay (days)	Surgical Operations	NEWBORNS		OUTPATIENT VISITS	
										Bassinets	Births	Emergency	Total
UNITED STATES	4,907	824,676	33,765,589	193,754,932	314,740,801	531,715	863,683	5.7	26,432,095	60,351	3,868,995	105,865,778	536,588,378
Nonmetropolitan	2,166	174,945	5,372,241	35,717,503	71,393,393	97,918	195,777	6.6	4,479,968	13,831	533,148	22,155,102	110,466,485
Metropolitan	2,741	649,731	28,393,348	158,037,429	243,347,408	433,797	667,906	5.6	21,952,127	46,520	3,335,847	83,710,676	426,121,893
CENSUS DIVISION 3, SOUTH ATLANTIC	730	152,052	6,453,744	36,338,028	57,259,963	99,941	157,492	5.6	5,168,553	10,597	694,845	20,100,193	78,526,967
Nonmetropolitan	288	32,640	1,122,394	7,260,223	13,203,205	19,888	36,164	6.5	919,760	2,282	104,986	4,558,055	18,537,204
Metropolitan	442	119,412	5,331,350	29,077,805	44,056,758	80,053	121,328	5.5	4,248,793	8,315	589,859	15,542,138	59,989,763
Delaware	5	1,853	83,047	502,238	803,839	1,376	2,203	6.0	81,663	112	11,286	268,517	1,484,918
Nonmetropolitan	2	447	14,284	126,228	238,132	346	652	8.8	11,579	25	1,616	54,152	370,083
Metropolitan	3	1,406	68,763	376,010	565,707	1,030	1,551	5.5	70,084	87	9,670	214,365	1,114,835
Dover	1	364	16,814	85,448	149,476	234	410	5.1	18,552	29	2,033	60,007	343,878
Wilmington-Newark	2	1,042	51,949	290,562	416,231	796	1,141	5.6	51,532	58	7,637	154,358	770,957
District of Columbia	10	3,372	131,906	903,469	1,235,917	2,474	3,385	6.8	98,280	198	12,583	337,851	1,419,048
Metropolitan	10	3,372	131,906	903,469	1,235,917	2,474	3,385	6.8	98,280	198	12,583	337,851	1,419,048
Washington	10	3,372	131,906	903,469	1,235,917	2,474	3,385	6.8	98,280	198	12,583	337,851	1,419,048
Florida	202	51,762	2,207,147	11,521,025	16,947,444	31,918	46,974	5.2	1,517,602	2,871	204,753	5,879,596	20,770,794
Nonmetropolitan	32	2,576	100,835	495,100	833,494	1,357	2,282	4.9	81,291	118	6,585	411,538	1,399,980
Metropolitan	170	49,186	2,106,312	11,025,925	16,113,950	30,561	44,692	5.2	1,436,311	2,753	198,168	5,468,058	19,370,814
Daytona Beach	7	1,657	62,490	286,981	465,153	786	1,275	4.6	43,628	60	3,955	235,005	831,904
Fort Lauderdale	17	5,072	205,369	1,065,227	1,553,643	2,920	4,256	5.2	117,418	227	20,408	575,226	1,825,822
Fort Myers-Cape Coral	5	1,788	72,253	355,423	542,237	1,232	1,889	4.9	53,202	104	7,490	146,731	604,174
Fort Pierce-Port St. Lucie	3	833	40,982	205,336	292,728	563	802	5.0	34,280	66	3,497	112,044	228,412
Fort Walton Beach	3	415	19,268	88,561	132,922	243	364	4.6	17,733	34	1,658	57,137	236,260
Gainesville	4	1,144	54,184	305,455	424,186	837	1,162	5.6	38,129	68	5,281	117,539	794,538
Jacksonville	10	3,233	137,376	713,285	1,094,118	2,047	3,143	5.2	119,509	242	15,451	449,262	1,350,429
Lakeland-Winter Haven	4	1,476	66,686	355,596	508,568	974	1,393	5.3	36,454	80	5,841	215,724	315,261
Melbourne-Titusville-Palm Bay	5	1,188	59,160	285,947	446,981	782	1,224	4.8	25,438	109	3,970	173,670	657,403
Miami	27	8,236	324,065	2,029,114	2,884,044	5,561	7,902	6.3	194,375	428	30,623	647,524	2,712,909
Naples	1	492	30,767	143,251	180,890	392	496	4.7	13,113	24	3,081	120,411	274,804
Ocala	2	533	35,250	161,251	226,869	442	621	4.6	22,221	40	2,434	106,225	186,651
Orlando	12	5,318	253,159	1,307,488	1,942,795	3,583	5,323	5.2	168,090	353	28,952	749,106	2,231,330
Panama City	2	547	22,266	103,913	159,144	284	436	4.7	17,730	44	2,410	75,882	239,463
Pensacola	6	1,634	58,969	319,110	478,310	874	1,310	5.4	42,173	67	5,012	180,609	886,184
Punta Gorda	3	722	25,694	119,518	176,482	328	483	4.7	23,765	10	1,075	50,179	193,020
Sarasota-Bradenton	7	2,140	86,574	472,736	645,426	1,297	1,768	5.5	49,611	75	5,725	223,697	739,184
Tallahassee	4	865	36,640	218,870	319,953	599	877	6.0	30,159	65	4,833	92,296	355,658
Tampa-St. Petersburg-Clearwater	33	8,471	352,934	1,723,596	2,512,092	4,720	6,880	4.9	254,796	450	31,910	787,899	3,410,112
West Palm Beach-Boca Raton	15	3,422	162,226	765,267	1,127,409	2,097	3,088	4.7	134,487	207	14,562	351,892	1,297,296
Georgia	147	24,113	903,663	5,484,805	9,295,145	15,064	25,542	6.1	781,897	2,039	130,673	3,149,115	12,015,054
Nonmetropolitan	83	9,106	251,138	1,918,757	3,524,096	5,253	9,650	7.6	208,247	625	30,465	999,790	3,883,894
Metropolitan	64	15,007	652,525	3,566,048	5,771,049	9,811	15,892	5.5	573,650	1,414	100,208	2,149,325	8,131,160
Albany	2	574	22,949	123,714	186,124	339	510	5.4	16,284	66	2,816	111,969	571,385
Athens	2	617	23,895	148,420	266,296	407	730	6.2	30,019	36	3,141	84,949	279,337
Atlanta	36	8,657	415,824	2,130,784	3,423,310	5,877	9,458	5.1	339,275	874	71,743	1,315,072	4,555,877
Augusta-Aiken	6	1,404	53,751	305,489	473,186	838	1,297	5.7	55,082	99	6,926	186,090	973,572
Chattanooga	2	307	6,876	79,423	155,038	217	425	11.6	9,311	15	927	36,411	114,101
Columbus	4	1,025	30,728	196,364	328,899	538	901	6.4	26,938	104	3,555	112,800	265,947
Macon	8	1,336	54,006	281,631	445,621	772	1,221	5.2	58,649	137	6,007	171,219	785,175
Savannah	4	1,087	44,496	300,223	492,575	823	1,350	6.7	38,092	83	5,093	130,815	585,766
Maryland	49	11,234	608,165	2,981,003	4,460,783	8,166	12,220	4.9	513,858	962	63,843	1,854,562	6,266,389
Nonmetropolitan	9	890	48,712	211,279	372,559	578	1,020	4.3	40,370	74	4,474	190,414	1,338,928
Metropolitan	40	10,344	559,453	2,769,724	4,088,224	7,588	11,200	5.0	473,488	888	59,369	1,664,148	4,927,461
Baltimore	23	6,690	362,517	1,823,597	2,630,429	4,996	7,205	5.0	311,149	508	33,756	1,033,418	2,892,613
Cumberland	2	422	16,759	108,483	210,120	297	576	6.5	9,232	12	1,053	56,331	328,030
Hagerstown	1	309	15,928	72,952	142,993	200	392	4.6	9,643	41	1,685	61,939	207,223
Washington	13	2,817	156,955	737,303	1,060,007	2,020	2,905	4.7	136,559	315	22,243	484,161	1,360,311
Wilmington-Newark	1	106	7,294	27,309	44,675	75	122	3.8	6,905	12	632	28,299	139,284

Table continues

MSAs

TABLE 8

U.S. CENSUS DIVISION 3, SOUTH ATLANTIC

U.S. Community Hospitals
(Nonfederal, short-term general and other special hospitals)

2001 Utilization, Personnel and Finances

FULL-TIME EQUIVALENT PERSONNEL					FULL-TIME EQUIV. TRAINEES			EXPENSES						
								LABOR				TOTAL		
Physicians and Dentists	Registered Nurses	Licensed Practical Nurses	Other Salaried Personnel	Total Personnel	Medical and Dental Residents	Other Trainees	Total Trainees	Payroll (in thousands)	Employee Benefits (in thousands)	Total (in thousands)	Percent of Total	Amount (in thousands)	Adjusted per Admission	Adjusted per Inpatient Day
70,153	956,577	126,143	2,828,126	3,980,999	77,440	5,751	83,191	$161,734,716	$34,640,089	$196,374,807	51.3	$383,082,895	$6,976.34	$1,217.14
8,081	142,404	36,781	476,073	663,339	1,719	697	2,416	22,294,816	5,051,240	27,346,046	53.3	51,353,805	4,803.37	719.31
62,072	814,173	89,362	2,352,053	3,317,660	75,721	5,054	80,775	139,439,900	29,588,849	169,028,761	51.0	331,729,090	7,501.70	1,363.19
9,461	182,434	22,499	501,033	715,427	11,386	717	12,103	27,873,562	5,825,461	33,699,030	50.7	66,532,757	6,542.46	1,161.94
1,087	29,293	6,918	91,502	128,800	479	88	567	4,271,842	982,210	5,254,052	52.7	9,968,847	4,863.51	755.03
8,374	153,141	15,581	409,531	586,627	10,907	629	11,536	23,601,720	4,843,251	28,444,978	50.3	56,563,910	6,966.30	1,283.89
207	2,820	210	7,979	11,216	217	0	217	491,038	128,758	619,796	59.1	1,049,014	7,971.78	1,305.01
7	462	59	1,348	1,876	0	0	0	75,344	17,299	92,643	57.2	161,988	5,958.30	680.25
200	2,358	151	6,631	9,340	217	0	217	415,694	111,459	527,153	59.4	887,026	8,496.09	1,568.00
10	496	55	1,491	2,052	0	0	0	78,807	25,003	103,810	60.4	171,748	5,839.18	1,149.00
190	1,862	96	5,140	7,288	217	0	217	336,888	86,456	423,343	59.2	715,278	9,538.19	1,718.46
1,086	4,577	292	13,576	19,531	991	104	1,095	1,048,122	160,929	1,209,051	56.0	2,157,226	11,773.26	1,745.45
1,086	4,577	292	13,576	19,531	991	104	1,095	1,048,122	160,929	1,209,051	56.0	2,157,226	11,773.26	1,745.45
1,086	4,577	292	13,576	19,531	991	104	1,095	1,048,122	160,929	1,209,051	56.0	2,157,226	11,773.26	1,745.45
2,093	55,402	7,003	152,011	216,509	2,786	118	2,904	8,434,984	1,789,247	10,224,232	49.9	20,475,866	6,257.98	1,208.20
71	2,203	493	6,519	9,286	4	17	21	331,772	73,430	405,205	51.6	785,490	4,598.46	942.41
2,022	53,199	6,510	145,492	207,223	2,782	101	2,883	8,103,212	1,715,816	9,819,027	49.9	19,690,376	6,349.39	1,221.95
76	1,229	194	3,807	5,306	48	3	51	224,709	49,520	274,231	51.0	537,931	5,278.85	1,156.46
173	4,828	565	12,207	17,773	56	1	57	733,484	142,967	876,450	49.0	1,788,883	5,941.12	1,151.41
130	1,684	244	5,591	7,649	15	0	15	285,714	51,038	336,752	52.7	638,951	5,812.88	1,178.36
11	969	89	2,277	3,346	4	0	4	136,424	32,982	169,406	50.9	332,580	5,669.91	1,136.14
10	415	99	982	1,506	2	0	2	50,208	10,760	60,968	47.8	127,543	4,314.15	959.54
19	1,645	163	4,688	6,515	10	0	10	233,230	51,105	284,334	44.1	645,215	8,617.57	1,521.07
133	4,606	288	11,673	16,700	196	8	204	545,188	136,496	681,684	48.4	1,407,474	6,582.21	1,286.40
19	1,361	272	4,345	5,997	0	17	17	204,814	43,381	248,195	52.2	475,830	4,968.47	935.63
82	1,067	110	4,075	5,334	98	6	104	241,422	49,503	290,924	53.5	543,404	5,841.24	1,215.72
433	8,900	1,019	23,698	34,050	1,500	29	1,529	1,536,887	310,085	1,846,973	50.1	3,683,470	7,819.30	1,277.19
0	755	80	1,745	2,580	0	0	0	108,721	22,193	130,914	50.4	259,939	6,690.66	1,437.00
0	810	34	1,916	2,760	0	0	0	110,717	24,328	135,046	50.2	268,833	5,417.29	1,184.97
241	7,630	872	19,965	28,708	235	9	244	1,051,806	257,359	1,309,166	52.5	2,493,429	6,654.57	1,283.42
1	452	97	1,554	2,104	0	0	0	79,344	18,588	97,932	49.4	198,105	5,844.32	1,244.82
90	1,544	233	4,191	6,058	0	0	0	198,431	37,378	235,808	47.1	500,306	5,656.18	1,045.99
20	529	76	1,393	2,018	13	2	15	82,957	19,965	102,921	50.0	205,705	5,425.85	1,165.59
29	2,082	361	5,444	7,916	7	0	7	296,549	63,824	360,373	47.6	756,579	6,408.65	1,172.22
53	967	190	2,964	4,174	30	0	30	165,300	28,599	193,899	55.4	350,136	6,588.68	1,094.33
411	8,828	1,147	24,753	35,139	491	23	514	1,282,083	264,205	1,546,287	48.1	3,217,719	6,229.97	1,280.89
91	2,898	377	8,224	11,590	77	3	80	535,225	101,539	636,764	50.6	1,258,346	5,236.50	1,116.14
1,170	28,326	4,502	77,395	111,393	985	136	1,121	4,123,868	890,062	5,013,929	51.0	9,839,984	6,507.71	1,058.62
284	7,132	2,203	23,215	32,834	133	39	172	1,015,674	236,764	1,252,435	52.5	2,385,964	5,120.61	677.04
886	21,194	2,299	54,180	78,559	852	97	949	3,108,194	653,298	3,761,494	50.5	7,454,021	7,125.55	1,291.62
40	720	82	2,066	2,007	74	7	81	117,087	24,470	141,556	50.6	270,682	8,150.80	1,502.66
2	851	50	2,295	3,198	0	0	0	132,721	19,039	151,760	58.1	261,316	6,361.78	981.30
310	13,250	1,193	32,277	47,030	131	72	203	1,917,492	394,762	2,312,254	49.7	4,656,659	6,993.36	1,360.28
380	2,071	381	5,005	7,897	400	0	400	285,887	74,739	360,626	51.2	704,627	8,329.81	1,489.11
2	237	84	856	1,179	0	0	0	40,466	9,379	49,845	56.0	89,064	6,625.30	574.47
2	942	150	2,799	3,893	38	0	38	121,513	27,522	149,035	47.8	312,024	6,197.83	948.69
25	1,672	196	4,848	6,741	111	0	111	258,714	60,445	319,160	53.2	600,085	6,878.72	1,346.63
125	1,442	163	3,984	5,714	98	18	116	234,314	42,944	277,258	50.4	550,563	7,953.35	1,117.72
1,564	15,595	758	47,579	65,496	1,332	167	1,499	2,696,835	495,127	3,191,961	50.3	6,345,349	6,935.37	1,422.47
54	953	108	3,964	5,079	0	2	2	183,393	40,527	223,920	50.3	445,300	5,155.60	1,195.25
1,510	14,042	650	40,615	60,417	1,002	105	1,407	2,510,442	454,000	2,000,041	50.0	5,000,040	7,120.00	1,440.10
1,412	10,229	405	30,138	42,184	1,280	165	1,445	1,735,833	305,122	2,040,955	49.5	4,125,802	7,846.41	1,568.49
18	484	36	1,275	1,813	0	0	0	67,164	17,859	85,023	57.5	147,862	4,584.59	703.70
9	364	43	1,315	1,731	0	0	0	74,217	17,860	92,077	60.9	151,079	4,839.18	1,056.55
66	3,433	155	10,333	13,987	52	0	52	613,824	108,987	722,812	50.9	1,420,299	6,246.78	1,339.90
5	132	11	554	702	0	0	0	22,403	4,771	27,174	49.4	55,007	4,623.62	1,231.27

Table continues

U.S. CENSUS DIVISION 3, SOUTH ATLANTIC CONTINUED

U.S. Community Hospitals
(Nonfederal, short-term general and other special hospitals)

2001 Utilization, Personnel and Finances

CLASSIFICATION	Hospitals	Beds	Admissions	Inpatient Days	Adjusted Patient Days	Average Daily Census	Adjusted Average Daily Census	Average Stay (days)	Surgical Operations	NEWBORNS Bassinets	NEWBORNS Births	OUTPATIENT VISITS Emergency	OUTPATIENT VISITS Total
North Carolina	111	23,755	973,451	5,959,143	9,840,634	16,330	26,961	6.1	749,805	1,581	110,585	3,230,198	13,430,676
Nonmetropolitan	61	8,001	286,209	1,912,673	3,548,520	5,244	9,722	6.7	219,944	597	27,912	1,152,556	4,385,018
Metropolitan	50	15,754	687,242	4,046,470	6,292,114	11,086	17,239	5.9	529,861	984	82,673	2,077,642	9,045,658
Asheville	2	801	39,083	210,199	292,365	576	801	5.4	38,174	30	3,599	97,431	474,277
Charlotte-Gastonia-Rock Hill	12	3,737	156,953	910,759	1,492,976	2,494	4,090	5.8	123,474	258	21,301	541,716	2,151,213
Fayetteville	1	537	27,647	166,017	240,095	455	658	6.0	26,724	48	3,930	91,898	366,119
Goldsboro	1	270	11,490	62,817	93,170	172	255	5.5	11,858	30	1,512	40,419	129,190
Greensboro—Winston-Salem—High Point	12	4,140	159,566	1,030,549	1,626,369	2,824	4,456	6.5	107,277	204	18,312	456,110	1,414,914
Greenville	1	731	32,263	199,913	255,565	548	700	6.2	17,612	42	3,477	55,620	249,667
Hickory-Morganton-Lenoir	5	1,085	37,081	272,076	472,142	745	1,294	7.3	33,537	82	4,259	177,740	804,522
Jacksonville	1	133	9,734	33,985	65,695	93	180	3.5	6,059	23	393	35,648	223,454
Raleigh-Durham-Chapel Hill	10	3,166	158,032	873,315	1,303,346	2,392	3,570	5.5	120,731	191	19,957	408,272	2,512,652
Rocky Mount	2	408	19,282	100,314	161,972	275	444	5.2	12,922	30	2,119	73,702	260,246
Wilmington	3	746	36,111	186,526	288,419	512	791	5.2	31,493	46	3,814	99,086	459,404
South Carolina	62	11,282	505,294	2,940,707	4,564,565	8,058	12,504	5.8	435,354	853	50,304	1,840,819	7,629,295
Nonmetropolitan	27	3,364	122,903	797,669	1,346,546	2,188	3,690	6.5	99,296	305	12,361	537,766	1,294,657
Metropolitan	35	7,918	382,391	2,143,038	3,218,019	5,870	8,814	5.6	336,058	548	37,943	1,303,053	6,334,638
Augusta-Aiken	2	309	12,600	56,525	83,940	155	230	4.5	7,897	18	1,031	58,245	62,638
Charleston-North Charleston	7	1,690	79,734	433,330	642,422	1,188	1,759	5.4	82,916	112	8,680	248,602	1,251,014
Charlotte-Gastonia-Rock Hill	1	276	14,680	63,980	91,416	175	250	4.4	13,241	25	1,628	50,803	130,070
Columbia	5	1,554	82,097	455,945	651,050	1,249	1,783	5.6	58,678	105	8,539	209,750	1,527,824
Florence	4	788	37,738	218,906	315,522	599	864	5.8	30,631	24	2,010	144,715	1,097,253
Greenville-Spartanburg-Anderson	12	2,493	120,399	684,401	1,054,578	1,874	2,889	5.7	109,063	183	12,387	428,290	1,777,616
Myrtle Beach	3	618	27,131	170,849	279,445	468	766	6.3	25,771	46	2,523	117,588	329,979
Sumter	1	190	8,012	59,102	99,646	162	273	7.4	7,861	35	1,145	45,060	158,244
Virginia	87	16,775	743,992	4,239,227	6,896,034	11,610	18,896	5.7	703,536	1,478	90,043	2,482,380	9,748,533
Nonmetropolitan	35	4,140	155,442	868,743	1,568,323	2,378	4,298	5.6	131,176	300	12,274	617,247	2,723,102
Metropolitan	52	12,635	588,550	3,370,484	5,327,711	9,232	14,598	5.7	572,360	1,178	77,769	1,865,133	7,025,431
Charlottesville	2	700	36,967	183,823	318,896	503	873	5.0	50,035	54	3,033	91,970	857,905
Danville	1	203	11,427	65,036	101,062	178	277	5.7	8,656	20	1,154	25,868	130,727
Johnson City-Kingsport-Bristol	1	135	5,338	21,511	45,702	59	125	4.0	8,582	12	726	30,436	91,985
Lynchburg	3	834	22,161	231,857	360,416	635	988	10.5	18,489	48	2,724	77,450	174,357
Norfolk-Virginia Beach-Newport News	16	3,418	152,986	927,296	1,546,368	2,539	4,238	6.1	147,698	289	19,444	584,779	2,189,931
Richmond-Petersburg	12	3,390	138,668	825,662	1,263,816	2,263	3,463	6.0	145,484	244	14,702	403,426	1,802,769
Roanoke	2	1,160	49,147	296,354	415,408	812	1,138	6.0	49,615	107	3,804	131,148	362,610
Washington	15	2,795	171,856	818,945	1,276,043	2,243	3,496	4.8	143,801	404	32,182	520,056	1,415,147
West Virginia	57	7,906	297,079	1,806,411	3,215,602	4,945	8,807	6.1	286,558	503	20,775	1,057,155	5,762,260
Nonmetropolitan	39	4,116	142,871	929,774	1,771,535	2,544	4,850	6.5	127,857	238	9,299	594,592	3,141,542
Metropolitan	18	3,790	154,208	876,637	1,444,067	2,401	3,957	5.7	158,701	265	11,476	462,563	2,620,718
Charleston	5	1,238	54,707	308,349	483,136	845	1,323	5.6	64,776	72	3,944	130,172	807,716
Cumberland	1	38	1,661	5,885	14,263	16	39	3.5	1,889	0	0	9,302	44,669
Huntington-Ashland	3	729	33,198	173,789	248,591	476	681	5.2	28,709	55	2,941	100,273	427,625
Parkersburg-Marietta	3	561	23,462	129,752	216,924	356	595	5.5	21,411	40	1,586	76,536	452,395
Steubenville-Weirton	1	238	7,987	40,434	81,590	111	224	5.1	5,589	21	348	27,402	188,238
Washington	2	214	9,880	48,715	94,079	133	258	4.9	11,633	21	1,067	53,926	183,592
Wheeling	3	772	23,313	169,713	305,484	464	837	7.3	24,694	56	1,590	64,952	516,483

TABLE 8

U.S. CENSUS DIVISION 3, SOUTH ATLANTIC CONTINUED

U.S. Community Hospitals
(Nonfederal, short-term general and other special hospitals)

2001 Utilization, Personnel and Finances

FULL-TIME EQUIVALENT PERSONNEL					FULL-TIME EQUIV. TRAINEES			EXPENSES						
								LABOR				TOTAL		
Physicians and Dentists	Registered Nurses	Licensed Practical Nurses	Other Salaried Personnel	Total Personnel	Medical and Dental Residents	Other Trainees	Total Trainees	Payroll (in thousands)	Employee Benefits (in thousands)	Total (in thousands)	Percent of Total	Amount (in thousands)	Adjusted per Admission	Adjusted per Inpatient Day
1,221	31,324	2,738	83,855	119,138	2,114	111	2,225	4,621,118	976,642	5,597,766	52.7	10,625,022	6,600.67	1,079.71
240	8,016	1,241	24,074	33,571	20	20	40	1,114,207	243,571	1,357,781	53.8	2,523,865	4,762.24	711.24
981	23,308	1,497	59,781	85,567	2,094	91	2,185	3,506,911	733,071	4,239,985	52.3	8,101,157	7,503.06	1,287.51
24	1,271	101	3,368	4,764	0	0	0	204,526	39,995	244,521	59.0	414,676	7,485.53	1,418.35
560	5,410	221	13,925	20,116	222	0	222	839,208	180,737	1,019,947	50.2	2,029,775	7,626.32	1,359.55
44	677	121	2,497	3,339	0	0	0	142,240	34,160	176,400	53.8	327,589	8,193.21	1,364.41
0	291	32	907	1,230	0	0	0	45,468	8,910	54,379	56.5	96,291	5,650.24	1,033.50
157	5,313	420	14,628	20,518	601	70	671	748,782	162,163	910,946	54.7	1,664,223	6,589.16	1,023.28
0	1,057	44	3,197	4,298	280	0	280	179,921	37,579	217,500	52.0	418,594	10,149.21	1,637.92
60	1,256	138	3,238	4,692	13	2	15	157,826	32,982	190,808	52.5	363,267	5,653.09	769.40
5	196	5	557	763	0	0	0	29,573	6,380	35,953	43.1	83,485	4,436.89	1,270.79
118	6,208	286	13,064	19,676	921	19	940	913,806	179,603	1,093,408	50.8	2,152,412	9,093.61	1,651.45
6	511	23	1,487	2,027	0	0	0	76,033	16,973	93,007	57.9	160,626	5,163.16	991.69
7	1,118	106	2,913	4,144	57	0	57	169,527	33,588	203,116	52.1	390,219	6,913.50	1,352.96
657	14,354	1,999	38,173	55,183	1,092	8	1,100	2,041,611	430,648	2,472,258	47.4	5,211,815	6,621.10	1,141.80
85	2,867	767	9,416	13,135	40	2	42	407,794	93,997	501,790	49.7	1,009,473	4,846.62	749.68
572	11,487	1,232	28,757	42,048	1,052	6	1,058	1,633,817	336,651	1,970,468	46.9	4,202,342	7,259.59	1,305.88
0	272	58	490	820	0	0	0	41,088	4,730	45,818	39.7	115,280	6,123.45	1,373.36
4	2,540	230	5,018	7,792	561	0	561	360,368	78,288	400,055	42.9	1,022,709	8,556.87	1,591.96
0	403	11	801	1,215	0	0	0	43,271	10,690	53,960	38.8	139,178	6,635.44	1,522.47
97	2,586	239	6,429	9,351	210	0	210	348,537	71,257	419,796	48.4	866,980	7,262.78	1,331.66
42	921	150	2,780	3,893	77	6	83	139,205	30,401	169,605	47.6	356,201	6,339.34	1,128.93
417	3,749	353	10,696	15,215	204	0	204	579,779	120,029	699,809	49.5	1,414,702	7,525.53	1,341.49
12	795	161	1,723	2,691	0	0	0	72,977	10,967	83,945	47.4	177,056	4,166.91	633.60
0	221	30	820	1,071	0	0	0	48,590	10,289	58,880	53.4	110,236	8,160.82	1,106.28
1,136	21,524	3,120	57,067	82,847	1,426	54	1,480	3,253,292	645,431	3,898,724	49.0	7,961,020	6,477.55	1,154.43
136	4,001	891	11,607	16,635	19	5	24	600,569	131,925	732,492	54.0	1,355,864	4,687.29	864.53
1,000	17,523	2,229	45,460	66,212	1,407	49	1,456	2,652,723	513,506	3,166,232	47.9	6,605,156	7,028.61	1,239.77
615	1,645	204	5,426	7,890	676	0	676	248,722	54,186	302,908	47.5	638,187	9,645.54	2,001.24
17	283	32	881	1,213	12	0	12	49,768	10,564	60,331	52.3	115,447	6,501.48	1,142.34
12	205	49	374	640	0	0	0	18,776	4,773	23,549	49.7	47,389	4,178.56	1,036.91
9	946	77	2,027	3,059	2	0	2	114,175	24,127	138,303	51.4	268,901	7,909.31	746.09
71	4,105	667	12,818	17,661	68	0	68	663,125	114,532	777,659	47.3	1,644,541	6,401.31	1,063.49
68	4,076	682	9,292	14,118	459	32	491	569,619	113,910	683,530	44.8	1,525,238	7,113.62	1,206.85
90	1,554	202	3,574	5,420	129	0	129	266,738	54,399	321,137	53.0	605,517	8,770.78	1,457.64
118	4,709	316	11,068	16,211	61	17	78	721,800	137,016	858,815	48.8	1,759,936	6,514.98	1,379.21
327	8,512	1,877	23,398	34,114	443	19	462	1,162,694	308,618	1,471,313	51.3	2,867,459	5,412.78	891.73
210	3,659	1,156	11,359	16,384	263	3	266	543,089	144,697	687,786	52.9	1,300,904	4,784.97	734.34
117	4,853	721	12,039	17,730	180	16	196	619,606	163,921	783,527	50.0	1,566,555	6,074.65	1,084.82
34	1,969	191	4,581	6,775	135	0	135	237,040	63,240	300,281	46.5	645,899	7,449.81	1,336.89
0	40	10	149	199	0	0	0	4,991	1,059	6,050	42.8	14,149	3,514.40	992.00
1	990	171	2,142	3,304	0	0	0	124,771	37,887	162,659	62.3	310,701	8,421.27	1,249.97
2	547	140	1,560	2,257	0	15	15	72,000	19,000	91,935	49.9	184,187	4,596.52	849.09
11	241	23	651	926	0	0	0	31,475	6,318	37,793	55.9	67,610	4,104.94	828.65
8	224	47	779	1,058	0	0	0	40,276	10,931	51,209	55.3	92,583	4,806.01	984.10
61	842	131	2,177	3,211	45	1	46	108,184	25,416	133,600	53.1	251,396	5,803.91	822.94

MSAs

TABLE 8

U.S. CENSUS DIVISION 4, EAST NORTH CENTRAL

U.S. Community Hospitals
(Nonfederal, short-term general and other special hospitals)

2001 Utilization, Personnel and Finances

CLASSIFICATION	Hospitals	Beds	Admissions	Inpatient Days	Adjusted Patient Days	Average Daily Census	Adjusted Average Daily Census	Average Stay (days)	Surgical Operations	NEWBORNS		OUTPATIENT VISITS	
										Bassinets	Births	Emergency	Total
UNITED STATES	4,907	824,676	33,765,589	193,754,932	314,740,801	531,715	863,683	5.7	26,432,095	60,351	3,868,995	105,865,778	536,588,378
Nonmetropolitan	2,166	174,945	5,372,241	35,717,503	71,393,393	97,918	195,777	6.6	4,479,968	13,831	533,148	22,155,102	110,466,485
Metropolitan	2,741	649,731	28,393,348	158,037,429	243,347,408	433,797	667,906	5.6	21,952,127	46,520	3,335,847	83,710,676	426,121,893
CENSUS DIVISION 4, EAST NORTH CENTRAL	734	130,407	5,418,071	29,208,239	51,807,036	80,136	142,071	5.4	4,484,800	10,363	600,441	17,712,357	105,053,844
Nonmetropolitan	294	25,657	796,776	4,964,288	11,486,986	13,601	31,463	6.2	737,174	2,191	82,511	3,591,132	20,135,183
Metropolitan	440	104,750	4,621,295	24,243,951	40,320,050	66,535	110,608	5.2	3,747,626	8,172	517,930	14,121,225	84,918,661
Illinois	192	36,834	1,559,357	8,215,380	13,367,705	22,627	36,774	5.3	1,124,467	2,843	173,967	4,582,408	25,269,913
Nonmetropolitan	72	6,632	190,314	1,250,645	2,553,909	3,432	6,992	6.6	151,881	458	16,178	783,362	4,149,871
Metropolitan	120	30,202	1,369,043	6,964,735	10,813,796	19,195	29,782	5.1	972,586	2,385	157,789	3,799,046	21,120,042
Bloomington-Normal	2	399	16,588	71,093	117,940	195	323	4.3	13,934	33	2,256	53,742	231,216
Champaign-Urbana	2	667	25,166	160,566	209,429	440	573	6.4	18,123	50	3,260	77,027	178,269
Chicago	84	22,021	1,053,568	5,248,313	7,990,504	14,492	22,048	5.0	694,557	1,801	124,956	2,797,009	15,679,667
Davenport-Moline-Rock Island	4	641	27,544	130,000	233,831	356	641	4.7	19,543	83	2,476	83,516	469,475
Decatur	2	522	20,211	104,193	224,820	286	616	5.2	20,708	34	1,736	64,000	366,591
Kankakee	2	607	17,893	127,231	198,945	349	545	7.1	18,794	41	1,720	69,408	445,002
Peoria-Pekin	5	1,241	51,570	282,249	471,826	773	1,292	5.5	53,930	74	5,227	148,295	1,511,264
Rockford	5	984	43,391	219,505	343,394	601	941	5.1	29,998	71	5,151	133,421	424,504
Springfield	3	1,108	46,061	254,268	367,353	696	1,006	5.5	41,237	60	3,877	110,707	604,424
St. Louis	11	2,012	67,051	367,317	655,754	1,007	1,797	5.5	61,762	138	7,130	261,921	1,209,630
Indiana	110	19,036	718,369	3,944,457	6,913,082	10,802	18,940	5.5	581,910	1,538	80,485	2,385,242	14,393,285
Nonmetropolitan	46	3,824	134,867	630,950	1,403,952	1,728	3,848	4.7	128,641	420	15,418	667,491	3,592,756
Metropolitan	64	15,212	583,502	3,313,507	5,509,130	9,074	15,092	5.7	453,269	1,118	65,067	1,717,751	10,800,529
Bloomington	1	811	17,687	222,442	316,614	609	867	12.6	8,808	40	2,041	52,155	309,786
Cincinnati	1	87	4,015	16,890	43,370	46	119	4.2	6,082	10	517	17,836	106,791
Elkhart-Goshen	2	450	19,421	92,174	156,797	252	430	4.7	11,408	39	3,201	70,875	599,979
Evansville-Henderson	4	1,143	40,506	227,747	347,921	624	953	5.6	18,369	47	3,588	108,889	510,843
Fort Wayne	9	1,551	64,445	352,289	586,686	964	1,606	5.5	45,715	134	7,767	191,858	869,986
Gary	8	2,530	95,668	512,317	801,555	1,403	2,196	5.4	56,372	231	8,098	219,951	1,179,876
Indianapolis	19	5,285	210,380	1,201,227	2,046,100	3,292	5,605	5.7	167,598	359	23,336	594,432	5,083,337
Kokomo	4	454	14,370	97,206	190,504	266	523	6.8	17,802	37	1,682	73,975	398,114
Lafayette	2	503	19,159	93,531	161,403	256	442	4.9	15,783	34	3,233	76,073	286,095
Louisville	6	668	25,477	136,487	267,486	373	732	5.4	31,858	51	2,643	102,162	455,471
Muncie	1	415	17,626	85,944	146,919	235	403	4.9	18,545	20	1,600	46,254	302,149
South Bend	3	754	31,648	158,112	247,314	433	678	5.0	33,532	57	5,011	93,583	243,926
Terre Haute	4	561	23,100	117,141	196,461	321	538	5.1	21,397	59	2,350	69,708	454,176
Michigan	145	25,630	1,122,004	6,108,896	11,824,789	16,736	32,397	5.4	1,023,833	1,975	126,846	3,753,945	25,984,089
Nonmetropolitan	59	4,648	147,757	941,280	2,734,052	2,572	7,492	6.4	167,102	381	15,589	702,158	4,787,363
Metropolitan	86	20,982	974,247	5,167,616	9,090,737	14,164	24,905	5.3	856,731	1,594	111,257	3,051,787	21,196,726
Ann Arbor	8	1,555	82,466	427,907	784,817	1,173	2,150	5.2	84,297	95	9,315	241,556	2,819,396
Benton Harbor	2	421	17,041	74,919	142,386	206	390	4.4	13,764	51	2,148	70,766	373,360
Detroit	41	10,409	506,352	2,606,570	4,426,298	7,143	12,127	5.1	433,220	793	54,579	1,559,980	10,095,853
Flint	3	1,281	64,685	322,909	517,488	885	1,418	5.0	39,547	103	6,869	196,131	1,571,457
Grand Rapids-Muskegon-Holland	11	2,587	115,350	600,611	1,120,662	1,645	3,069	5.2	111,077	295	17,834	357,631	2,030,932
Jackson	2	472	17,917	85,276	185,001	234	507	4.8	14,093	24	1,993	64,777	361,366
Kalamazoo-Battle Creek	8	1,441	55,218	334,512	631,978	918	1,732	6.1	51,425	107	7,116	207,358	1,291,402
Lansing-East Lansing	5	1,132	47,336	302,921	619,659	831	1,698	6.4	42,156	56	5,943	184,859	1,313,347
Saginaw-Bay City-Midland	6	1,684	67,882	411,991	662,448	1,129	1,814	6.1	67,152	70	5,460	168,729	1,339,613

Table continues

TABLE 8

U.S. CENSUS DIVISION 4, EAST NORTH CENTRAL

U.S. Community Hospitals
(Nonfederal, short-term general and other special hospitals)

2001 Utilization, Personnel and Finances

FULL-TIME EQUIVALENT PERSONNEL					FULL-TIME EQUIV. TRAINEES			EXPENSES						
								LABOR				TOTAL		
Physicians and Dentists	Registered Nurses	Licensed Practical Nurses	Other Salaried Personnel	Total Personnel	Medical and Dental Residents	Other Trainees	Total Trainees	Payroll (in thousands)	Employee Benefits (in thousands)	Total (in thousands)	Percent of Total	Amount (in thousands)	Adjusted per Admission	Adjusted per Inpatient Day
70,153	956,577	126,143	2,828,126	3,980,999	77,440	5,751	83,191	$161,734,716	$34,640,089	$196,374,807	51.3	$383,082,895	$6,976.34	$1,217.14
8,081	142,404	36,781	476,073	663,339	1,719	697	2,416	22,294,816	5,051,240	27,346,046	53.3	51,353,805	4,803.37	719.31
62,072	814,173	89,362	2,352,053	3,317,660	75,721	5,054	80,775	139,439,900	29,588,849	169,028,761	51.0	331,729,090	7,501.70	1,363.19
15,061	163,209	16,815	495,051	690,136	15,688	1,435	17,123	28,030,243	5,921,591	33,951,834	51.7	65,691,366	6,906.48	1,268.00
1,580	23,126	4,366	78,577	107,649	189	325	514	3,774,952	909,544	4,684,492	53.4	8,766,858	4,966.24	763.20
13,481	140,083	12,449	416,474	582,487	15,499	1,110	16,609	24,255,291	5,012,047	29,267,342	51.4	56,924,507	7,348.65	1,411.82
4,660	44,900	3,339	137,847	190,746	5,372	181	5,553	7,774,824	1,592,930	9,367,750	51.2	18,304,829	7,233.23	1,369.33
286	5,234	1,103	17,562	24,185	49	18	67	781,988	186,766	968,754	50.7	1,911,781	4,901.74	748.57
4,374	39,666	2,236	120,285	166,561	5,323	163	5,486	6,992,836	1,406,164	8,398,996	51.2	16,393,048	7,658.03	1,515.94
48	571	34	1,619	2,272	0	5	5	75,250	18,395	93,645	50.2	186,709	6,783.52	1,583.09
3	678	33	1,681	2,395	16	0	16	92,471	17,945	110,416	46.3	238,671	7,093.59	1,139.63
3,708	30,394	1,271	91,192	126,565	4,875	133	5,008	5,538,942	1,080,153	6,619,092	51.2	12,927,133	8,001.63	1,617.81
33	563	43	2,179	2,818	0	0	0	105,455	23,288	128,743	52.0	247,439	5,082.23	1,058.19
29	423	158	2,142	2,752	15	0	15	86,623	20,595	107,218	52.3	205,065	4,647.27	912.13
30	464	55	1,359	1,908	37	3	40	76,130	15,960	92,089	49.4	186,565	6,403.46	937.77
178	1,954	90	5,208	7,430	160	0	160	296,445	64,220	360,665	52.1	691,994	7,957.89	1,466.63
283	1,673	181	4,994	7,131	0	0	0	232,877	51,327	284,203	53.6	530,171	7,820.21	1,540.91
23	1,103	195	4,372	5,783	210	22	232	232,511	51,326	283,838	49.6	572,343	8,636.40	1,558.02
39	1,753	176	5,539	7,507	10	0	10	256,132	62,955	319,087	52.6	606,957	5,015.76	925.59
1,209	21,468	3,160	68,258	94,095	792	139	931	3,586,162	805,723	4,391,886	52.0	8,446,387	6,650.62	1,221.80
297	3,880	845	13,960	18,982	21	52	73	646,249	154,293	800,541	54.6	1,465,693	5,069.51	1,043.98
912	17,588	2,315	54,298	75,113	771	87	858	2,939,913	651,430	3,591,345	51.4	6,980,694	7,116.65	1,267.11
66	540	41	1,750	2,397	116	3	119	87,945	18,230	106,175	55.8	190,215	7,555.70	600.78
0	92	25	394	511	0	0	0	19,364	4,261	23,625	54.5	43,382	4,207.76	1,000.28
29	673	55	1,572	2,329	0	0	0	88,737	25,611	114,347	53.7	213,077	6,418.57	1,358.94
95	1,159	95	3,850	5,199	46	0	46	193,814	39,774	233,588	53.3	438,432	6,921.77	1,260.15
17	1,910	236	6,559	8,722	0	8	8	284,853	67,650	352,503	53.3	661,157	6,170.85	1,126.94
157	2,527	205	7,156	10,045	107	7	114	429,407	99,629	529,035	52.1	1,016,004	6,711.57	1,267.54
418	6,709	1,053	21,742	29,922	339	68	407	1,226,865	259,924	1,486,791	50.4	2,950,479	8,290.75	1,442.00
18	428	97	1,605	2,148	8	0	8	66,591	15,472	82,063	52.2	157,346	5,583.62	825.95
10	673	65	1,583	2,331	0	0	0	90,330	23,724	114,054	53.9	211,653	6,283.69	1,311.34
15	598	101	2,314	3,028	0	1	1	110,097	19,396	129,492	53.5	242,247	4,500.55	905.64
10	502	108	1,276	1,896	70	0	70	78,292	15,253	93,545	48.5	192,866	6,400.90	1,312.73
57	1,055	59	2,498	3,669	66	0	66	166,421	39,805	206,226	48.7	423,773	8,567.65	1,713.50
20	722	175	1,999	2,916	19	0	19	97,196	22,704	119,901	49.9	240,064	6,125.33	1,221.94
3,930	34,053	3,982	104,300	146,265	3,619	283	3,902	6,002,614	1,252,891	7,255,506	52.2	13,891,062	6,602.07	1,174.74
472	4,572	977	16,646	22,667	38	16	54	800,986	197,217	998,202	55.4	1,801,247	5,041.37	658.82
3,458	29,481	3,005	87,654	123,598	3,581	267	3,848	5,201,627	1,055,674	6,257,304	51.8	12,089,815	6,921.31	1,329.90
75	3,285	140	9,760	13,260	840	2	842	587,382	149,610	736,993	51.5	1,429,768	9,239.09	1,821.78
5	517	60	2,095	2,677	0	0	0	79,139	22,525	101,664	54.7	185,783	5,734.92	1,304.78
2,452	14,779	657	42,757	60,645	2,065	247	2,312	2,600,792	478,099	3,078,892	51.2	6,009,760	6,922.51	1,357.74
144	1,797	203	4,755	6,899	335	0	335	337,602	73,020	410,622	55.5	739,323	7,134.19	1,428.68
389	3,518	1,252	10,809	15,968	155	3	158	591,625	116,321	707,945	52.1	1,358,249	5,828.47	1,212.01
13	380	77	1,618	2,088	0	0	0	88,474	16,377	104,852	50.3	208,308	5,346.72	1,125.98
75	1,707	140	4,818	6,746	0	0	0	286,699	65,277	351,976	47.7	738,655	7,288.08	1,168.80
173	1,656	115	4,980	6,924	144	3	147	300,733	53,030	353,763	55.6	636,655	6,275.24	1,027.43
132	1,842	355	6,062	8,391	42	12	54	329,182	81,415	410,597	52.4	783,314	6,930.45	1,182.45

Table continues

MSAs

TABLE 8

U.S. CENSUS DIVISION 4, EAST NORTH CENTRAL CONTINUED

U.S. Community Hospitals
(Nonfederal, short-term general and other special hospitals)

2001 Utilization, Personnel and Finances

CLASSIFICATION	Hospitals	Beds	Admissions	Inpatient Days	Adjusted Patient Days	Average Daily Census	Adjusted Average Daily Census	Average Stay (days)	Surgical Operations	NEWBORNS		OUTPATIENT VISITS	
										Bassinets	Births	Emergency	Total
Ohio	166	33,310	1,439,252	7,483,873	13,023,704	20,505	35,683	5.2	1,211,012	2,668	151,371	5,124,561	28,377,274
Nonmetropolitan	52	4,874	181,106	899,983	1,915,137	2,466	5,246	5.0	168,933	544	20,937	923,159	4,393,169
Metropolitan	114	28,436	1,258,146	6,583,890	11,108,567	18,039	30,437	5.2	1,042,079	2,124	130,434	4,201,402	23,984,105
Akron	7	1,762	88,350	486,167	812,037	1,331	2,224	5.5	67,953	132	8,740	281,898	1,646,745
Canton-Massillon	5	1,357	56,994	306,244	531,544	838	1,457	5.4	45,544	111	5,043	181,310	1,235,904
Cincinnati	14	3,365	167,576	809,713	1,311,517	2,219	3,595	4.8	140,572	242	19,218	474,743	2,410,984
Cleveland-Lorain-Elyria	34	8,371	331,788	1,980,829	3,365,033	5,427	9,221	6.0	320,008	547	31,374	1,072,011	8,034,661
Columbus	13	4,169	211,658	955,561	1,588,364	2,618	4,354	4.5	156,204	295	24,881	742,409	3,491,355
Dayton-Springfield	10	2,729	123,132	616,109	1,032,617	1,689	2,827	5.0	117,489	261	13,772	439,171	2,313,923
Hamilton-Middletown	4	541	31,211	120,807	237,162	331	649	3.9	19,197	74	4,531	143,087	465,045
Lima	3	623	29,129	137,266	258,496	377	708	4.7	18,404	66	2,837	113,989	629,464
Mansfield	3	490	17,383	102,553	197,352	281	540	5.9	13,423	51	1,911	95,011	277,465
Parkersburg-Marietta	2	248	8,565	37,934	79,299	103	217	4.4	6,999	21	657	38,340	221,995
Steubenville-Weirton	1	355	11,654	74,234	112,324	203	308	6.4	6,598	17	573	43,264	210,076
Toledo	8	2,401	97,524	527,461	850,810	1,445	2,332	5.4	75,375	158	9,819	304,853	1,667,379
Wheeling	3	321	8,538	68,285	135,458	187	371	8.0	6,324	10	341	27,713	235,744
Youngstown-Warren	7	1,704	74,644	360,727	596,554	990	1,634	4.8	47,989	139	6,737	243,603	1,143,365
Wisconsin	121	15,597	579,089	3,455,633	6,677,756	9,466	18,277	6.0	543,578	1,339	67,772	1,866,201	11,029,283
Nonmetropolitan	65	5,679	142,732	1,241,430	2,879,936	3,403	7,885	8.7	120,617	388	14,389	514,962	3,212,024
Metropolitan	56	9,918	436,357	2,214,203	3,797,820	6,063	10,392	5.1	422,961	951	53,383	1,351,239	7,817,259
Appleton-Oshkosh-Neenah	6	763	35,114	149,812	281,798	411	772	4.3	49,743	90	5,189	98,003	429,679
Duluth-Superior	1	38	1,041	3,492	9,185	10	25	3.4	1,009	0	0	14,429	53,702
Eau Claire	5	682	22,523	140,314	278,694	384	763	6.2	17,326	51	2,287	62,581	340,816
Green Bay	3	575	27,649	117,286	215,347	322	590	4.2	32,319	54	4,095	112,886	517,699
Janesville-Beloit	3	477	14,966	116,138	200,126	319	547	7.8	13,683	33	2,036	149,236	775,059
Kenosha	2	194	10,517	41,802	103,301	115	283	4.0	10,593	31	1,832	52,447	383,419
La Crosse	2	501	22,786	115,605	184,380	316	504	5.1	17,607	46	2,187	41,312	189,463
Madison	4	1,170	54,262	277,260	415,352	758	1,136	5.1	73,882	79	6,626	107,711	800,049
Milwaukee-Waukesha	19	4,233	198,182	984,221	1,618,451	2,693	4,427	5.0	160,599	440	22,953	550,228	3,513,782
Minneapolis-St. Paul	4	117	4,693	15,350	37,034	42	102	3.3	4,751	23	691	14,204	80,116
Racine	3	455	19,191	111,402	211,850	306	580	5.8	15,317	39	2,298	82,787	472,191
Sheboygan	3	498	11,792	85,236	158,379	233	433	7.2	13,787	37	1,742	40,029	172,033
Wausau	1	215	13,641	56,285	83,923	154	230	4.1	12,345	28	1,447	25,386	89,251

U.S. CENSUS DIVISION 4, EAST NORTH CENTRAL CONTINUED

U.S. Community Hospitals
(Nonfederal, short-term general and other special hospitals)

2001 Utilization, Personnel and Finances

FULL-TIME EQUIVALENT PERSONNEL					FULL-TIME EQUIV. TRAINEES			EXPENSES						
								LABOR				TOTAL		
Physicians and Dentists	Registered Nurses	Licensed Practical Nurses	Other Salaried Personnel	Total Personnel	Medical and Dental Residents	Other Trainees	Total Trainees	Payroll (in thousands)	Employee Benefits (in thousands)	Total (in thousands)	Percent of Total	Amount (in thousands)	Adjusted per Admission	Adjusted per Inpatient Day
4,684	46,026	5,018	131,466	187,194	5,248	274	5,522	7,752,934	1,579,701	9,332,641	52.2	17,866,115	7,064.48	1,371.82
259	5,488	944	16,803	23,494	78	22	100	828,263	203,914	1,032,179	53.0	1,948,865	4,889.14	1,017.61
4,425	40,538	4,074	114,663	163,700	5,170	252	5,422	6,924,671	1,375,787	8,300,462	52.1	15,917,250	7,471.51	1,432.88
198	3,315	540	7,896	11,949	376	34	410	459,374	91,944	551,318	51.9	1,062,284	7,086.00	1,308.17
93	1,687	273	5,113	7,166	158	6	164	266,847	59,388	326,236	53.7	607,218	6,233.12	1,142.37
440	5,215	234	12,542	18,431	816	99	915	761,370	133,922	895,292	47.1	1,899,741	6,901.20	1,448.51
1,713	11,248	1,310	33,504	47,775	2,059	21	2,080	2,342,404	443,936	2,786,344	56.0	4,978,876	8,769.97	1,479.59
551	6,382	258	19,938	27,129	757	12	769	1,078,296	227,342	1,305,639	47.9	2,728,401	7,717.51	1,717.74
1,132	3,875	284	12,082	17,373	447	8	455	655,113	122,868	777,981	53.2	1,461,862	7,054.33	1,415.69
11	1,006	70	2,163	3,250	0	0	0	113,326	20,550	133,877	50.6	264,712	4,280.18	1,116.17
14	866	162	2,575	3,617	2	0	2	137,061	36,281	173,341	54.1	320,356	5,828.35	1,239.31
5	508	135	1,785	2,433	0	0	0	88,309	24,760	113,069	55.4	203,966	6,092.17	1,033.51
3	233	65	796	1,097	3	0	3	39,699	10,951	50,650	54.3	93,279	5,225.12	1,176.29
36	396	41	1,148	1,621	21	2	23	56,139	11,860	67,999	51.2	132,690	7,524.70	1,181.32
83	3,322	318	9,046	12,769	405	68	473	551,589	109,298	660,888	51.7	1,277,448	8,284.89	1,501.45
18	288	56	719	1,081	0	0	0	34,528	6,817	41,345	54.1	76,467	4,577.50	564.51
128	2,197	328	5,356	8,009	126	2	128	340,614	75,868	416,483	51.4	809,951	6,604.73	1,357.72
578	16,762	1,316	53,180	71,836	657	558	1,215	2,913,709	690,315	3,604,051	50.2	7,182,972	6,664.31	1,075.66
266	3,952	497	13,606	18,321	3	217	220	717,465	167,354	884,816	54.0	1,639,272	4,963.76	569.20
312	12,810	819	39,574	53,515	654	341	995	2,196,244	522,991	2,719,235	40.1	5,540,700	7,415.54	1,459.71
24	800	00	2,593	3,514	0	0	0	165,137	36,425	201,562	53.3	377,841	5,714.31	1,340.82
0	30	7	117	154	0	0	0	6,172	1,278	7,450	60.5	12,315	4,497.96	1,340.82
2	648	45	1,951	2,646	0	0	0	92,844	21,265	114,109	55.6	205,394	5,067.20	736.99
55	1,044	113	2,808	4,020	0	0	0	178,386	35,830	214,215	57.3	374,115	7,203.53	1,737.27
34	688	69	1,940	2,731	16	2	18	114,392	25,599	139,991	54.1	258,980	10,192.43	1,294.08
40	301	29	1,108	1,478	0	0	0	69,146	15,262	84,408	55.0	153,562	5,902.84	1,486.55
7	596	69	2,329	3,001	23	0	23	107,669	33,165	140,834	56.8	248,088	6,914.56	1,345.52
17	1,624	64	5,041	6,746	458	332	790	303,831	84,489	388,320	50.7	765,406	9,590.95	1,842.79
129	5,742	222	17,213	23,306	157	7	164	946,728	221,205	1,167,932	44.5	2,624,523	7,984.17	1,621.63
0	121	8	416	545	0	0	0	21,017	3,861	24,878	49.3	50,464	4,382.83	1,362.64
0	567	56	1,859	2,482	0	0	0	89,045	19,305	108,351	50.4	214,842	5,857.51	1,014.12
2	335	33	1,038	1,408	0	0	0	45,928	10,622	56,550	50.3	112,379	5,132.64	709.56
2	305	16	1,161	1,484	0	0	0	55,950	14,685	70,635	48.4	145,791	7,168.03	1,737.20

TABLE 8

U.S. CENSUS DIVISION 5, EAST SOUTH CENTRAL

U.S. Community Hospitals
(Nonfederal, short-term general and other special hospitals)

2001 Utilization, Personnel and Finances

CLASSIFICATION	Hospitals	Beds	Admissions	Inpatient Days	Adjusted Patient Days	Average Daily Census	Adjusted Average Daily Census	Average Stay (days)	Surgical Operations	NEWBORNS Bassinets	NEWBORNS Births	OUTPATIENT VISITS Emergency	OUTPATIENT VISITS Total
UNITED STATES	4,907	824,676	33,765,589	193,754,932	314,740,801	531,715	863,683	5.7	26,432,095	60,351	3,868,995	105,865,778	536,588,378
Nonmetropolitan	2,166	174,945	5,372,241	35,717,503	71,393,393	97,918	195,777	6.6	4,479,968	13,831	533,148	22,155,102	110,466,485
Metropolitan	2,741	649,731	28,393,348	158,037,429	243,347,408	433,797	667,906	5.6	21,952,127	46,520	3,335,847	83,710,676	426,121,893
CENSUS DIVISION 5, EAST SOUTH CENTRAL	429	65,898	2,467,417	13,998,816	22,865,383	38,392	62,705	5.7	1,926,290	4,472	227,383	8,156,784	30,102,877
Nonmetropolitan	260	25,831	818,966	5,053,527	9,167,578	13,834	25,117	6.2	610,873	1,796	68,493	3,332,432	11,811,952
Metropolitan	169	40,067	1,648,451	8,945,289	13,697,805	24,558	37,588	5.4	1,315,417	2,676	158,890	4,824,352	18,290,925
Alabama	107	16,627	684,923	3,570,273	5,613,045	9,783	15,376	5.2	484,083	1,328	55,794	1,959,967	7,786,063
Nonmetropolitan	50	4,061	133,383	733,414	1,354,360	2,007	3,709	5.5	101,337	334	11,110	529,926	1,859,308
Metropolitan	57	12,566	551,540	2,836,859	4,258,685	7,776	11,667	5.1	382,746	994	44,684	1,430,041	5,926,755
Anniston	3	428	21,389	90,878	146,454	249	401	4.2	14,733	28	1,807	85,690	198,989
Auburn-Opelika	1	292	15,745	71,946	117,320	197	321	4.6	9,525	28	1,429	40,167	87,972
Birmingham	17	4,556	192,819	1,001,820	1,462,367	2,748	4,006	5.2	138,243	273	14,881	461,844	2,171,757
Decatur	4	525	17,260	78,565	111,719	216	306	4.6	13,855	30	1,813	74,085	217,287
Dothan	3	630	33,918	139,642	222,095	382	608	4.1	20,348	73	2,162	89,734	460,936
Florence	3	593	25,016	190,006	272,509	521	747	7.6	23,100	66	2,037	89,295	261,571
Gadsden	2	538	21,988	109,042	156,439	299	429	5.0	17,876	47	1,471	53,012	197,443
Huntsville	4	1,074	48,899	225,377	359,880	618	985	4.6	34,925	100	4,409	154,128	601,586
Mobile	10	2,164	87,763	483,494	752,480	1,324	2,062	5.5	61,715	187	7,037	175,936	990,579
Montgomery	8	1,147	52,093	260,256	413,759	713	1,134	5.0	28,690	116	4,639	98,566	369,237
Tuscaloosa	2	619	34,650	185,833	243,663	509	668	5.4	19,736	46	2,999	107,584	369,398
Kentucky	103	15,001	594,899	3,315,218	5,572,292	9,081	15,270	5.6	526,436	1,034	52,818	1,985,284	8,677,388
Nonmetropolitan	71	7,756	271,091	1,550,121	2,828,813	4,243	7,747	5.7	221,172	550	21,194	1,022,607	4,903,451
Metropolitan	32	7,245	323,808	1,765,097	2,743,479	4,838	7,523	5.5	305,264	484	31,624	962,677	3,773,937
Cincinnati	5	867	44,075	204,477	317,590	560	869	4.6	27,982	77	4,840	168,164	585,035
Clarksville-Hopkinsville	1	151	5,754	24,578	51,714	67	142	4.3	5,181	18	670	22,666	76,502
Evansville-Henderson	1	209	8,158	35,148	57,541	96	158	4.3	10,819	12	836	28,055	164,267
Huntington-Ashland	2	580	29,558	134,502	208,133	368	570	4.6	32,145	29	1,505	92,474	357,607
Lexington	12	2,030	80,444	469,058	735,348	1,288	2,020	5.8	72,445	129	8,530	207,386	1,101,502
Louisville	10	3,063	136,735	818,967	1,251,228	2,244	3,430	6.0	136,730	185	13,324	366,426	1,223,079
Owensboro	1	345	19,084	78,367	121,925	215	334	4.1	19,962	34	1,919	77,506	265,945
Mississippi	96	13,670	436,100	2,990,906	4,835,570	8,192	13,248	6.9	270,609	863	42,049	1,501,052	4,102,499
Nonmetropolitan	76	8,333	251,249	1,850,209	3,128,416	5,068	8,571	7.4	140,855	535	22,687	945,776	2,385,233
Metropolitan	20	5,337	184,851	1,140,697	1,707,154	3,124	4,677	6.2	129,754	328	19,362	555,276	1,717,266
Biloxi-Gulfport-Pascagoula	7	1,359	52,099	276,057	431,942	755	1,184	5.3	47,556	129	4,349	193,586	811,708
Hattiesburg	2	748	32,959	175,662	264,504	481	725	5.3	16,232	35	3,475	117,619	215,622
Jackson	10	2,911	91,218	601,791	885,108	1,649	2,424	6.6	61,208	140	10,213	211,522	618,059
Memphis	1	319	8,575	87,187	125,600	239	344	10.2	4,758	24	1,325	32,549	71,877
Tennessee	123	20,600	751,495	4,122,419	6,844,476	11,336	18,811	5.5	645,162	1,247	76,722	2,710,481	9,536,927
Nonmetropolitan	63	5,681	163,243	919,783	1,855,989	2,516	5,090	5.6	147,509	377	13,502	834,123	2,663,960
Metropolitan	60	14,919	588,252	3,202,636	4,988,487	8,820	13,721	5.4	497,653	870	63,220	1,876,358	6,872,967
Chattanooga	6	1,581	61,350	316,908	484,103	869	1,326	5.2	62,391	59	6,410	194,195	693,677
Clarksville-Hopkinsville	1	194	10,985	48,316	85,278	132	234	4.4	5,332	16	1,347	42,085	112,561
Jackson	2	758	27,544	141,873	223,825	389	613	5.2	24,057	42	3,293	73,046	168,855
Johnson City-Kingsport-Bristol	11	2,024	64,187	351,336	572,732	962	1,570	5.5	60,911	136	5,406	259,101	937,262
Knoxville	10	2,520	91,035	508,509	841,314	1,394	2,304	5.6	97,472	158	11,446	333,696	1,191,246
Memphis	12	3,508	147,175	924,785	1,307,047	2,578	3,635	6.3	87,310	202	18,018	421,958	1,324,749
Nashville	18	4,334	185,976	910,909	1,474,188	2,496	4,039	4.9	160,180	257	17,300	552,277	2,444,617

TABLE 8

U.S. CENSUS DIVISION 5, EAST SOUTH CENTRAL

U.S. Community Hospitals
(Nonfederal, short-term general and other special hospitals)

2001 Utilization, Personnel and Finances

FULL-TIME EQUIVALENT PERSONNEL					FULL-TIME EQUIV. TRAINEES			EXPENSES						
								LABOR				TOTAL		
Physicians and Dentists	Registered Nurses	Licensed Practical Nurses	Other Salaried Personnel	Total Personnel	Medical and Dental Residents	Other Trainees	Total Trainees	Payroll (in thousands)	Employee Benefits (in thousands)	Total (in thousands)	Percent of Total	Amount (in thousands)	Adjusted per Admission	Adjusted per Inpatient Day
70,153	956,577	126,143	2,828,126	3,980,999	77,440	5,751	83,191	$161,734,716	$34,640,089	$196,374,807	51.3	$383,082,895	$6,976.34	$1,217.14
8,081	142,404	36,781	476,073	663,339	1,719	697	2,416	22,294,816	5,051,240	27,346,046	53.3	51,353,805	4,803.37	719.31
62,072	814,173	89,362	2,352,053	3,317,660	75,721	5,054	80,775	139,439,900	29,588,849	169,028,761	51.0	331,729,090	7,501.70	1,363.19
1,715	64,152	12,623	190,173	268,663	2,094	549	2,643	9,342,181	2,030,236	11,372,415	49.1	23,153,846	5,688.45	1,012.62
679	18,590	5,658	58,998	83,925	92	56	148	2,621,866	610,292	3,232,154	51.6	6,263,433	4,129.60	683.22
1,036	45,562	6,965	131,175	184,738	2,002	493	2,495	6,720,316	1,419,945	8,140,261	48.2	16,890,413	6,614.32	1,233.07
519	17,216	3,251	47,532	68,518	863	62	925	2,286,777	499,746	2,786,520	49.2	5,664,284	5,174.74	1,009.13
134	2,773	708	8,775	12,390	33	18	51	356,746	78,425	435,167	52.4	831,047	3,277.05	613.61
385	14,443	2,543	38,757	56,128	830	44	874	1,930,031	421,321	2,351,353	48.6	4,833,237	5,746.96	1,134.91
4	525	87	1,086	1,702	13	0	13	56,764	12,634	69,399	50.3	137,899	3,874.10	941.58
4	422	43	1,222	1,691	0	0	0	54,671	9,179	63,850	49.8	128,332	4,998.34	1,093.87
150	5,541	762	14,402	20,855	681	7	688	743,385	165,994	909,378	46.8	1,943,513	6,694.45	1,329.02
25	421	90	1,293	1,829	49	0	49	62,695	16,780	79,476	49.3	161,082	6,412.50	1,441.85
27	722	248	2,335	3,332	3	9	12	111,299	22,587	133,886	50.5	264,873	4,901.52	1,192.61
7	603	207	2,058	2,875	2	0	2	89,810	21,904	111,713	54.7	204,081	5,363.22	748.90
0	544	65	1,224	1,833	0	0	0	52,634	11,229	63,863	43.7	145,973	4,623.94	933.10
31	1,446	192	3,172	4,841	1	0	1	185,165	44,477	229,643	50.4	455,274	5,002.11	1,265.07
76	2,271	520	6,818	9,685	28	0	28	295,719	65,599	361,318	48.4	746,481	5,575.83	992.03
55	1,140	155	3,030	4,380	53	6	59	155,085	32,172	187,257	49.4	378,858	4,576.73	915.65
6	808	174	2,117	3,105	0	22	22	122,803	18,767	141,570	53.0	266,871	5,863.24	1,095.25
443	15,507	2,693	46,921	65,564	142	54	196	2,293,180	488,393	2,781,571	48.5	5,731,886	5,649.52	1,028.64
242	6,524	1,703	20,124	28,593	46	30	76	949,437	222,914	1,172,351	51.4	2,279,729	4,487.78	805.90
201	8,983	990	26,797	36,971	96	24	120	1,343,743	265,479	1,609,220	46.6	3,452,157	6,814.46	1,258.31
69	995	115	2,814	3,993	82	13	95	171,383	34,700	206,082	53.0	388,644	5,598.77	1,223.73
0	144	43	409	596	0	0	0	18,692	4,110	22,802	40.8	55,873	4,614.91	1,080.42
4	302	36	1,190	1,532	0	0	0	37,535	8,116	45,650	71.7	63,653	4,765.90	1,106.23
26	719	147	1,895	2,787	9	0	9	109,427	27,476	136,902	50.3	271,967	5,946.85	1,306.70
59	3,034	241	6,966	10,300	5	2	7	355,120	70,586	425,706	44.6	955,441	7,503.48	1,299.30
39	3,330	343	12,106	15,818	0	9	9	589,335	106,933	696,268	44.4	1,567,296	7,500.57	1,252.61
4	459	65	1,417	1,945	0	0	0	62,251	13,559	75,810	50.8	149,283	5,027.87	1,224.38
319	11,279	2,344	32,428	46,370	360	20	380	1,495,040	338,917	1,833,957	50.7	3,614,545	5,135.81	747.49
234	5,557	1,647	17,943	25,381	2	6	8	772,746	185,259	958,005	50.7	1,888,247	4,454.07	603.58
85	5,722	697	14,485	20,989	358	14	372	722,293	153,658	875,952	50.7	1,726,297	6,168.54	1,011.21
17	1,713	126	3,772	5,628	0	0	0	207,420	41,202	248,623	50.9	488,710	5,976.71	1,131.42
31	855	162	2,619	3,667	0	0	0	111,941	29,125	141,065	50.9	277,324	5,597.31	1,048.47
37	2,943	354	7,490	10,824	358	14	372	376,626	77,063	453,690	50.5	897,698	6,591.66	1,014.22
0	211	55	604	870	0	0	0	26,307	6,268	32,574	52.1	62,565	5,064.77	498.13
434	20,150	4,335	63,292	88,211	729	413	1,142	3,267,185	703,181	3,970,367	48.8	8,143,131	6,476.41	1,189.74
69	3,736	1,600	12,156	17,561	11	2	13	542,936	123,694	666,631	52.7	1,264,410	3,817.72	681.26
365	16,414	2,735	51,136	70,650	718	411	1,129	2,724,249	579,487	3,303,736	48.0	6,070,721	7,427.10	1,378.92
37	2,127	200	5,686	8,086	135	1	136	287,337	62,162	349,500	49.0	713,101	7,497.48	1,473.03
2	256	79	680	1,017	0	0	0	35,835	7,797	43,632	52.4	83,263	4,294.35	876.07
34	843	179	2,373	3,429	0	0	0	121,261	30,015	151,276	51.1	295,912	6,808.21	1,322.07
4	1,833	348	4,883	7,060	0	0	0	248,613	56,271	304,885	45.4	671,582	6,260.90	1,172.59
98	2,710	760	9,042	12,610	123	12	135	495,054	102,274	597,328	49.5	1,206,749	8,103.39	1,434.36
120	2,742	311	14,640	17,813	91	398	489	703,423	141,173	844,500	47.0	1,775,649	8,488.70	1,358.52
70	5,903	822	13,832	20,627	369	0	369	832,726	179,794	1,012,519	47.5	2,132,466	7,041.79	1,446.54

MSAs

TABLE 8

U.S. CENSUS DIVISION 6, WEST NORTH CENTRAL

U.S. Community Hospitals
(Nonfederal, short-term general and other special hospitals)

2001 Utilization, Personnel and Finances

CLASSIFICATION	Hospitals	Beds	Admissions	Inpatient Days	Adjusted Patient Days	Average Daily Census	Adjusted Average Daily Census	Average Stay (days)	Surgical Operations	NEWBORNS Bassinets	NEWBORNS Births	OUTPATIENT VISITS Emergency	OUTPATIENT VISITS Total
UNITED STATES	4,907	824,676	33,765,589	193,754,932	314,740,801	531,715	863,683	5.7	26,432,095	60,351	3,868,995	105,865,778	536,588,378
Nonmetropolitan	2,166	174,945	5,372,241	35,717,503	71,393,393	97,918	195,777	6.6	4,479,968	13,831	533,148	22,155,102	110,466,485
Metropolitan	2,741	649,731	28,393,348	158,037,429	243,347,408	433,797	667,906	5.6	21,952,127	46,520	3,335,847	83,710,676	426,121,893
CENSUS DIVISION 6, WEST NORTH CENTRAL	673	75,020	2,481,753	16,650,444	30,070,524	45,663	82,460	6.7	2,032,147	5,267	261,796	6,937,436	44,674,726
Nonmetropolitan	492	33,322	736,111	6,978,301	14,543,009	19,156	39,909	9.5	620,263	2,586	73,869	2,586,701	18,191,469
Metropolitan	181	41,698	1,745,642	9,672,143	15,527,515	26,507	42,551	5.5	1,411,884	2,681	187,927	4,350,735	26,483,257
Iowa	116	11,538	370,885	2,491,172	5,115,263	6,829	14,017	6.7	396,899	819	37,628	1,063,304	9,399,353
Nonmetropolitan	95	5,987	143,655	1,254,095	3,042,204	3,438	8,337	8.7	139,982	447	13,054	485,235	4,494,396
Metropolitan	21	5,551	227,230	1,237,077	2,073,059	3,391	5,680	5.4	256,917	372	24,574	578,069	4,904,957
Cedar Rapids	2	741	27,926	160,048	293,531	439	804	5.7	36,616	55	3,689	90,283	491,881
Davenport-Moline-Rock Island	2	525	20,781	115,435	185,802	316	509	5.6	13,788	32	2,600	61,732	220,410
Des Moines	6	1,503	69,516	361,615	559,887	991	1,533	5.2	55,106	120	8,145	173,715	1,557,514
Dubuque	2	511	15,631	84,486	139,403	232	382	5.4	15,288	42	1,623	46,155	125,922
Iowa City	2	924	31,864	219,044	348,379	600	955	6.9	85,107	38	2,609	53,195	1,008,019
Omaha	2	306	12,498	67,064	107,501	184	295	5.4	13,683	20	1,065	45,534	149,203
Sioux City	2	469	23,629	113,752	174,436	312	478	4.8	17,426	30	2,540	49,523	412,270
Waterloo-Cedar Falls	3	572	25,385	115,633	264,120	317	724	4.6	19,903	35	2,303	57,932	939,738
Kansas	133	11,211	322,067	2,175,989	3,918,816	5,962	10,741	6.8	248,738	800	37,847	907,083	5,394,028
Nonmetropolitan	105	6,170	133,149	1,149,211	2,347,731	3,147	6,436	8.6	101,274	504	12,305	396,014	2,865,064
Metropolitan	28	5,041	188,918	1,026,778	1,571,085	2,815	4,305	5.4	147,464	296	25,542	511,069	2,528,964
Kansas City	13	2,088	78,444	421,063	663,063	1,153	1,817	5.4	76,193	163	11,893	209,486	1,190,572
Lawrence	1	126	6,948	29,905	72,352	82	198	4.3	4,764	13	1,061	29,043	143,112
Topeka	3	626	24,259	117,269	217,128	322	595	4.8	19,890	42	3,092	81,272	420,890
Wichita	11	2,201	79,267	458,541	618,542	1,258	1,695	5.8	46,617	78	9,496	191,268	774,390
Minnesota	133	16,508	586,016	4,102,576	7,274,559	11,235	19,929	7.0	443,246	1,317	67,706	1,506,825	8,565,860
Nonmetropolitan	88	6,976	126,018	1,677,005	3,341,139	4,590	9,154	13.3	113,072	494	15,619	483,206	2,690,820
Metropolitan	45	9,532	459,998	2,425,571	3,933,420	6,645	10,775	5.3	330,174	823	52,087	1,023,619	5,875,040
Duluth-Superior	8	1,200	40,709	301,196	513,439	826	1,405	7.4	39,582	89	3,185	74,411	453,144
Grand Forks	2	289	2,412	78,710	230,596	215	632	32.6	1,652	17	187	3,219	62,715
Minneapolis-St. Paul	28	5,970	323,743	1,471,967	2,284,210	4,032	6,258	4.5	237,024	619	43,662	820,197	4,386,810
Rochester	3	1,195	70,099	345,493	515,233	946	1,412	4.9	38,384	47	2,417	78,147	610,307
St. Cloud	4	878	23,035	228,205	389,942	626	1,068	9.9	13,532	51	2,636	47,645	362,064
Missouri	117	19,257	800,648	4,219,659	7,215,107	11,561	19,766	5.3	599,128	1,225	75,350	2,443,744	14,198,807
Nonmetropolitan	57	4,550	173,001	868,935	1,764,112	2,384	4,832	5.0	136,156	425	16,212	728,510	4,631,365
Metropolitan	60	14,707	627,647	3,350,724	5,450,995	9,177	14,934	5.3	462,972	800	59,138	1,715,234	9,567,442
Columbia	4	970	33,527	191,830	284,853	526	782	5.7	29,888	46	3,168	60,004	775,106
Joplin	4	764	37,158	173,856	310,891	476	852	4.7	24,108	52	3,446	137,651	758,169
Kansas City	21	3,748	150,661	864,965	1,380,917	2,370	3,782	5.7	112,590	206	15,751	523,902	2,424,267
Springfield	3	1,361	63,459	312,020	568,015	855	1,556	4.9	46,981	60	6,110	155,605	1,385,360
St. Joseph	1	495	16,924	67,630	105,184	185	288	4.0	7,197	20	1,532	41,085	458,765
St. Louis	27	7,369	325,918	1,740,423	2,801,135	4,765	7,674	5.3	242,208	416	29,131	796,987	3,765,775
Nebraska	84	8,324	206,700	1,826,566	3,327,744	5,003	9,116	8.8	197,546	627	24,313	545,607	3,429,842
Nonmetropolitan	70	4,449	86,420	881,749	1,900,993	2,414	5,208	10.2	75,262	392	9,409	263,216	1,804,878
Metropolitan	14	3,875	120,280	944,817	1,426,751	2,589	3,908	7.9	122,284	235	14,904	282,391	1,624,964
Lincoln	3	1,042	35,318	246,531	356,963	676	978	7.0	26,476	85	4,567	80,326	374,450
Omaha	11	2,833	84,962	698,286	1,069,788	1,913	2,930	8.2	95,808	150	10,337	202,065	1,250,514
North Dakota	40	3,717	91,530	787,722	1,484,643	2,160	4,064	8.6	69,532	231	8,691	259,673	1,858,738
Nonmetropolitan	33	2,216	29,287	453,037	911,568	1,243	2,494	15.5	21,957	126	2,694	115,541	753,213
Metropolitan	7	1,501	62,243	334,685	573,075	917	1,570	5.4	47,575	105	5,997	144,132	1,105,525
Bismarck	2	494	18,792	96,245	186,524	263	511	5.1	17,036	15	1,670	29,723	602,881
Fargo-Moorhead	3	653	31,378	154,687	217,345	424	596	4.9	20,159	66	3,089	80,614	415,386
Grand Forks	2	354	12,073	83,753	169,206	230	463	6.9	10,380	24	1,238	33,795	87,258
South Dakota	50	4,465	103,907	1,046,760	1,734,392	2,913	4,827	10.1	77,058	248	10,261	211,200	1,828,098
Nonmetropolitan	44	2,974	44,581	694,269	1,235,262	1,940	3,448	15.6	32,560	198	4,576	114,979	951,733
Metropolitan	6	1,491	59,326	352,491	499,130	973	1,379	5.9	44,498	50	5,685	96,221	876,365
Rapid City	1	363	16,894	88,431	123,197	242	338	5.2	8,140	12	1,918	39,306	137,002
Sioux Falls	5	1,128	42,432	264,060	375,933	731	1,041	6.2	36,358	38	3,767	56,915	739,363

TABLE 8

U.S. CENSUS DIVISION 6, WEST NORTH CENTRAL

U.S. Community Hospitals
(Nonfederal, short-term general and other special hospitals)

2001 Utilization, Personnel and Finances

FULL-TIME EQUIVALENT PERSONNEL					FULL-TIME EQUIV. TRAINEES			EXPENSES						
								LABOR				TOTAL		
Physicians and Dentists	Registered Nurses	Licensed Practical Nurses	Other Salaried Personnel	Total Personnel	Medical and Dental Residents	Other Trainees	Total Trainees	Payroll (in thousands)	Employee Benefits (in thousands)	Total (in thousands)	Percent of Total	Amount (in thousands)	Adjusted per Admission	Adjusted per Inpatient Day
70,153	956,577	126,143	2,828,126	3,980,999	77,440	5,751	83,191	$161,734,716	$34,640,089	$196,374,807	51.3	$383,082,895	$6,976.34	$1,217.14
8,081	142,404	36,781	476,073	663,339	1,719	697	2,416	22,294,816	5,051,240	27,346,046	53.3	51,353,805	4,803.37	719.31
62,072	814,173	89,362	2,352,053	3,317,660	75,721	5,054	80,775	139,439,900	29,588,849	169,028,761	51.0	331,729,090	7,501.70	1,363.19
5,123	75,737	11,403	232,476	324,739	2,717	217	2,934	12,429,211	2,489,447	14,918,660	52.1	28,645,889	6,545.99	952.62
1,437	22,193	6,054	77,377	107,061	88	55	143	3,399,458	702,455	4,101,917	54.3	7,554,266	4,832.28	519.44
3,686	53,544	5,349	155,099	217,678	2,629	162	2,791	9,029,753	1,786,993	10,816,743	51.3	21,091,624	7,498.43	1,358.34
781	12,029	1,310	38,592	52,712	587	28	615	1,786,524	406,206	2,192,730	52.2	4,202,394	5,838.26	821.54
260	4,842	803	15,781	21,686	25	0	25	664,880	147,208	812,090	53.9	1,505,601	4,474.60	494.90
521	7,187	507	22,811	31,026	562	28	590	1,121,644	258,998	1,380,640	51.2	2,696,793	7,035.25	1,300.88
6	956	93	2,322	3,377	0	17	17	116,636	28,311	144,947	51.0	284,336	5,622.39	968.67
2	622	30	1,609	2,263	8	0	8	89,612	20,237	109,849	49.0	224,271	6,647.44	1,207.05
257	2,031	78	7,512	9,878	175	0	175	326,851	73,012	399,862	50.6	790,419	7,291.69	1,411.75
13	520	12	1,301	1,846	0	0	0	61,930	12,157	74,087	49.8	148,688	5,599.44	1,066.60
71	1,478	30	4,505	6,084	358	9	367	240,192	68,834	309,026	50.3	614,862	12,088.83	1,764.92
11	333	26	861	1,231	0	2	2	54,107	10,251	64,358	56.9	113,206	5,647.87	1,053.07
60	635	72	2,406	3,173	0	0	0	108,075	21,908	129,983	52.7	246,461	6,749.58	1,412.90
101	612	166	2,295	3,174	21	0	21	124,242	21,287	140,520	54.1	274,551	4,847.21	1,039.49
494	8,925	1,356	29,118	39,893	14	35	49	1,434,260	271,554	1,705,813	51.9	3,285,567	5,801.02	838.41
163	3,739	821	13,136	17,859	1	35	36	555,601	109,338	664,939	54.8	1,212,769	4,582.89	516.57
331	5,186	535	15,982	22,034	13	0	13	878,659	162,217	1,040,874	50.2	2,072,798	6,869.32	1,319.34
81	2,254	117	6,377	8,829	0	0	0	349,452	66,915	416,368	48.7	855,349	6,646.58	1,290.00
13	182	22	545	762	0	0	0	34,187	5,960	40,147	52.4	76,657	4,560.19	1,059.50
164	826	221	2,625	3,836	0	0	0	160,767	25,250	186,016	56.5	329,502	7,064.35	1,517.55
73	1,924	175	6,435	8,607	13	0	13	334,253	64,092	398,343	49.1	811,290	7,402.01	1,311.62
950	16,483	2,776	50,409	70,618	441	74	515	3,250,472	678,610	3,929,087	55.6	7,067,072	7,104.17	971.48
236	3,644	1,387	14,077	19,344	7	9	16	659,777	143,048	802,828	56.5	1,420,541	5,296.06	425.17
714	12,839	1,389	36,332	51,274	434	65	499	2,590,695	535,562	3,126,259	55.4	5,646,531	7,771.68	1,435.53
73	1,077	264	3,492	4,906	1	0	1	211,348	51,315	262,664	54.8	479,037	7,314.21	933.00
0	87	69	373	529	0	0	0	15,475	2,961	18,436	62.8	29,354	4,164.21	127.29
408	9,234	677	26,223	36,542	326	49	375	1,933,547	394,557	2,328,105	55.8	4,174,388	8,201.43	1,827.50
197	1,690	175	4,090	6,152	86	16	102	307,146	62,347	369,492	52.6	702,625	6,512.36	1,363.70
36	751	204	2,154	3,145	21	0	21	123,179	24,383	147,562	56.5	261,128	7,031.85	669.66
1,498	24,587	3,469	69,664	99,218	1,556	39	1,595	3,772,222	706,619	4,478,842	49.1	9,118,865	6,611.00	1,263.86
403	4,674	1,511	15,335	21,923	42	0	42	710,747	145,668	856,417	51.1	1,674,532	4,722.87	949.22
1,095	19,913	1,958	54,329	77,295	1,514	39	1,553	3,061,474	560,951	3,622,425	48.7	7,444,333	7,264.25	1,365.68
24	1,317	239	3,880	5,460	301	0	301	184,952	40,270	225,221	42.8	525,791	10,416.03	1,845.83
188	1,166	205	2,903	4,462	10	0	10	187,712	36,913	224,626	55.9	402,142	6,072.63	1,293.51
197	4,993	431	12,707	18,328	169	18	187	758,983	136,744	895,727	50.3	1,781,134	7,564.26	1,289.82
119	1,878	200	7,351	9,548	24	1	25	336,448	65,277	401,725	50.9	789,704	6,844.55	1,300.20
50	504	154	1,461	2,177	0	0	0	100,253	17,506	117,759	57.2	206,044	7,827.81	1,958.89
509	10,055	729	26,027	37,320	1,010	20	1,030	1,493,127	264,241	1,757,367	47.0	3,739,520	7,043.43	1,335.00
420	7,301	1,060	22,492	31,585	50	40	90	1,115,567	230,879	1,346,445	50.9	2,645,027	7,158.16	794.84
158	2,746	890	9,631	13,425	13	11	24	429,427	83,379	512,806	54.4	941,820	5,061.83	495.44
262	4,558	479	12,861	18,160	37	29	66	686,140	147,500	833,639	48.9	1,703,207	9,284.36	1,193.77
60	1,413	187	3,911	5,571	7	0	7	186,683	41,636	228,319	50.4	453,391	9,113.74	1,270.13
202	3,145	292	8,950	12,589	30	29	59	499,457	105,864	605,320	48.4	1,249,817	9,347.85	1,168.28
836	2,937	785	11,039	15,597	53	1	54	565,625	98,008	663,632	54.4	1,220,687	6,894.28	822.21
164	1,062	413	4,070	[illegible]	0	0	0	175,020	30,345	205,364	58.1	350,519	5,212.00	387.81
672	1,875	372	6,660	9,579	53	1	54	390,605	67,662	458,268	52.8	867,169	7,938.34	1,513.19
145	672	175	2,146	3,138	0	0	0	134,067	16,871	[illegible]	[illegible]	[illegible]	7,441.30	1,446.91
333	879	140	2,463	3,815	53	1	54	130,584	25,480	156,065	43.6	358,170	8,141.15	1,647.93
194	324	57	2,051	2,626	0	0	0	125,954	25,311	151,265	63.3	239,115	8,252.47	1,413.16
144	3,472	338	11,162	15,116	16	0	16	504,542	97,572	602,111	54.4	1,106,277	6,537.47	637.85
53	1,486	229	5,038	6,806	0	0	0	204,006	43,469	247,473	55.6	445,484	5,209.31	360.64
91	1,986	109	6,124	8,310	16	0	16	300,536	54,103	354,638	53.7	660,792	7,894.39	1,323.89
2	528	54	1,615	2,199	16	0	16	84,045	9,184	93,228	51.4	181,316	7,703.76	1,471.75
89	1,458	55	4,509	6,111	0	0	0	216,491	44,920	261,410	54.5	479,477	7,968.96	1,275.43

MSAs

Table 8

U.S. CENSUS DIVISION 7, WEST SOUTH CENTRAL

U.S. Community Hospitals
(Nonfederal, short-term general and other special hospitals)

2001 Utilization, Personnel and Finances

CLASSIFICATION	Hospitals	Beds	Admissions	Inpatient Days	Adjusted Patient Days	Average Daily Census	Adjusted Average Daily Census	Average Stay (days)	Surgical Operations	NEWBORNS Bassinets	NEWBORNS Births	OUTPATIENT VISITS Emergency	OUTPATIENT VISITS Total
UNITED STATES	4,907	824,676	33,765,589	193,754,932	314,740,801	531,715	863,683	5.7	26,432,095	60,351	3,868,995	105,865,778	536,588,378
Nonmetropolitan	2,166	174,945	5,372,241	35,717,503	71,393,393	97,918	195,777	6.6	4,479,968	13,831	533,148	22,155,102	110,466,485
Metropolitan	2,741	649,731	28,393,348	158,037,429	243,347,408	433,797	667,906	5.6	21,952,127	46,520	3,335,847	83,710,676	426,121,893
CENSUS DIVISION 7, WEST SOUTH CENTRAL	727	95,071	3,949,513	20,782,167	32,381,612	56,975	88,801	5.3	2,789,736	7,645	509,537	12,453,535	50,578,007
Nonmetropolitan	333	19,063	662,914	3,289,111	6,238,208	9,009	17,108	5.0	397,825	1,550	59,178	2,599,955	10,881,145
Metropolitan	394	76,008	3,286,599	17,493,056	26,143,404	47,966	71,693	5.3	2,391,911	6,095	450,359	9,853,580	39,696,862
Arkansas	83	9,535	371,080	2,034,589	3,465,655	5,579	9,510	5.5	260,895	767	36,863	1,152,995	4,493,774
Nonmetropolitan	55	4,281	146,382	801,892	1,607,551	2,200	4,416	5.5	92,812	326	12,341	558,196	2,120,376
Metropolitan	28	5,254	224,698	1,232,697	1,858,104	3,379	5,094	5.5	168,083	441	24,522	594,799	2,373,398
Fayetteville-Springdale-Rogers	6	520	27,980	125,085	189,144	344	521	4.5	16,162	73	4,753	85,389	182,154
Fort Smith	4	870	39,140	209,191	295,756	574	810	5.3	43,173	71	3,719	119,640	263,508
Jonesboro	3	470	21,953	121,406	195,470	333	535	5.5	17,565	32	2,149	60,986	231,111
Little Rock-North Little Rock	13	2,919	117,753	677,718	1,029,381	1,856	2,821	5.8	78,623	229	11,856	273,873	1,509,662
Memphis	1	119	4,851	24,202	39,035	66	107	5.0	5,790	11	648	18,000	31,272
Pine Bluff	1	356	13,021	75,095	109,318	206	300	5.8	6,770	25	1,397	36,911	155,691
Louisiana	125	17,975	682,586	3,736,536	5,811,983	10,237	15,930	5.5	458,751	1,244	63,248	2,267,490	10,060,381
Nonmetropolitan	49	3,105	108,454	586,784	1,030,010	1,607	2,824	5.4	64,427	172	7,222	441,053	1,536,251
Metropolitan	76	14,870	574,132	3,149,752	4,781,973	8,630	13,106	5.5	394,324	1,072	56,026	1,826,437	8,524,130
Alexandria	5	753	33,579	174,511	276,589	478	758	5.2	21,102	65	3,253	137,722	448,278
Baton Rouge	9	2,091	82,817	449,996	699,370	1,236	1,920	5.4	67,114	125	10,089	255,365	842,397
Houma	5	735	31,142	135,059	224,598	370	614	4.3	26,560	72	3,247	114,085	417,445
Lafayette	11	1,554	56,619	295,632	461,086	809	1,264	5.2	42,845	133	6,625	210,253	668,418
Lake Charles	8	924	35,473	178,910	277,959	492	762	5.0	23,152	90	3,313	103,427	405,104
Monroe	5	1,040	42,951	243,239	342,387	666	938	5.7	21,579	101	3,824	107,177	427,379
New Orleans	24	5,992	212,547	1,258,977	1,882,623	3,445	5,157	5.9	144,391	350	20,073	739,561	4,303,858
Shreveport-Bossier City	9	1,781	79,004	413,428	617,361	1,134	1,693	5.2	47,581	136	5,602	158,847	1,011,251
Oklahoma	108	11,207	434,831	2,360,979	3,745,543	6,463	10,271	5.4	294,169	888	43,053	1,226,716	4,569,904
Nonmetropolitan	68	4,097	133,541	708,174	1,292,728	1,936	3,547	5.3	83,684	380	12,402	484,710	1,585,143
Metropolitan	40	7,110	301,290	1,652,805	2,452,815	4,527	6,724	5.5	210,485	508	30,651	742,006	2,984,761
Enid	2	360	12,202	80,753	119,892	222	329	6.6	6,379	40	1,154	30,315	102,510
Fort Smith	1	41	1,054	4,865	11,689	13	32	4.6	1,184	0	0	4,460	23,903
Lawton	2	441	13,643	79,685	140,680	218	386	5.8	9,965	37	1,483	44,457	154,785
Oklahoma City	20	3,686	161,319	889,501	1,307,230	2,437	3,584	5.5	100,303	270	15,896	431,703	1,711,324
Tulsa	15	2,582	113,072	598,001	873,324	1,637	2,393	5.3	92,654	161	12,118	231,071	992,239
Texas	411	56,354	2,461,016	12,650,063	19,358,431	34,696	53,090	5.1	1,775,921	4,746	366,373	7,806,334	31,453,948
Nonmetropolitan	161	7,580	274,537	1,192,261	2,307,919	3,266	6,321	4.3	156,902	672	27,213	1,115,996	5,639,375
Metropolitan	250	48,774	2,186,479	11,457,802	17,050,512	31,430	46,769	5.2	1,619,019	4,074	339,160	6,690,338	25,814,573
Abilene	2	576	22,281	118,388	182,512	324	500	5.3	13,670	46	2,753	64,774	190,012
Amarillo	4	853	40,602	207,757	288,994	569	792	5.1	29,578	50	4,369	95,650	316,384
Austin-San Marcos	15	2,212	103,598	538,402	849,512	1,474	2,328	5.2	88,048	219	22,383	464,805	1,263,074
Beaumont-Port Arthur	11	1,887	67,930	373,687	546,382	1,024	1,497	5.5	41,250	108	6,413	164,303	639,247
Brazoria	3	234	9,304	35,378	81,495	97	224	3.8	8,451	32	1,232	49,022	145,767
Brownsville-Harlingen-San Benito	5	810	47,637	204,089	284,467	559	779	4.3	24,364	72	9,343	93,312	342,334
Bryan-College Station	2	428	19,774	95,503	143,316	262	393	4.8	15,317	60	3,307	67,835	259,299
Corpus Christi	9	1,660	75,663	409,841	603,320	1,123	1,653	5.4	53,231	132	10,004	189,271	747,501
Dallas	43	7,897	371,963	1,877,722	2,777,590	5,144	7,609	5.0	270,807	733	65,491	1,259,855	4,236,730
El Paso	8	1,699	75,044	379,293	557,779	1,040	1,528	5.1	41,505	194	15,443	212,352	1,149,501
Fort Worth-Arlington	23	3,655	177,511	927,482	1,401,121	2,540	3,838	5.2	139,912	360	30,556	680,388	2,111,150
Galveston-Texas City	3	984	39,172	216,725	352,667	594	966	5.5	34,390	50	5,722	109,926	905,441
Houston	51	11,078	493,577	2,674,198	3,893,747	7,370	10,726	5.4	369,105	851	75,938	1,270,945	5,498,092
Killeen-Temple	4	800	33,958	168,638	369,835	462	1,012	5.0	27,250	40	4,271	114,379	1,720,797
Laredo	2	426	23,066	112,292	171,239	307	469	4.9	16,051	85	6,283	59,288	221,323
Longview-Marshall	4	647	29,900	141,601	217,830	389	597	4.7	19,559	66	3,414	125,944	321,426
Lubbock	6	2,201	72,932	422,910	637,542	1,158	1,747	5.8	43,334	64	6,380	216,410	1,021,849
McAllen-Edinburg-Mission	7	1,344	71,495	366,545	478,622	1,005	1,310	5.1	36,833	104	14,740	114,575	349,778
Odessa-Midland	4	741	31,865	108,745	240,245	462	667	5.3	29,216	81	4,828	115,055	355,071
San Angelo	2	371	19,408	83,006	133,321	227	365	4.3	15,445	39	2,041	62,686	239,957
San Antonio	21	4,217	198,818	1,006,502	1,439,933	2,755	3,945	5.1	177,299	420	28,836	565,122	1,808,799
Sherman-Denison	3	568	23,826	132,794	204,023	363	559	5.6	12,041	46	2,106	170,177	363,007
Texarkana	4	586	26,572	149,622	219,914	410	602	5.6	13,882	50	2,341	98,913	288,781
Tyler	5	928	44,183	244,934	356,015	671	976	5.5	30,040	54	3,263	120,127	627,024
Victoria	3	794	22,918	116,313	170,544	318	467	5.1	21,249	55	2,058	57,152	181,379
Waco	2	720	25,211	182,190	285,953	499	783	7.2	26,489	51	3,614	80,627	347,736
Wichita Falls	4	458	18,271	103,245	159,594	284	437	5.7	20,703	12	2,031	67,445	163,114

TABLE 8

U.S. CENSUS DIVISION 7, WEST SOUTH CENTRAL

U.S. Community Hospitals
(Nonfederal, short-term general and other special hospitals)

2001 Utilization, Personnel and Finances

FULL-TIME EQUIVALENT PERSONNEL					FULL-TIME EQUIV. TRAINEES			EXPENSES						
								LABOR				TOTAL		
Physicians and Dentists	Registered Nurses	Licensed Practical Nurses	Other Salaried Personnel	Total Personnel	Medical and Dental Residents	Other Trainees	Total Trainees	Payroll (in thousands)	Employee Benefits (in thousands)	Total (in thousands)	Percent of Total	Amount (in thousands)	Adjusted per Admission	Adjusted per Inpatient Day
70,153	956,577	126,143	2,828,126	3,980,999	77,440	5,751	83,191	$161,734,716	$34,640,089	$196,374,807	51.3	$383,082,895	$6,976.34	$1,217.14
8,081	142,404	36,781	476,073	663,339	1,719	697	2,416	22,294,816	5,051,240	27,346,046	53.3	51,353,805	4,803.37	719.31
62,072	814,173	89,362	2,352,053	3,317,660	75,721	5,054	80,775	139,439,900	29,588,849	169,028,761	51.0	331,729,090	7,501.70	1,363.19
3,114	102,300	23,418	297,953	426,785	5,101	1,105	6,206	15,645,793	3,239,999	18,885,793	48.3	39,110,488	6,270.56	1,207.80
447	13,760	7,297	49,064	70,568	22	40	62	2,071,296	442,975	2,514,273	51.7	4,865,726	3,905.96	779.99
2,667	88,540	16,121	248,889	356,217	5,079	1,065	6,144	13,574,496	2,797,025	16,371,520	47.8	34,244,762	6,860.70	1,309.88
295	10,093	3,231	27,541	41,160	12	1	13	1,266,622	275,893	1,542,519	47.5	3,249,944	5,321.56	937.76
184	3,467	1,628	10,348	15,627	3	0	3	443,168	98,366	541,537	50.5	1,073,324	4,027.12	667.68
111	6,626	1,603	17,193	25,533	9	1	10	823,454	177,526	1,000,982	46.0	2,176,620	6,323.91	1,171.42
48	647	212	2,147	3,054	0	0	0	90,659	17,592	108,251	52.6	205,659	4,788.23	1,087.32
1	1,072	353	2,656	4,082	0	0	0	117,511	30,077	147,590	48.9	301,955	5,316.29	1,020.96
0	552	222	1,423	2,197	0	0	0	58,897	14,992	73,890	40.3	183,406	5,056.96	938.28
59	3,916	668	9,884	14,527	9	1	10	492,618	105,309	597,927	44.9	1,332,810	7,347.64	1,294.77
2	107	53	225	387	0	0	0	17,930	2,078	20,008	50.7	39,501	5,048.70	1,011.94
1	332	95	858	1,286	0	0	0	45,838	7,478	53,316	47.1	113,289	5,976.74	1,036.33
1,019	17,584	3,730	54,384	76,717	802	117	919	2,545,537	526,259	3,071,799	49.3	6,231,829	5,806.37	1,072.24
106	2,260	1,014	8,180	11,560	6	32	38	342,336	67,141	409,481	53.4	766,347	3,955.52	744.02
913	15,324	2,716	46,204	65,157	796	85	881	2,203,200	459,118	2,662,318	48.7	5,465,482	6,214.07	1,142.93
45	863	171	2,710	3,789	30	0	30	121,213	26,213	147,426	50.3	293,227	5,497.02	1,060.16
249	2,123	298	6,088	8,758	108	0	108	319,657	55,795	375,452	47.9	784,476	6,085.88	1,121.69
40	734	139	2,468	3,381	8	2	10	116,158	28,584	144,742	49.4	293,053	5,638.88	1,304.79
71	1,488	460	4,451	6,470	67	6	73	209,864	43,290	253,153	49.0	516,656	5,821.61	1,120.52
24	967	198	2,619	3,808	12	9	21	107,358	22,477	129,836	49.8	260,673	4,660.61	937.81
63	1,119	255	2,984	4,421	34	0	34	138,297	33,963	172,260	45.2	381,390	6,225.15	1,113.92
247	6,227	955	19,051	26,480	245	43	288	956,634	196,553	1,153,189	48.3	2,386,563	7,431.84	1,267.68
174	1,803	240	5,833	8,050	292	25	317	234,018	52,242	286,260	52.1	549,443	4,646.53	889.99
560	10,264	2,807	35,704	49,335	361	46	407	1,519,605	300,350	1,819,954	48.9	3,722,315	5,343.38	993.80
131	2,765	1,383	10,793	15,072	10	7	17	420,930	89,438	510,368	53.2	959,358	3,901.88	742.12
429	7,499	1,424	24,911	34,263	351	39	390	1,098,675	210,912	1,309,586	47.1	2,702,957	6,129.67	1,126.44
0	270	80	968	1,334	0	0	0	40,848	5,856	46,704	45.2	103,417	5,732.35	862.59
2	42	19	163	226	0	0	0	4,291	925	5,216	54.4	9,580	3,783.58	819.58
60	241	206	1,438	1,945	0	0	0	64,812	12,472	77,284	44.4	173,897	7,195.06	1,236.12
117	4,170	692	12,173	17,152	155	28	183	600,222	115,440	715,661	47.6	1,503,480	6,286.50	1,150.13
242	2,768	427	10,169	13,606	196	11	207	388,502	76,219	464,721	47.8	972,582	5,829.12	1,113.66
1,240	64,359	13,650	180,324	259,573	3,926	941	4,867	10,314,029	2,137,497	12,451,521	48.1	25,906,400	6,717.51	1,338.25
26	5,268	3,272	19,743	28,309	3	1	4	864,862	188,028	1,052,887	50.9	2,066,697	3,830.17	895.48
1,214	59,091	10,378	160,581	231,264	3,923	940	4,863	9,449,167	1,949,469	11,398,634	47.8	23,839,703	7,187.20	1,398.18
0	656	202	1,909	2,767	0	37	37	87,348	16,367	103,714	47.1	220,319	6,440.93	1,207.15
9	1,210	169	2,518	3,906	0	0	0	143,729	28,978	172,707	44.4	389,083	6,730.73	1,346.34
54	2,947	361	6,791	10,153	105	0	105	437,144	73,231	510,374	49.1	1,039,591	6,122.70	1,220.70
15	1,790	308	4,002	6,205	16	2	18	222,743	42,044	264,787	48.6	544,433	5,347.75	996.43
0	179	56	623	858	0	0	0	31,753	7,682	39,435	47.7	82,695	3,807.48	1,014.72
20	798	314	2,738	3,870	15	0	15	153,529	43,181	196,711	50.9	386,268	5,771.40	1,357.87
0	551	218	1,624	2,393	0	0	0	66,360	16,378	82,738	48.6	170,271	5,739.80	1,188.08
7	1,643	422	4,803	6,875	115	0	115	253,893	51,687	305,580	46.7	654,041	5,813.80	1,084.07
200	10,792	1,066	27,120	39,178	1,037	25	1,062	1,727,769	302,647	2,030,417	46.8	1,300,040	7,590.01	1,561.08
12	1,547	104	4,873	6,596	0	0	0	266,341	55,435	321,776	43.4	740,750	6,677.82	1,328.04
24	5,216	894	12,893	19,027	232	0	232	767,699	160,698	928,397	49.3	1,884,526	6,823.52	1,345.01
0	1,353	169	3,859	5,381	601	0	601	187,701	30,020	220,528	41.0	552,689	8,740.52	1,567.17
686	14,089	1,892	42,472	59,139	740	605	1,345	2,568,478	557,772	3,126,249	49.8	6,274,395	8,600.27	1,611.40
0	923	190	2,802	3,915	294	256	550	327,072	82,055	409,127	62.9	650,586	8,788.14	1,760.12
0	392	103	1,572	2,007	0	0	0	67,537	13,804	81,430	45.3	179,916	5,119.12	1,050.67
0	793	118	2,144	3,055	0	7	7	102,190	24,832	127,022	49.1	258,954	5,536.64	1,188.79
35	2,224	407	5,775	8,441	64	5	69	353,300	87,045	441,033	46.1	956,972	8,623.70	1,501.03
0	1,471	454	3,604	5,529	0	0	0	192,615	27,389	220,005	46.9	468,804	4,900.63	979.49
1	938	198	2,182	3,319	0	0	0	112,371	42,186	154,557	45.1	342,674	7,469.08	1,408.76
0	366	110	1,288	1,764	0	0	0	57,824	14,156	71,981	46.6	154,411	4,954.64	1,158.19
31	4,933	1,031	11,655	17,650	684	0	684	697,692	127,813	825,504	42.1	1,958,682	6,792.82	1,360.26
19	738	181	1,903	2,841	1	0	1	101,038	20,370	121,409	48.3	251,343	6,868.60	1,231.93
0	715	190	1,869	2,774	0	3	3	96,367	18,029	114,396	48.3	236,712	5,826.62	1,076.39
73	1,174	292	4,960	6,499	19	0	19	203,107	53,270	256,376	46.6	550,381	8,516.14	1,545.95
1	649	356	1,264	2,270	0	0	0	68,898	14,539	83,436	49.5	168,531	5,012.38	988.20
27	620	191	1,882	2,720	0	0	0	88,287	14,151	102,439	45.3	225,953	5,762.92	790.17
0	384	232	1,456	2,072	0	0	0	66,471	14,014	80,486	50.1	160,679	5,412.80	1,006.80

MSAs

TABLE 8

U.S. CENSUS DIVISION 8, MOUNTAIN

U.S. Community Hospitals
(Nonfederal, short-term general and other special hospitals)

2001 Utilization, Personnel and Finances

MSAs

CLASSIFICATION	Hospitals	Beds	Admissions	Inpatient Days	Adjusted Patient Days	Average Daily Census	Adjusted Average Daily Census	Average Stay (days)	Surgical Operations	NEWBORNS		OUTPATIENT VISITS	
										Bassinets	Births	Emergency	Total
UNITED STATES	4,907	824,676	33,765,589	193,754,932	314,740,801	531,715	863,683	5.7	26,432,095	60,351	3,868,995	105,865,778	536,588,378
Nonmetropolitan	2,166	174,945	5,372,241	35,717,503	71,393,393	97,918	195,777	6.6	4,479,968	13,831	533,148	22,155,102	110,466,485
Metropolitan	2,741	649,731	28,393,348	158,037,429	243,347,408	433,797	667,906	5.6	21,952,127	46,520	3,335,847	83,710,676	426,121,893
CENSUS DIVISION 8, MOUNTAIN	345	42,116	1,825,214	9,432,684	15,633,399	25,844	42,844	5.2	1,364,705	3,817	277,576	5,444,391	28,044,288
Nonmetropolitan	205	12,323	339,991	2,413,981	5,095,430	6,614	13,971	7.1	279,475	1,148	49,355	1,444,004	7,527,156
Metropolitan	140	29,793	1,485,223	7,018,703	10,537,969	19,230	28,873	4.7	1,085,230	2,669	228,221	4,000,387	20,517,132
Arizona	61	10,732	562,824	2,520,301	3,697,592	6,904	10,129	4.5	356,918	995	80,408	1,401,509	5,071,628
Nonmetropolitan	15	915	41,233	177,721	364,948	487	1,002	4.3	29,622	74	5,373	160,345	715,648
Metropolitan	46	9,817	521,591	2,342,580	3,332,644	6,417	9,127	4.5	327,296	921	75,035	1,241,164	4,355,980
Flagstaff	2	262	11,110	56,808	90,855	155	248	5.1	7,037	23	1,748	32,767	73,058
Las Vegas	3	415	18,680	82,299	123,965	225	340	4.4	13,456	24	1,789	62,459	180,700
Phoenix-Mesa	30	6,821	364,381	1,631,038	2,280,320	4,468	6,245	4.5	227,095	707	55,513	831,343	2,484,124
Tucson	10	2,043	111,059	505,057	737,731	1,384	2,021	4.5	69,922	148	12,802	265,319	1,469,413
Yuma	1	276	16,361	67,378	99,773	185	273	4.1	9,786	19	3,183	49,276	148,685
Colorado	66	9,442	413,605	2,111,549	3,630,040	5,785	9,952	5.1	325,599	790	61,708	1,380,740	6,912,525
Nonmetropolitan	35	1,832	45,351	348,255	887,312	954	2,436	7.7	47,611	161	6,446	219,100	1,356,695
Metropolitan	31	7,610	368,254	1,763,294	2,742,728	4,831	7,516	4.8	277,988	629	55,262	1,161,640	5,555,830
Boulder-Longmont	3	399	22,988	90,600	164,655	248	451	3.9	18,158	57	5,102	101,603	608,160
Colorado Springs	2	823	46,703	200,052	312,007	549	854	4.3	35,846	69	6,030	122,164	552,930
Denver	17	4,470	221,654	1,073,468	1,644,366	2,941	4,506	4.8	168,249	336	34,463	623,694	2,690,785
Fort Collins-Loveland	3	402	22,284	95,033	158,998	260	436	4.3	14,049	54	3,398	70,261	397,510
Grand Junction	3	741	17,344	135,518	209,208	371	574	7.8	14,796	45	1,942	134,219	648,582
Greeley	1	276	14,654	60,922	91,916	167	252	4.2	10,817	23	2,094	43,051	312,386
Pueblo	2	499	22,627	107,701	161,578	295	443	4.8	16,073	45	2,233	66,648	345,477
Idaho	40	3,439	122,510	682,010	1,184,542	1,868	3,249	5.6	98,948	281	19,672	411,533	2,640,078
Nonmetropolitan	33	2,087	65,250	409,716	751,760	1,121	2,062	6.3	50,667	187	9,994	242,840	1,117,931
Metropolitan	7	1,352	57,260	272,294	432,782	747	1,187	4.8	48,281	94	9,678	168,693	1,522,147
Boise City	5	1,029	49,452	206,213	323,136	566	886	4.2	41,921	72	8,021	128,426	1,275,910
Pocatello	2	323	7,808	66,081	109,646	181	301	8.5	6,360	22	1,657	40,267	246,237
Montana	53	4,463	103,346	1,058,079	2,043,046	2,898	5,599	10.2	69,318	277	9,766	276,175	2,648,345
Nonmetropolitan	48	3,035	49,517	698,086	1,448,926	1,912	3,971	14.1	30,041	178	4,767	172,864	1,169,409
Metropolitan	5	1,428	53,829	359,993	594,120	986	1,628	6.7	39,277	99	4,999	103,311	1,478,936
Billings	2	624	25,558	165,747	319,249	454	875	6.5	19,900	36	2,141	40,547	1,002,625
Great Falls	1	479	13,211	118,578	161,752	325	443	9.0	8,249	42	1,303	28,640	132,073
Missoula	2	325	15,060	75,668	113,119	207	310	5.0	11,128	21	1,555	34,124	344,238
Nevada	24	4,099	207,844	1,019,835	1,480,737	2,795	4,059	4.9	168,175	250	28,040	548,798	2,126,113
Nonmetropolitan	9	532	14,444	82,776	204,622	228	560	5.7	12,801	40	2,095	78,419	388,531
Metropolitan	15	3,567	193,400	937,059	1,276,115	2,567	3,499	4.8	155,374	210	25,945	470,379	1,737,582
Las Vegas	11	2,652	151,738	731,339	979,266	2,003	2,685	4.8	127,197	144	20,424	353,288	1,292,101
Reno	4	915	41,662	205,720	296,849	564	814	4.9	28,177	66	5,521	117,091	445,481
New Mexico	35	3,584	164,461	758,923	1,336,780	2,079	3,662	4.6	123,442	417	24,884	528,979	3,409,228
Nonmetropolitan	22	1,498	57,552	238,892	468,266	654	1,283	4.2	46,177	191	8,844	251,453	1,180,868
Metropolitan	13	2,086	106,909	520,031	868,514	1,425	2,379	4.9	77,265	226	16,040	277,526	2,228,360
Albuquerque	10	1,537	79,704	408,575	692,618	1,120	1,897	5.1	59,119	153	11,547	191,993	1,866,232
Las Cruces	1	297	14,284	67,904	102,297	186	280	4.8	10,839	40	2,560	29,627	195,678
Santa Fe	2	252	12,921	43,552	73,599	119	202	3.4	7,307	33	1,933	55,906	166,450
Utah	42	4,437	203,037	902,313	1,522,042	2,474	4,170	4.4	182,117	623	47,319	699,934	4,418,349
Nonmetropolitan	21	908	36,410	158,048	344,250	434	943	4.3	34,912	173	8,064	181,568	987,361
Metropolitan	21	3,529	166,627	744,265	1,177,792	2,040	3,227	4.5	147,205	450	39,255	518,366	3,430,988
Flagstaff	1	33	418	5,529	13,284	15	36	13.2	810	3	129	2,125	11,386
Provo-Orem	5	655	35,977	128,409	208,902	352	573	3.6	26,538	111	10,428	109,517	595,788
Salt Lake City-Ogden	15	2,841	130,232	610,327	955,606	1,673	2,618	4.7	119,857	336	28,698	406,724	2,823,814
Wyoming	24	1,920	47,587	379,674	738,620	1,041	2,024	8.0	40,188	184	5,779	196,723	818,022
Nonmetropolitan	22	1,516	30,234	300,487	625,346	824	1,714	9.9	27,644	144	3,772	137,415	610,713
Metropolitan	2	404	17,353	79,187	113,274	217	310	4.6	12,544	40	2,007	59,308	207,309
Casper	1	205	8,618	37,632	53,238	103	146	4.4	5,674	24	918	32,086	76,048
Cheyenne	1	199	8,735	41,555	60,036	114	164	4.8	6,870	16	1,089	27,222	131,261

U.S. CENSUS DIVISION 8, MOUNTAIN

U.S. Community Hospitals
(Nonfederal, short-term general and other special hospitals)

2001 Utilization, Personnel and Finances

FULL-TIME EQUIVALENT PERSONNEL					FULL-TIME EQUIV. TRAINEES			EXPENSES						
								LABOR				TOTAL		
Physicians and Dentists	Registered Nurses	Licensed Practical Nurses	Other Salaried Personnel	Total Personnel	Medical and Dental Residents	Other Trainees	Total Trainees	Payroll (in thousands)	Employee Benefits (in thousands)	Total (in thousands)	Percent of Total	Amount (in thousands)	Adjusted per Admission	Adjusted per Inpatient Day
70,153	956,577	126,143	2,828,126	3,980,999	77,440	5,751	83,191	$161,734,716	$34,640,089	$196,374,807	51.3	$383,082,895	$6,976.34	$1,217.14
8,081	142,404	36,781	476,073	663,339	1,719	697	2,416	22,294,816	5,051,240	27,346,046	53.3	51,353,805	4,803.37	719.31
62,072	814,173	89,362	2,352,053	3,317,660	75,721	5,054	80,775	139,439,900	29,588,849	169,028,761	51.0	331,729,090	7,501.70	1,363.19
2,719	47,791	5,794	142,261	198,565	2,085	203	2,288	8,082,066	1,675,234	9,757,292	50.8	19,222,843	6,521.35	1,229.60
563	9,746	1,865	32,794	44,968	25	34	59	1,518,603	346,408	1,865,004	53.6	3,478,625	4,847.99	682.70
2,156	38,045	3,929	109,467	153,597	2,060	169	2,229	6,563,463	1,328,826	7,892,288	50.1	15,744,218	7,059.75	1,494.05
447	12,328	1,300	35,202	49,277	778	53	831	2,050,959	409,672	2,460,631	49.3	4,986,268	6,053.23	1,348.52
34	1,028	127	3,289	4,478	0	10	10	151,835	33,004	184,839	51.6	358,560	4,371.40	982.50
413	11,300	1,173	31,913	44,799	778	43	821	1,899,124	376,668	2,275,792	49.2	4,627,708	6,239.22	1,388.60
3	362	8	870	1,243	0	0	0	59,397	13,457	72,855	49.4	147,382	8,259.02	1,622.17
10	440	70	1,258	1,778	2	0	2	58,517	13,580	72,097	49.3	146,203	5,194.80	1,179.39
270	7,479	787	21,460	29,996	677	33	710	1,319,128	257,439	1,576,567	48.9	3,226,606	6,348.25	1,414.98
130	2,641	273	7,138	10,182	99	10	109	406,929	80,561	487,489	49.5	983,950	6,028.00	1,333.75
0	378	35	1,187	1,600	0	0	0	55,153	11,631	66,784	54.0	123,567	5,100.40	1,238.48
646	12,230	964	34,911	48,751	612	57	669	2,154,655	416,860	2,571,514	52.0	4,948,616	7,258.24	1,363.24
90	1,373	309	5,237	7,009	4	2	6	251,962	56,305	308,264	53.0	581,833	5,361.08	655.73
556	10,857	655	29,674	41,742	608	55	663	1,902,693	360,556	2,263,250	51.8	4,366,783	7,617.40	1,592.13
32	755	49	2,140	2,976	0	0	0	123,637	22,696	146,333	54.6	267,787	6,374.83	1,626.35
66	1,147	62	3,667	4,942	147	26	173	192,275	37,228	229,504	50.8	451,341	6,187.33	1,446.57
358	6,501	327	16,260	23,446	339	23	362	1,165,494	208,572	1,374,067	51.7	2,657,466	7,819.59	1,616.10
16	684	41	1,869	2,610	18	0	18	104,935	26,708	131,642	51.7	254,855	7,238.14	1,602.88
78	877	101	2,660	3,716	48	6	54	164,609	34,904	199,513	51.4	387,998	14,269.88	1,854.60
0	316	18	1,196	1,530	36	0	36	67,060	13,412	80,471	49.2	163,722	7,405.20	1,781.21
6	577	57	1,882	2,522	20	0	20	84,684	17,036	101,720	55.4	183,615	5,407.58	1,136.38
144	3,371	624	10,835	14,974	9	11	20	563,388	128,316	691,705	52.6	1,313,950	6,186.76	1,109.25
53	1,759	402	5,302	7,516	8	11	19	262,834	62,454	325,289	54.7	595,173	4,931.46	791.71
91	1,612	222	5,533	7,458	1	0	1	300,554	65,863	366,416	51.0	718,777	7,839.04	1,660.83
80	1,371	122	4,771	6,344	1	0	1	259,155	56,003	315,157	50.8	620,666	7,899.84	1,920.76
11	241	100	762	1,114	0	0	0	41,399	9,860	51,259	52.2	98,111	7,475.10	894.79
405	2,989	666	10,647	14,707	2	3	5	555,874	119,389	675,263	55.5	1,216,570	6,115.45	595.47
109	1,523	377	5,598	7,607	1	3	4	240,164	54,254	294,418	56.1	524,727	4,709.54	362.15
296	1,466	289	5,049	7,100	1	0	1	315,710	65,135	380,845	55.0	691,843	7,905.33	1,164.48
226	684	175	2,689	3,774	1	0	1	164,661	33,482	198,143	55.8	355,062	7,568.36	1,112.18
5	326	50	1,097	1,478	0	0	0	63,140	15,210	78,350	54.0	145,000	8,046.19	896.44
65	456	64	1,263	1,848	0	0	0	87,908	16,443	104,352	54.4	191,781	8,493.01	1,695.39
127	4,746	481	12,210	17,564	199	6	205	822,994	168,495	991,489	47.5	2,087,682	7,015.34	1,409.89
24	382	49	1,577	2,032	0	0	0	79,792	18,822	98,615	50.8	194,197	5,635.77	949.05
103	4,364	432	10,633	15,532	199	6	205	743,201	149,673	892,874	47.2	1,893,485	7,196.00	1,483.79
77	3,359	346	7,557	11,339	184	4	188	547,578	113,325	660,903	46.2	1,429,264	7,039.81	1,459.53
20	1,005	[illegible]	3,070	4,193	15	2	17	195,023	30,348	231,971	50.0	404,220	7,723.62	1,563.83
565	4,703	705	15,004	20,977	224	18	242	768,755	171,274	940,026	50.3	1,868,614	6,346.89	1,307.85
141	1,616	275	5,311	7,343	10	7	17	229,963	51,521	281,481	52.7	533,814	4,557.92	1,139.98
424	3,087	430	9,693	13,634	214	11	225	538,792	119,753	658,545	49.3	1,334,800	7,528.65	1,536.88
387	2,455	381	7,665	10,888	190	5	195	431,760	90,593	522,353	50.0	1,045,322	7,804.11	1,509.23
13	356	9	1,087	1,465	12	6	18	59,263	12,579	71,842	44.1	162,979	7,573.73	1,593.20
24	276	40	941	1,281	12	0	12	47,770	16,581	64,350	50.9	126,499	5,794.19	1,718.76
317	5,816	759	18,206	25,098	261	54	315	924,488	205,626	1,130,114	50.4	2,242,551	6,414.42	1,473.38
46	953	172	2,789	3,960	2	0	2	139,013	32,157	171,170	51.9	329,665	4,178.53	957.67
271	4,863	587	15,417	21,138	259	54	313	785,475	173,469	958,944	50.1	1,912,887	7,066.03	1,624.13
1	19	9	74	103	0	0	0	2,299	495	2,794	54.4	5,132	5,111.59	386.33
52	953	89	2,423	3,517	30	11	41	125,010	26,450	151,460	51.2	295,777	4,897.22	1,415.87
218	3,891	489	12,920	17,518	229	43	272	658,166	146,524	804,690	49.9	1,611,977	7,701.20	1,686.86
68	1,608	295	5,246	7,217	0	1	1	240,952	55,601	296,550	53.1	558,591	6,260.82	756.26
66	1,112	154	3,691	5,023	0	1	1	163,039	37,891	200,928	55.7	360,655	5,599.54	576.73
2	496	141	1,555	2,194	0	0	0	77,913	17,709	95,622	48.3	197,935	7,977.39	1,747.40
2	285	113	741	1,141	0	0	0	40,716	11,092	51,807	46.2	112,020	9,187.98	2,104.13
0	211	28	814	1,053	0	0	0	37,197	6,618	43,815	51.0	85,915	6,807.87	1,431.06

MSAs

TABLE 8

U.S. CENSUS DIVISION 9, PACIFIC

U.S. Community Hospitals
(Nonfederal, short-term general and other special hospitals)

2001 Utilization, Personnel and Finances

										NEWBORNS		OUTPATIENT VISITS	
CLASSIFICATION	Hospitals	Beds	Admissions	Inpatient Days	Adjusted Patient Days	Average Daily Census	Adjusted Average Daily Census	Average Stay (days)	Surgical Operations	Bassinets	Births	Emergency	Total
UNITED STATES	4,907	824,676	33,765,589	193,754,932	314,740,801	531,715	863,683	5.7	26,432,095	60,351	3,868,995	105,865,778	536,588,378
Nonmetropolitan	2,166	174,945	5,372,241	35,717,503	71,393,393	97,918	195,777	6.6	4,479,968	13,831	533,148	22,155,102	110,466,485
Metropolitan	2,741	649,731	28,393,348	158,037,429	243,347,408	433,797	667,906	5.6	21,952,127	46,520	3,335,847	83,710,676	426,121,893
CENSUS DIVISION 9, PACIFIC	570	96,010	4,347,642	22,968,771	34,737,704	62,964	95,249	5.3	3,046,220	7,540	630,251	13,916,852	70,193,381
Nonmetropolitan	137	8,682	292,944	1,744,232	3,402,333	4,776	9,326	6.0	305,358	784	38,174	1,397,313	7,138,149
Metropolitan	433	87,328	4,054,698	21,224,539	31,335,371	58,188	85,923	5.2	2,740,862	6,756	592,077	12,519,539	63,055,232
Alaska	19	1,442	49,065	303,092	523,103	830	1,433	6.2	53,737	131	7,448	205,595	1,387,626
Nonmetropolitan	16	779	21,029	150,468	291,550	411	799	7.2	21,662	82	3,079	96,176	649,588
Metropolitan	3	663	28,036	152,624	231,553	419	634	5.4	32,075	49	4,369	109,419	738,038
Anchorage	3	663	28,036	152,624	231,553	419	634	5.4	32,075	49	4,369	109,419	738,038
California	384	73,291	3,332,839	17,835,799	25,907,882	48,906	71,055	5.4	2,152,812	5,402	493,383	10,262,726	48,547,534
Nonmetropolitan	40	2,315	78,889	460,548	921,714	1,262	2,526	5.8	80,874	194	10,337	471,595	2,525,740
Metropolitan	344	70,976	3,253,950	17,375,251	24,986,168	47,644	68,529	5.3	2,071,938	5,208	483,046	9,791,131	46,021,794
Bakersfield	10	1,355	58,572	328,529	524,095	899	1,436	5.6	35,764	81	9,031	151,495	646,568
Chico-Paradise	4	519	27,606	131,275	208,511	360	571	4.8	19,665	33	2,572	110,390	641,116
Fresno	15	1,938	91,832	489,446	785,744	1,341	2,152	5.3	84,516	151	14,839	421,271	2,255,544
Los Angeles-Long Beach	102	23,907	1,043,019	5,845,562	7,994,908	16,012	21,902	5.6	633,351	1,597	151,868	2,901,074	11,510,163
Merced	3	320	7,342	39,470	70,887	148	263	5.4	4,698	40	1,644	30,686	144,087
Modesto	4	1,118	46,337	305,404	450,973	838	1,236	6.6	30,017	77	8,231	188,283	373,146
Oakland	19	5,070	240,306	1,318,105	1,924,921	3,611	5,275	5.5	131,622	640	38,611	735,112	3,668,689
Orange County	31	5,740	262,922	1,238,572	1,725,847	3,394	4,728	4.7	186,147	370	34,431	739,218	2,847,027
Redding	3	581	20,660	127,301	175,185	349	479	6.2	15,210	11	1,840	81,939	416,119
Riverside-San Bernardino	32	5,993	326,251	1,529,285	2,209,914	4,191	6,057	4.7	178,126	462	45,346	934,004	3,253,995
Sacramento	13	3,357	174,909	899,386	1,288,115	2,464	3,529	5.1	108,185	267	25,692	436,397	3,360,367
Salinas	4	592	35,738	166,843	229,954	457	630	4.7	20,881	80	6,466	117,724	570,703
San Diego	20	5,310	254,421	1,370,655	1,989,372	3,755	5,452	5.4	162,690	399	39,439	644,921	2,666,834
San Francisco	19	4,344	177,706	1,152,851	1,704,930	3,160	4,671	6.5	127,333	152	18,336	680,068	4,972,419
San Jose	12	3,379	155,937	743,954	1,076,983	2,038	2,954	4.8	104,980	304	32,521	416,207	3,283,948
San Luis Obispo-Atascadero-Paso Robles	5	478	18,402	88,556	137,795	244	378	4.8	13,376	36	2,334	99,517	456,953
Santa Barbara-Santa Maria-Lompoc	7	921	39,148	228,175	357,383	625	979	5.8	31,054	82	6,044	108,044	375,692
Santa Cruz-Watsonville	3	435	21,580	92,931	129,501	254	355	4.3	10,810	32	1,751	95,361	298,286
Santa Rosa	9	1,070	45,831	214,255	358,344	586	982	4.7	35,697	51	5,664	152,470	763,775
Stockton-Lodi	7	1,084	52,858	266,581	406,678	731	1,114	5.0	34,689	75	8,993	250,971	1,289,479
Vallejo-Fairfield-Napa	6	897	39,409	180,939	295,863	496	810	4.6	29,952	73	6,355	116,691	509,828
Ventura	8	1,484	62,755	361,277	541,488	989	1,484	5.8	43,239	120	10,867	170,938	873,429
Visalia-Tulare-Porterville	4	732	29,623	168,769	257,743	463	706	5.7	16,016	35	6,509	130,118	523,881
Yolo	2	151	7,723	26,281	51,603	72	141	3.4	5,535	26	1,640	52,777	257,991
Yuba City	2	201	13,063	60,849	89,431	167	245	4.7	8,385	14	2,022	25,455	61,755
Hawaii	23	3,235	108,252	879,258	1,383,171	2,406	3,788	8.1	83,627	215	10,007	287,017	3,167,587
Nonmetropolitan	10	1,017	29,390	273,715	435,545	748	1,192	9.3	20,884	62	3,835	73,119	289,547
Metropolitan	13	2,218	78,862	605,543	947,626	1,658	2,596	7.7	62,743	153	6,172	213,898	2,878,040
Honolulu	13	2,218	78,862	605,543	947,626	1,658	2,596	7.7	62,743	153	6,172	213,898	2,878,040
Oregon	60	6,660	334,862	1,449,556	2,552,423	3,971	6,994	4.3	280,424	723	45,279	1,098,201	7,658,130
Nonmetropolitan	31	1,953	85,577	379,080	754,846	1,039	2,070	4.4	72,276	216	9,922	365,661	1,819,932
Metropolitan	29	4,707	249,285	1,070,476	1,797,577	2,932	4,924	4.3	208,148	507	35,357	732,540	5,838,198
Corvalis	1	145	8,109	31,740	48,888	87	134	3.9	6,922	24	1,048	17,542	189,124
Eugene-Springfield	4	585	31,187	128,231	195,487	351	536	4.1	26,196	54	3,613	91,790	334,661
Medford-Ashland	3	434	22,320	91,590	146,542	250	401	4.1	15,718	34	2,273	61,802	874,253
Portland-Vancouver	17	3,026	164,925	716,976	1,234,077	1,964	3,380	4.3	143,022	337	23,611	468,212	4,008,946
Salem	4	517	22,744	101,939	172,583	280	473	4.5	16,290	58	4,812	93,194	431,214
Washington	84	11,382	522,624	2,501,066	4,371,125	6,851	11,979	4.8	475,620	1,069	74,134	2,063,313	9,432,504
Nonmetropolitan	40	2,618	78,059	480,421	998,678	1,316	2,739	6.2	109,662	230	11,001	390,762	1,853,342
Metropolitan	44	8,764	444,565	2,020,645	3,372,447	5,535	9,240	4.5	365,958	839	63,133	1,672,551	7,579,162
Bellingham	1	208	13,724	56,233	85,650	154	235	4.1	8,240	30	1,921	46,784	95,020
Bremerton	1	239	12,267	46,132	71,879	126	197	3.8	10,753	18	1,655	48,913	127,005
Olympia	2	412	21,089	84,937	136,215	233	373	4.0	21,103	27	2,733	70,313	325,086
Portland-Vancouver	1	334	21,097	77,496	148,868	212	408	3.7	16,037	50	4,754	87,252	235,643
Richland-Kennewick-Pasco	4	392	17,112	74,257	152,173	203	418	4.3	14,059	53	3,619	83,493	230,668
Seattle-Bellevue-Everett	20	4,372	229,629	1,076,625	1,779,511	2,948	4,874	4.7	183,323	463	30,086	799,234	4,105,668
Spokane	6	1,284	55,056	287,894	430,131	789	1,179	5.2	56,792	59	6,119	104,600	452,893
Tacoma	5	1,022	53,028	234,347	427,100	643	1,169	4.4	42,955	82	8,179	315,810	1,482,827
Yakima	4	501	21,563	82,724	140,920	227	387	3.8	12,696	57	4,067	116,152	524,352

TABLE 8

U.S. CENSUS DIVISION 9, PACIFIC

U.S. Community Hospitals
(Nonfederal, short-term general and other special hospitals)

2001 Utilization, Personnel and Finances

FULL-TIME EQUIVALENT PERSONNEL					FULL-TIME EQUIV. TRAINEES			EXPENSES						
								LABOR				TOTAL		
Physicians and Dentists	Registered Nurses	Licensed Practical Nurses	Other Salaried Personnel	Total Personnel	Medical and Dental Residents	Other Trainees	Total Trainees	Payroll (in thousands)	Employee Benefits (in thousands)	Total (in thousands)	Percent of Total	Amount (in thousands)	Adjusted per Admission	Adjusted per Inpatient Day
70,153	956,577	126,143	2,828,126	3,980,999	77,440	5,751	83,191	$161,734,716	$34,640,089	$196,374,807	51.3	$383,082,895	$6,976.34	$1,217.14
8,081	142,404	36,781	476,073	663,339	1,719	697	2,416	22,294,816	5,051,240	27,346,046	53.3	51,353,805	4,803.37	719.31
62,072	814,173	89,362	2,352,053	3,317,660	75,721	5,054	80,775	139,439,900	29,588,849	169,028,761	51.0	331,729,090	7,501.70	1,363.19
7,934	118,413	13,081	337,711	477,139	8,547	639	9,186	21,894,053	5,297,045	27,191,103	51.3	52,988,296	7,990.08	1,525.38
479	8,330	1,438	27,841	38,088	38	87	125	1,562,316	405,582	1,967,898	54.8	3,588,084	6,144.71	1,054.60
7,455	110,083	11,643	309,870	439,051	8,509	552	9,061	20,331,736	4,891,463	25,223,205	51.1	49,400,212	8,168.26	1,576.50
111	1,983	237	5,606	7,937	33	28	61	391,004	91,076	482,079	52.5	918,695	10,859.27	1,756.24
72	794	128	2,807	3,801	2	9	11	190,110	46,885	236,994	53.6	441,934	10,507.47	1,515.81
39	1,189	109	2,799	4,136	31	19	50	200,894	44,191	245,085	51.4	476,761	11,207.09	2,058.97
39	1,189	109	2,799	4,136	31	19	50	200,894	44,191	245,085	51.4	476,761	11,207.09	2,058.97
5,920	85,961	10,387	243,654	345,922	7,102	384	7,486	16,078,731	3,953,526	20,032,263	50.6	39,559,377	8,143.67	1,526.92
90	2,341	526	7,821	10,778	6	32	38	408,418	123,298	531,717	53.7	990,668	6,259.35	1,074.81
5,830	83,620	9,861	235,833	335,144	7,096	352	7,448	15,670,313	3,830,229	19,500,546	50.6	38,568,709	8,207.13	1,543.60
107	1,230	197	4,165	5,699	110	5	115	227,780	60,050	287,829	50.5	569,413	6,358.39	1,086.47
14	680	129	2,378	3,201	4	0	4	127,978	33,327	161,305	52.7	306,371	7,028.80	1,469.33
133	2,734	305	7,913	11,085	140	5	145	447,890	97,957	545,847	52.2	1,044,969	6,946.59	1,329.91
2,639	27,465	3,293	76,109	109,506	3,076	74	3,150	4,948,641	1,154,874	6,103,519	49.4	12,360,396	8,600.65	1,546.03
9	210	38	728	985	2	0	2	26,911	5,901	32,812	57.5	57,034	4,513.24	804.57
7	1,608	131	3,401	5,147	4	0	4	175,914	52,954	228,868	49.8	459,662	7,049.71	1,019.27
433	5,955	620	16,141	23,149	466	57	523	1,390,462	344,030	1,734,494	54.7	3,173,658	9,073.84	1,648.72
129	6,653	669	18,171	25,622	148	6	154	1,063,245	266,594	1,329,837	47.7	2,789,478	7,571.15	1,616.30
17	738	70	1,658	2,483	23	0	23	101,993	22,984	124,977	49.0	254,917	9,547.46	1,455.13
964	6,965	1,006	20,568	29,503	416	28	444	1,135,124	259,276	1,394,399	47.8	2,917,157	6,139.91	1,320.03
345	5,357	558	14,573	20,833	559	25	584	1,079,805	252,494	1,332,299	50.7	2,625,928	10,461.45	2,038.58
46	884	166	2,801	3,897	36	0	36	200,662	91,478	292,140	58.6	498,766	10,200.33	2,168.98
285	5,737	593	16,637	23,252	660	26	686	1,028,794	238,908	1,267,705	50.5	2,510,524	6,795.98	1,261.97
306	5,179	598	14,746	20,829	288	59	347	1,259,931	277,142	1,537,074	51.5	2,985,394	11,159.14	1,751.04
122	4,568	327	12,330	17,347	931	52	983	1,034,585	309,386	1,343,971	52.5	2,560,601	11,322.58	2,377.57
10	509	73	1,273	1,865	1	0	1	76,820	18,412	95,231	48.4	196,719	6,639.62	1,427.62
16	901	95	2,512	3,524	47	1	48	165,580	34,088	199,669	49.9	399,957	6,829.06	1,119.13
5	428	50	1,146	1,629	1	0	1	87,461	10,410	100,879	54.2	197,355	6,271.40	1,523.96
55	868	149	2,811	3,883	59	10	69	198,774	62,238	261,012	52.6	496,506	6,375.02	1,385.56
79	1,163	136	3,933	5,311	76	1	77	228,028	59,765	287,792	55.2	520,987	6,399.62	1,281.08
29	849	91	2,865	3,834	13	0	13	173,662	43,669	217,332	52.1	417,312	6,501.40	1,410.49
48	1,771	228	4,734	6,781	27	0	27	268,203	65,965	334,170	48.9	683,214	7,293.53	1,261.73
9	713	223	2,636	3,581	4	3	7	117,207	36,536	153,743	53.3	288,267	6,205.69	1,118.43
16	168	29	550	763	3	0	3	59,827	12,605	72,432	52.8	137,184	8,673.19	2,658.45
7	287	87	1,054	1,435	2	0	2	45,033	10,176	55,210	47.2	116,940	6,232.49	1,307.60
246	3,430	487	10,381	14,544	38	17	55	687,341	155,543	842,884	53.1	1,587,146	9,203.41	1,147.47
35	744	183	2,219	3,181	9	8	17	130,720	30,747	161,467	53.5	302,035	6,078.76	693.47
211	2,686	304	8,162	11,363	29	9	38	556,621	124,796	681,417	53.0	1,285,111	10,468.06	1,356.14
211	2,686	304	8,162	11,363	29	9	38	556,621	124,796	681,417	53.0	1,285,111	10,468.06	1,356.14
606	11,266	575	28,805	41,252	573	46	610	1,002,194	432,910	2,115,102	53.5	3,951,387	6,648.56	1,548.09
122	2,279	198	7,263	9,862	3	2	5	395,845	103,881	499,723	56.3	887,948	5,259.02	1,176.33
484	8,987	377	21,542	31,390	570	44	614	1,286,349	329,029	1,615,379	52.7	3,063,439	7,199.98	1,704.20
26	218	6	741	991	0	0	0	48,942	11,716	60,659	56.1	108,089	8,651.00	2,210.90
21	1,147	80	2,579	3,827	0	2	2	150,802	37,716	188,518	53.6	351,528	7,163.51	1,798.22
30	695	33	1,940	2,698	0	0	0	103,257	34,111	137,368	54.0	254,577	7,086.75	1,737.23
384	6,282	200	14,333	21,199	570	42	612	861,004	214,403	1,075,407	51.0	2,095,551	7,267.56	1,698.07
20	645	58	1,949	2,675	0	0	0	122,344	31,083	153,427	60.5	253,694	6,398.17	1,469.98
1,051	15,773	1,395	40,266	67,404	801	164	965	3,054,782	663,990	3,718,775	53.3	6,971,691	7,555.73	1,594.94
160	2,172	403	7,731	10,466	18	36	54	437,223	100,771	537,997	55.7	965,498	5,918.06	660.70
891	13,601	992	11,504	57,010	783	128	911	2,617,559	563,219	3,180,778	53.0	6,006,192	7,927.60	1,780.96
4	339	6	902	1,251	0	0	0	60,094	14,087	74,181	53.3	139,216	6,660.11	1,625.41
0	0	0	1,054	1,054	0	0	0	54,663	12,728	67,391	57.9	116,346	6,087.28	1,618.64
19	424	9	1,643	2,095	18	0	18	101,462	21,360	122,822	52.5	233,866	6,883.07	1,716.89
35	691	33	1,497	2,256	18	0	18	109,837	24,190	134,027	57.8	231,959	5,723.57	1,558.15
15	463	48	1,310	1,836	0	0	0	82,697	16,638	99,335	52.9	187,773	5,535.75	1,233.94
575	7,706	429	23,263	31,973	458	118	576	1,479,406	315,844	1,795,250	51.6	3,482,412	8,878.40	1,956.95
135	1,829	179	5,293	7,436	250	6	256	328,591	69,386	397,978	59.0	673,984	8,162.09	1,566.93
86	1,578	208	4,856	6,728	39	4	43	298,731	64,297	363,027	52.4	692,658	7,102.80	1,621.77
22	571	80	1,716	2,389	0	0	0	102,078	24,689	126,767	51.1	247,978	6,727.01	1,759.71

MSAs

Glossary

This glossary explains specific terms as they are used in the tables and text of Hospital Statistics

Adjusted average daily census: An estimate of the average number of patients (both inpatients and outpatients) receiving care each day during the reporting period, which is usually 12 months. The figure is derived by dividing the number of inpatient day equivalents (also called adjusted inpatient days) by the number of days in the reporting period.

Adjusted inpatient days: An aggregate figure reflecting the number of days of inpatient care, plus an estimate of the volume of outpatient services, expressed in units equivalent to an inpatient day in terms of level of effort. The figure is derived by first multiplying the number of outpatient visits by the ratio of outpatient revenue per outpatient visit to inpatient revenue per inpatient day. The product (which represents the number of patient days attributable to outpatient services) is then added to the number of *inpatient days*. Originally, the purpose of this calculation was to summarize overall productivity and calculate a unit cost that would include both inpatient and outpatient activities.

Formula 1:

$$\frac{\text{total expenses}}{\text{inpatient days} + \text{outpatient visits}\left(\dfrac{\text{outpatient revenue per outpatient visit}}{\text{inpatient revenue per inpatient day}}\right)}$$

However, the value of this calculation has changed over the years as the outpatient share of total revenue has grown and third-party payers have exerted a greater influence on pricing.

Admissions: The number of patients, excluding newborns, accepted for inpatient service during the reporting period; the number includes patients who visit the emergency room and are later admitted for inpatient service.

Adult day care program: Program providing supervision, medical and psychological care, and social activities for older adults who live at home or in another family setting, but cannot be alone or prefer to be with others during the day. May include intake assessment, health monitoring, occupational therapy, personal care, noon meal, and transportation services.

Acute long term care: Providers specialized acute hospital care to medically complex patients who are critically ill, have multisystem complications and/or failure, and require hospitalization averaging 25 days, in a facility offering specialized treatment programs and therapeutic intervention on a 24 hour/7day a week basis.

Alcoholism-drug abuse or dependency inpatient care: Provides diagnosis and therapeutic services to patients with alcoholism or other drug dependencies. Includes care for inpatient/residential treatment for patients whose course of treatment involves more intensive care than provided in an outpatient setting or where patient requires supervised withdrawal.

Alcoholism-drug abuse or dependency outpatient services: Organized hospital services that provide medical care and/or rehabilitative treatment services to outpatients for whom the primary diagnosis is alcoholism or other chemical dependency.

Ambulance services: Provision of ambulance services to the ill and injured who require medical attention on a scheduled or unscheduled basis.

Angioplasty: The reconstruction or restructuring of a blood vessel by operative means or by nonsurgical techniques such as balloon dilation or laser.

Arthritis treatment center: Specifically equipped and staffed center for the diagnosis and treatment of arthritis and other joint disorders.

Assisted living: A special combination of housing, supportive services, personalized assistance and health care designed to respond to the individual needs of those who need help in activities of daily living and instrumental activities of daily living. Supportive services are available, 24 hours a day, to meet scheduled and unscheduled needs, in a way that promotes maximum independence and dignity for each resident and encourages the involvement of a resident's family, neighbor and friends.

Auxiliary: A volunteer community organization formed to assist the hospital in carrying out its purpose and to serve as a link between the institution and the community.

Average daily census: The average number of people served on an inpatient basis on a single day during the reporting period; the figure is calculated by dividing the number of inpatient days by the number of days in the reporting period.

Beds: The average number of beds, cribs, and pediatric bassinets set up and staffed for use for inpatients on the last day of the reporting period.

Bed-size category: Hospitals are categorized by the number of beds set up and staffed for use at the end of the reporting period. The eight categories in Hospital Statistics are: 6 to 24 beds; 25 to 49; 50 to 99; 100 to 199; 200 to 299; 300 to 399; 400 to 499; and 500 or more.

Birthing room-LDR room-LDRP room: A single-room type of maternity care with a more homelike setting for families than the traditional three-room unit(labor/delivery/recovery) with a separate postpartum area. A birthing room combines labor and delivery in one room. An LDR room accommodates three stages in the birthing process—labor, delivery, and recovery. An LDRP room accommodates all four stages of the birth process—labor, delivery, recovery, and postpartum.

Births: Total number of infants born in the hospital during the reporting period. Births do not include infants transferred from other institutions, and are excluded from admission and discharge figures.

Breast cancer screening/mammograms: Mammography screening - The use of breast x-ray to detect unsuspected breast cancer in asymptomatic women. Diagnostic mammography - The x-ray imaging of breast tissue in symptomatic women who are considered to have a substantial likelihood of having breast cancer already.

Burn care: Provides care to severely burned patients. Severely burned patients are those with any of the following: (1) second-degree burns of more than 25% total body surface area for adults or 20% total body surface area for children: (2) third-degree burns of more than 10% total body surface area; (3) any severe burns of the hands, face, eyes, ears, or feet; or (4) all inhalation injuries, electrical burns, complicated burn injuries involving fractures and other major traumas, and all other poor risk factors.

Capitation: An at-risk payment arrangement in which a health care organization receives a fixed, prearranged payment and in turn guarantees to deliver or arrange all medically necessary care required by enrollees in the capitated plan. Specified by contractual agreements between the payer and the organization, the amount of the fixed payment reflects an actuarial assessment of the services required by enrollees and the costs of providing these services.

Cardiac catheterization laboratory: Facilities offering special diagnostic procedures for cardiac patients. Available procedures must include, but need not be limited to, introduction of a catheter into the interior of the heart by way of a vein or artery or by direct needle puncture. Procedures must be performed in a laboratory or a special procedure room.

Cardiac intensive care: Provides patient care of a more specialized nature than the usual medical and surgical care, on the basis of physicians' orders and approved nursing care plans. The unit is staffed with specially trained nursing personnel and contains monitoring and specialized support or treatment equipment for patients who, because of heart seizure, open-heart surgery, or other life-threatening conditions, require intensified, comprehensive observation and care. May include myocardial infarction, pulmonary care, and heart transplant units.

Case management: A system of assessment, treatment planning, referral and follow-up that ensures the provision of comprehensive and continuous services and the coordination of payment and reimbursement for care.

Children wellness program: A program that encourages improved health status and a healthful lifestyle of children through health education, exercise, nutrition and health promotion.

Chiropractic services: An organized clinical service including spinal manipulation or adjustment and related diagnostic and therapeutic services.

Closed physician-hospital organization (Closed PHO): A joint venture between the hospital and physicians who have been selected on the basis of cost-effectiveness and/or high quality. The PHO can act as a unified agent in managed care contracting, own a managed care plan, own and operate ambulatory care centers or ancillary services projects, or provide administrative services to physician members.

Community hospitals: All nonfederal, short-term general, and special hospitals whose facilities and services are available to the public. (Special hospitals include obstetrics and gynecology; eye, ear, nose, and throat; rehabilitation; orthopedic; and other individually described specialty services.) Short-term general and special childrens hospitals are also considered to be community hospitals.

A hospital may include a nursing-home-type unit and still be classified as short-term, provided that the majority of its patients are admitted to units where the average length of stay is less than 30 days. Therefore, statistics for community hospitals often include some data about such nursing-home-type units. An example is furnished by Montana, where in 1995 63.6 percent of all hospitals classified as community hospitals include nursing-home-type units. Expense, revenue, utilization, and personnel data for these hospitals include data about their nursing-home-type units. Thus, total admissions to Montana community hospitals in 1995 were 96,154; total inpatient days, 997,759; total expenses, $791,806,393; and total payroll expenses, $352,583,331. If nursing-home-type unit data were excluded, these same items would be 94,034; 457,340; 752,567,865; and $328,911841, respectively.

Note that before 1972, hospital units of institutions such as prison and college infirmaries were included in the category of community hospitals. Including these units made this category equivalent to the short-term general and other special hospitals category. Although these hospital units are few in number and small in size, this change in definition should be taken into consideration when comparing data.

Community outreach: A program that systematically interacts with the community to identify those in need of services, alerting persons and their families to the availability of services, locating needed services, and enabling persons to enter the service delivery system.

Complementary Medicine Services: Organized hospital services or formal arrangements to providers that provide care or treatment not based solely on traditional western allopathic medical teachings as instructed in most U.S. medical schools. Includes any of the following: acupuncture, chiropractic, homeopathy, osteopathy, diet and lifestyle changes, herbal medicine, message therapy, etc.

Control: The type of organization responsible for establishing policy concerning the overall operation of hospitals. The three major categories are government (including federal, state, and local); nongovernment (nonprofit); and investor-owned (for-profit).

Crisis prevention: Services provided in order to promote physical and mental well being and the early identification of disease and ill health prior to the onset and recognition of symptoms so as to permit early treatment.

CT scanner: Computed tomographic scanner for head or whole body scans.

Deduction from revenue: The difference between revenue at full established rates (gross) and the payment actually received from payers (net).

Dental Services: An organized dental service or dentists on staff, not necessarily involving special facilities, providing dental or oral services to inpatients or outpatients.

Diagnostic radioisotope facility: The use of radioactive isotopes (Radiopharmaceuticals) as tracers or indicators to detect an abnormal condition or disease.

Emergency department: Hospital facilities for the provision of unscheduled outpatient services to patients whose conditions require immediate care.

Emergency room visits: The number of visits to the emergency unit. When emergency outpatients are admitted to the inpatient areas of the hospital, they are counted as emergency room visits and subsequently, as inpatient admissions.

Enabling services: A program that is designed to help the patient access health care services by offering any of the following: linguistic services, transportation services, and/or referrals to local social services agencies.

Enrollment assistance services: A program that provides enrollment assistance for patients who are potentially eligible for public health insurance programs such as Medicaid, State Children's Health Insurance, or local/state indigent care programs. The specific services offered could include explanation of benefits, assist applicants in completing the application and locating all relevant documents, conduct eligibility interviews, and/or forward applications and documentation to state/local social service or health agency.

Equity model: An arrangement that allows established practitioners to become shareholders in a professional corporation in exchange for tangible and intangible assets of their existing practices.

Expenses: Includes all expenses for the reporting period including payroll, non-payroll, bad debt, and all nonoperating expenses. *Payroll expenses* include all salaries and wages. *Non-payroll expenses* are all professional fees and those salary expenditures excluded from payroll. *Labor related expenses* are defined as payroll expenses plus employee benefits. *Non-labor related expenses* are all other non-payroll expenses. *Bad debt* has been reclassified from a "reduction in revenue" to an expense in accordance with the revised AICPA Audit Guide. However, for purposes of historical consistency, the expense total that appears throughout *Hospital Statistics does not include "bad debt" as an expense item.* Note: Financial data may not add due to rounding.

Extracorporeal shock wave lithotripter (ESWL): A medical device used for treating stones in the kidney or ureter. The device disintegrates kidney stones noninvasively through the transmission of acoustic shock waves directed at the stones.

Fitness center: Provides exercise, testing, or evaluation programs and fitness activities to the community and hospital employees.

Foundation: A corporation, organized as a hospital affiliate or subsidiary, that purchases both tangible and intangible assets of one or more medical group practices. Physicians remain in a separate corporate entity but sign a professional services agreement with the foundation.

General medical-surgical care: Provides acute care to patients in medical and surgical units on the basis of physicians' orders and approved nursing care plans.

Geriatric services: The branch of medicine dealing with the physiology of aging and the diagnosis and treatment of disease affecting the aged. Services could include: Adult day care; Alzheimer's diagnostic-assessment services; Comprehensive geriatric assessment; Emergency response system; Geriatric acute care unit; and/or Geriatric clinics.

Government, nonfederal, state, local: Controlled by an agency of state, county, or city government.

Gross inpatient revenue: Revenue from services rendered to inpatients at full established rates (also known as "charges").

Gross outpatient revenue: Revenue from services rendered to outpatients at full established rates.

Group practice without walls: In this organization, the hospital sponsors the formation of a physician group or provides capital to physicians to establish one. The group shares administrative expenses, although the physicians remain independent practitioners.

Group Purchasing Organization: An organization whose primary function is to negotiate contracts for the purpose of purchasing for members of the group or has a central supply site for its members.

Health fair: Community health education events that focus on the prevention of disease and promotion of health through such activities as audiovisual exhibits and free diagnostic services.

Health information center: Education which is directed at increasing the information of individuals and populations. It is intended to increase the ability to make informed personal, family and community health decisions by providing consumers with informed choices about health matters with the objective of improving health status.

Health maintenance organization (HMO): A health care organization that acts as both insurer and provider of comprehensive but specified medical services in return for prospective per capita (capitation) payments.

Health screening: A preliminary procedure such as a test or examination to detect the most characteristic sign or signs of a disorder that may require further investigation.

Hemodialysis: Provision of equipment and personnel for the treatment of renal insufficiency on an inpatient or outpatient basis.

HIV-AIDS services: (could include). *HIV-AIDS unit* - Special unit or team designated and equipped specifically for diagnosis, treatment, continuing care planning, and counseling services for HIV-AIDS patients and their families. *General inpatient care for HIV-AIDS* - Inpatient diagnosis and treatment for human immunodeficiency virus and acquired immunodeficiency syndrome patients, but dedicated unit is not available. *Specialized outpatient program for HIV-AIDS* - Special outpatient program providing diagnostic, treatment, continuing care planning, and counseling for HIV-AIDS patients and their families.

Home health services: Service providing nursing, therapy, and health-related homemaker or social services in the patient's home.

Hospice: A program providing palliative care, chiefly medical relief of pain and supportive services, addressing the emotional, social, financial, and legal needs of terminally ill patients and their families. Care can be provided in a variety of settings, both inpatient and at home.

Hospital district or authority: A political subdivision of a state, county, or city created solely for the purpose of establishing and maintaining medical care or health-related care institutions.

Hospitals in a network: Hospitals participating in a group that may include other hospitals, physicians, other providers, insurers, and/or community agencies that work together to coordinate and deliver a broad spectrum of services to the community.

Hospitals in a system: Hospitals belonging to a corporate body that owns and/or manages health provider facilities or health-related subsidiaries; the system may also own non-health-related facilities.

Hospital unit: The hospital operation, excluding activity pertaining to nursing-home-type unit (as described below), for the following items: Admissions, Beds, FTEs (full-time, part-time, and total), Inpatient Days, Length of Stay, Net Revenue, and Total Expense.

Hospital unit of institutions: A hospital unit that is not open to the public and is contained within a nonhospital unit. An example is an infirmary that is contained within a college.

Indemnity fee for service: The traditional type of health insurance, in which the insured is reimbursed for covered expenses without regard to choice of provider. Payment up to a stated limit may be made either to the individual incurring and claiming the expense, or directly to providers.

Independent practice association (IPA): An IPA is a legal entity that holds managed care contracts and contracts with physicians, usually in solo practice, to provide care either on a fee-for-services or capitated basis. The purpose of an IPA is to assist solo physicians in obtaining managed care contracts.

Inpatient days: The number of adult and pediatric days of care, excluding newborn days of care, rendered during the entire reporting period.

Inpatient surgeries: Surgical services provided to patients who remain in the hospital overnight.

Insurance product: In tables 3 through 6, insurance product refers to a hospital-owned insurance product.

Integrated salary model: In this arrangement, physicians are salaried by the hospital or other entity of a health system to provide medical services for primary care and specialty care.

Intermediate nursing care: Provides health-related services (skilled nursing care and social services) to residents with a variety of physical conditions or functional disabilities. These residents do not require the care provided by a hospital or skilled nursing facility, but do need supervision and support services.

Investor-owned, for-profit: Investor-owned, for-profit hospitals are those controlled on a for-profit basis by an individual, partnership, or profit-making corporation.

Labor-related expenses: Payroll expenses plus employee benefits. *Non-labor-related expenses refers* to all other nonpayroll expenses, such as interest depreciation, supplies, purchased services, professional fees, and others.

Length of stay (LOS): LOS refers to the average number of days a patient stays at the facility. Short-term hospitals are those where the average LOS is less than 30 days. Long-term hospitals are those where the average LOS is 30 days or more. The figure is derived by dividing the number of inpatient days by the number of admissions.

Note that this publication carries two LOS variables: *total facility length of stay and hospital unit length of stay. Total facility* includes admissions and inpatient days from nursing-home-type units under control of the hospital. In *hospital unit length of stay*, nursing home utilization is subtracted.

Licensed practical nurse (LPN): A nurse who has graduated from an approved school of practical (vocational) nursing and works under the supervision of registered nurses and/or physicians.

Long-term: Hospitals are classified either short-term or long-term according to the average length of stay (LOS). A long-term hospital is one in which the average LOS is 30 days or more.

Magnetic resonance imaging (MRI): The use of a uniform magnetic field and radio frequencies to study tissue and structure of the body. This procedure enables the visualization of biochemical activity of the cell in vivo without the use of ionizing radiation, radioisotopic substances, or high-frequency sound.

Managed care: A term covering a broad spectrum of arrangements for health care delivery and financing, including managed indemnity plans (MIP), health maintenance organizations (HMO), preferred provider organizations (PPO), point-of-service plans (POS), and direct contracting arrangements between employers and providers.

Managed care contract: A contract between the hospital and a managed care organization.

Management services organization (MSO): A corporation owned by the hospital or a physician/hospital joint venture that provides management services to one or more medical group practices. As part of a full-service management agreement, the MSO purchases the tangible assets of the practices and leases them back, employs all non-physician staff, and provides all supplies/administrative systems for a fee.

Meals on wheels: A hospital sponsored program which delivers meals to people, usually the elderly, who are unable to prepare their own meals. Low cost, nutritional meals are delivered to individuals' homes on a regular basis.

Medical surgical intensive care: Provides patient care of a more intensive nature than the usual medical and surgical care, on the basis of physicians' orders and approved nursing care plans. These units are staffed with specially trained nursing personnel and contain monitoring and specialized support equipment for patients who, because of shock, trauma, or other life-threatening conditions, require intensified, comprehensive observation and care. Includes mixed intensive care units.

Neonatal intensive care: A unit that must be separate from the newborn nursery providing intensive care to all sick infants including those with the very lowest birth weights (less than 1500 grams). NICU has potential for providing mechanical ventilation, neonatal surgery, and special care for the sickest infants born in the hospital or transferred from another institution. A full-time neonatologist serves as director of the NICU.

Neonatal intermediate care: A unit that must be separate from the normal newborn nursery and that provides intermediate and/or recovery care and some specialized services, including immediate resuscitation, intravenous therapy, and capacity for prolonged oxygen therapy and monitoring.

Net patient revenue: The estimated net realizable amounts from patients, third-party payers, and others for services rendered. The number includes estimated retroactive adjustments called for by agreements with third-party payers; retroactive adjustments are accrued on an estimated basis in the period the related services are rendered and then adjusted later as final settlements are determined.

Net total revenue: Net patient revenue plus all other revenue, including contributions, endowment revenue, governmental grants, and all other payments not made on behalf of individual patients.

Nongovernment, nonprofit: Hospitals that are nongovernment, nonprofit are controlled by not-for-profit organizations, including religious organizations (Catholic hospitals, for example), fraternal societies, and others.

Nursing-home-type unit/facility: A unit/facility that primarily offers the following type of services to a majority of all admissions:

- *Skilled nursing*: The provision of medical and nursing care services, health-related services, and social services under the supervision of a registered nurse on a 24-hour basis.
- *Intermediate care*: The provision, on a regular basis, of health-related care and services to individuals who do not require the degree of care or treatment that a skilled nursing unit is designed to provide.
- *Personal care*: The provision of general supervision and direct personal care services for residents who require assistance in activities of daily living but who do not need nursing services or inpatient care. Medical and nursing services are available as needed.

- *Sheltered/residential care*: The provision of general supervision and protective services for residents who do not need nursing services or continuous personal care services in the conduct of daily life. Medical and nursing services are available as needed.

Nutrition programs: Those services within a health care facility which are designed to provide inexpensive, nutritionally sound meals to patients.

Obstetrics: Levels should be designated: (1) unit provides services for uncomplicated maternity and newborn cases; (2) unit provides services for uncomplicated cases, the majority of complicated problems, and special neonatal services; and (3) unit provides services for all serious illnesses and abnormalities and is supervised by a full-time maternal/fetal specialist.

Occupational health services: Includes services designed to protect the safety of employees from hazards in the work environment.

Oncology services: An organized program for the treatment of cancer by the use of drugs or chemicals.

Open heart surgery: Heart surgery where the chest has been opened and the blood recirculated and oxygenated with the proper equipment and the necessary staff to perform the surgery.

Open physician hospital organization (Open PHO): A joint venture between the hospital and all members of the medical staff who wish to participate. The open PHO can act as a unified agent in managed care contracting, own a managed care plan, own and operate ambulatory care centers or ancillary services projects, or provide administrative services to physician members.

Osteopathic hospitals: Osteopathic medicine is a medical practice based on a theory that diseases are due chiefly to a loss of structural integrity, which can be restored by manipulation of the neuro-muscular and skeletal systems, supplemented by therapeutic measures (such as medicine or surgery).

Other Intensive Care: A distinct intensive care unit that is not one of the following types: medical/surgical, cardiac, pediatric and neonatal.

Other long term care: Provision of long term care other than skilled nursing care or intermediate care. This can include residential care-elderly housing services for those who do not require daily medical or nursing services, but may require some assistance in the activities of daily living, or sheltered care facilities for developmentally disabled.

Other special care: Provides care to patients requiring care more intensive than that provided in the acute area, yet not sufficiently intensive to require admission to an intensive care unit. Patients admitted to this area are usually transferred here from an intensive care unit once their condition has improved. These units are sometimes referred to as definitive observation, step-down, or progressive care units.

Outpatient care: Treatment provided to patients who do not remain in the hospital for overnight care. Hospitals may deliver outpatient care on site or through a facility owned and operated by the hospital, but physically separate from the hospital. In addition to treating minor illnesses or injuries, a free-standing center will stabilize seriously ill or injured patients before transporting them to a hospital. Laboratory and radiology services are usually available.

Outpatient care center (Freestanding): A facility owned and operated by the hospital, but physically separate from the hospital, that provides various medical treatments on an outpatient basis only. In addition to treating minor illnesses or injuries, the center will stabilize seriously ill or injured patients before transporting them to a hospital. Laboratory and radiology services are usually available.

Outpatient care center-services (Hospital-based): Organized hospital health care services offered by appointment on an ambulatory basis. Services may include outpatient surgery, examination, diagnosis, and treatment of a variety of medical conditions on a nonemergency basis, and laboratory and other diagnostic testing as ordered by staff or outside physician referral.

Outpatient surgeries: Scheduled surgical services provided to patients who do not remain in the hospital overnight. In the AHA Annual Survey, outpatient surgery may be performed in operating suites also used for inpatient surgery, specially designated surgical suites for outpatient surgery, or procedure rooms within an outpatient care facility.

Outpatient visit: A visit by a patient who is not lodged in the hospital while receiving medical, dental, or other services. Each visit an outpatient makes to a discrete unit constitutes one visit regardless of the number of diagnostic and/or therapeutic treatments that the patient receives. Total outpatient visits should include all clinic visits, referred visits, observation services, outpatient surgeries, and emergency room visits.

Pain management: A hospital wide formalized program that includes staff education for the management of chronic and acute pain based on guidelines and protocols like those developed by the Agency for Health Care Policy Research, etc.

Palliative care program: An organized program providing specialized medical care, drugs or therapies for the management of acute or chronic pain and/or the control of symptoms administered by specially trained physicians and other clinicians; and supportive care services, such as counseling on advanced directives, spiritual care, and social services, to patients with advanced disease and their families.

Patient education center: Written goals and objectives for the patient and/or family related to therapeutic regimens, medical procedures, and self care.

Patient representative services: Organized hospital services providing personnel through whom patients and staff can seek solutions to institutional problems affecting the delivery of high-quality care and services.

Payroll expenses: Includes all salaries and wages. All professional fees and salary expenditures excluded from payroll, such as employee benefits, are defined as nonpayroll expenses and are included in total expenses.

Pediatric intensive care: Provides care to pediatric patients that is of a more intensive nature than that usually provided to pediatric patients. The unit is staffed with specially trained personnel and contains monitoring and specialized support equipment for treatment of patients who, because of shock, trauma, or other life-threatening conditions, require intensified, comprehensive observation and care.

Pediatric medical-surgical care: Provides acute care to pediatric patients on the basis of physicians' orders and approved nursing care plans.

Personnel: Number of persons on the hospital payroll at the end of the reporting period. Personnel are recorded in *Hospital Statistics* as full-time equivalents (FTEs), which are calculated by adding the number of full-time personnel to one-half the number of part-time personnel, excluding medical and dental residents, interns, and other trainees. *Per 100 adjusted census* indicates the ratio of personnel to adjusted average daily census, calculated on a per-100 basis.

Physical rehabilitation inpatient care: Provides care encompassing a comprehensive array of restoration services for the disabled and all support services necessary to help patients attain their maximum functional capacity.

Physical rehabilitation outpatient services: Outpatient program providing medical, health-related, therapy, social, and/or vocational services to help disabled persons attain or retain their maximum functional capacity.

Population: Population refers to the residential population of the United States. This includes both civilian and military personnel. Note that population is being used to calculate the values *for community health indicators per 1000 population.*

Positron emission tomography scanner (PET): A nuclear medicine imaging technology which uses radioactive (positron emitting) isotopes created in a cyclotron or generator and computers to produce composite pictures of the brain and heart at work. PET scanning produces sectional images depicting metabolic activity or blood flow rather than anatomy.

Preferred provider organization (PPO): A pre-set arrangement in which purchasers and providers agree to furnish specified health services to a group of employees/patients.

Primary care department: A unit or clinic within the hospital that provides primary care services (e.g. general pediatric care, general internal medicine, family practice, gynecology) through hospital-salaried medical and/or nursing staff, focusing on evaluating and diagnosing medical problems and providing medical treatment on an outpatient basis.

Psychiatric child-adolescent services: Provides care to emotionally disturbed children and adolescents, including those admitted for diagnosis and those admitted for treatment.

Psychiatric consultation-liaison services: Provides organized psychiatric consultation/liaison services to nonpsychiatric hospital staff and/or departments on psychological aspects of medical care that may be generic or specific to individual patients.

Psychiatric education services: Provides psychiatric educational services to community agencies and workers such as schools, police, courts, public health nurses, welfare agencies, clergy, and so forth. The purpose is to expand the mental health knowledge and competence of personnel not working in the mental health field and to promote good mental health through improved understanding, attitudes, and behavioral patterns.

Psychiatric emergency services: Services of facilities available on a 24-hour basis to provide immediate unscheduled outpatient care, diagnosis, evaluation, crisis intervention, and assistance to persons suffering acute emotional or mental distress.

Psychiatric geriatric services: Provides care to emotionally disturbed elderly patients, including those admitted for diagnosis and those admitted for treatment.

Psychiatric inpatient care: Provides acute or long-term care to emotionally disturbed patients, including patients admitted for diagnosis and those admitted for treatment of psychiatric problems, on the basis of physicians' orders and approved nursing care plans. Long-term care may include intensive supervision to the chronically mentally ill, mentally disordered, or other mentally incompetent persons.

Psychiatric outpatient services: Provides medical care, including diagnosis and treatment, of psychiatric outpatients.

Psychiatric partial hospitalization program: Organized hospital services of intensive day/evening outpatient services of three hours of more duration, distinguished from other outpatient visits of one hour.

Radiation therapy: The branch of medicine concerned with radioactive substances and using various techniques of visualization, with the diagnosis and treatment of disease using any of the various sources of radiant energy. Services could include: megavoltage radiation therapy; radioactive implants; stereotactic radiosurgery; therapeutic radioisotope facility; X-ray radiation therapy.

Registered nurse (RN): A nurse who has graduated from an approved school of nursing and who is currently registered by the state. RNs are responsible for the nature and quality of all nursing care that patients receive. In these tables, the number of RNs does not include those registered nurses more appropriately reported in other occupational categories, such as facility administrators, which are listed under *all other personnel* (Tables 1 and 2).

Rehabilitation services: A wide array of restoration services for disabled and recuperating patients, including all support services necessary to help them attain their maximum functional capacity.

Reproductive health (could include): *Fertility counseling* - A service that counsels and educates on infertility problems and includes laboratory and surgical workup and management for individuals having problems conceiving children. *In vitro fertilization* - Program providing for the induction of fertilization of a surgically removed ovum by donated sperm in a culture medium followed by a short incubation period. The embryo is then reimplanted in the womb.

Retirement housing: A facility which provides social activities to senior citizens, usually retired persons, who do not require health care but some short-term skilled nursing care may be provided. A retirement center may furnish housing and may also have acute hospital and long-term care facilities, or it may arrange for acute and long term care through affiliated institutions.

Rural: A rural hospital is located outside a metropolitan statistical area (MSA), as designated by the U.S. Office of Management and Budget, which is a geographically defined, integrated social and economic unit with a large population nucleus.

Single photon emission computerized tomography (SPECT): A nuclear medicine imaging technology that combines existing technology of gamma camera imaging with computed tomographic imaging technology to provide a more precise and clear image.

Skilled nursing care: Provides non-acute medical and skilled nursing care services, therapy, and social services under the supervision of a licensed registered nurse on a 24-hour basis.

Sleep Center: Specially equipped and staffed center for the diagnosis and treatment of sleep disorders.

Social work services (could include): Organized services that are properly directed and sufficiently staffed by qualified individuals who provide assistance and counseling to patients and their families in dealing with social, emotional, and environmental problems associated with illness or disability, often in the context of financial or discharge planning coordination.

Sports medicine: Provision of diagnostic screening and assessment and clinical and rehabilitation services for the prevention and treatment of sports-related injuries.

Support groups: A hospital sponsored program which allows a group of individuals with the same or similar problems who meet periodically to share experiences, problems, and solutions in order to support each other.

Surgical operations: Those surgical operations, whether major or minor, performed in the operating room(s). A surgical operation involving more than one surgical procedure is still considered only one surgical operation.

Tobacco treatment/cessation program: Organized hospital services with the purpose of ending tobacco-use habits of patients addicted to tobacco/nicotine.

Teen outreach services: A program focusing on the teenager which encourages an improved health status and a healthful lifestyle including physical, emotional, mental, social, spiritual and economic health through education, exercise, nutrition and health promotion.

Transplant services: The branch of medicine that transfers an organ or tissue from one person to another or from one body part to another to replace a diseased structure or to restore function or to change appearance. Services could include: Bone marrow transplant program; kidney transplant; organ transplant (other than kidney); tissue transplant.

Transportation to health facilities: A long-term care support service designed to assist the mobility of the elderly. Some programs offer improved financial access by offering reduced rates and barrier-free buses or vans with ramps and lifts to assist the elderly or handicapped; others offer subsidies for public transport systems or operate mini-bus services exclusively for use by senior citizens.

Trauma center (certified): A facility to provide emergency and specialized intensive care to critically ill and injured patients. **Level 1:** A regional resource trauma center, which is capable of providing total care for every aspect of injury and plays a leadership role in trauma research and education. **Level 2:** A community trauma center, which is capable of providing trauma care to all but the most severely injured patients who require highly specialized care. **Level 3:** A rural trauma hospital, which is capable of providing care to a large number of injury victims and can resuscitate and stabilize more severely injured patients so that they can be transported to Level 1 or 2 facilities.

Ultrasound: The use of acoustic waves above the range of 20,000 cycles per second to visualize internal body structures.

Urban: An urban hospital is located inside a Metropolitan Statistical Area (MSA), designated by the U.S. Office of Management and Budget, which is a geographically defined, integrated social and economic unit with a large population base.

Urgent care center: A facility that provides care and treatment for problems that are not life-threatening but require attention over the short term. These units function like emergency rooms but are separate from hospitals with which they may have backup affiliation arrangements.

Volunteer services department: An organized hospital department responsible for coordinating the services of volunteers working within the institution.

Women's health center/services: An area set aside for coordinated education and treatment services specifically for and promoted to women as provided by this special unit. Services may or may not include obstetrics but include a range of services other than OB.

2001 AHA Annual Survey
Health Forum, L.L.C.

Please return to:
AHA Annual Survey
One North Franklin, 29th Floor
Chicago, Illinois 60606

Please return by:

A. REPORTING PERIOD (please refer to the instructions and definitions on the reverse side of this page)

Report data for a full 12-month period, preferably your last completed fiscal year (365 days). (Be consistent in using the same reporting period for responses throughout various sections of this survey.)

1. Reporting Period used (beginning and ending date) .... __ / __ / __ to __ / __ / __
   (Month / Day / Year to Month / Day / Year)

2. a. Were you in operation 12 full months at the end of your reporting period .... YES ☐ NO ☐
   b. Number of days open during reporting period .... ☐

3. Indicate the beginning of your current fiscal year .... __ / __ / __
   (Month / Day / Year)

B. ORGANIZATIONAL STRUCTURE

1. CONTROL

Indicate the type of organization that is responsible for establishing policy for overall operation of your hospital. CHECK ONLY ONE:

Government, nonfederal
- ☐ 12 State
- ☐ 13 County
- ☐ 14 City
- ☐ 15 City-County
- ☐ 16 Hospital district or authority

Nongovernment, not-for profit (NFP)
- ☐ 21 Church-operated
- ☐ 23 Other not-for-profit (including NFP Corporation)

Investor-owned, for-profit
- ☐ 31 Individual
- ☐ 32 Partnership
- ☐ 33 Corporation

Government, federal
- ☐ 41 Air Force
- ☐ 42 Army
- ☐ 43 Navy
- ☐ 44 Public Health Service
- ☐ 45 Veterans' Affairs
- ☐ 46 Federal other than 41-45 or 47-48
- ☐ 47 PHS Indian Service
- ☐ 48 Department of Justice

2. SERVICE

Indicate the ONE category that BEST describes your hospital or the type of service it provides to the MAJORITY of admissions:

- ☐ 10 General medical and surgical
- ☐ 11 Hospital unit of an institution (prison hospital, college infirmary)
- ☐ 12 Hospital unit within an institution for the mentally retarded
- ☐ 22 Psychiatric
- ☐ 33 Tuberculosis and other respiratory diseases
- ☐ 44 Obstetrics and gynecology
- ☐ 45 Eye, ear, nose, and throat
- ☐ 46 Rehabilitation
- ☐ 47 Orthopedic
- ☐ 48 Chronic disease
- ☐ 62 Institution for mentally retarded
- ☐ 82 Alcoholism and other chemical dependency
- ☐ 49 Other-specify treatment area: ____________

3. OTHER

a. Does your hospital restrict admissions primarily to children? .... YES ☐ NO ☐

b. Is your hospital primarily osteopathic? .... YES ☐ NO ☐

GENERAL INSTRUCTIONS

A copy of the 2001 Annual Survey questionnaire is enclosed. Please check and correct any label information as printed on the front of the survey. Return the original completed copy in the enclosed return envelope to the American Hospital Association and retain the photocopy in your files for reference. Also, please forward a photocopy of the completed questionnaire to your state hospital association.

Requested return date is listed on the cover page, but if additional time is necessary to complete the survey, please complete page 16, listing the expected return date and fax it to the Annual Survey staff at 1 800/530-9092. If you prefer, you may notify us by calling 1 800/530-9092.

Report utilization and financial information for a full 12-month period, preferably your fiscal year as the reporting period.

Make an entry for every item on the form. Enter "NA" only if data are not available. Enter "0" if zero is appropriate.

If assistance is needed, please contact the American Hospital Association Annual Survey staff at 1 800/530-9092. You may also contact your state hospital association or other state agency if so directed by survey return instructions.

INSTRUCTIONS AND DEFINITIONS FOR THE 2001 ANNUAL SURVEY

HOSPITAL. For purposes of this survey, a hospital is defined as the organization or corporate entity licensed or registered as a hospital by a state to provide diagnostic and therapeutic patient services for a variety of medical conditions, both surgical and nonsurgical.

SECTION A
REPORTING PERIOD
Instructions

Record the beginning and ending dates of the reporting period in a six-digit number: for example, January 1, 2001, should be shown as 01/01/01. Number of days should equal the time span between the two dates that the hospital was open. If you are reporting for less than 365 days, utilization and finances should be presented for days reported only.

SECTION B
ORGANIZATIONAL STRUCTURE
Instructions and Definitions

1. CONTROL

Check the box to the left of the type of organization that is responsible for establishing policy for overall operation of the hospital.

Government, nonfederal.

State. Controlled by an agency of state government.

County. Controlled by an agency of county government.

City. Controlled by an agency of municipal government.

City-County. Controlled jointly by agencies of municipal and county governments.

Hospital district or authority. Controlled by a political subdivision of a state, county, or city created solely for the purpose of establishing and maintaining medical care or health-related care institutions.

2. SERVICE

Indicate the ONE category that best describes the type of service that your hospital provides to the majority of admissions.

General medical and surgical. Provides diagnostic and therapeutic services to patients for a variety of medical conditions, both surgical and nonsurgical.

Hospital unit of an institution. Provides diagnostic and therapeutic services to patients in an institution.

Hospital unit within an institution for the mentally retarded. Provides diagnostic and therapeutic services to patients in an institution for the mentally retarded.

Psychiatric. Provides diagnostic and therapeutic services to patients with mental or emotional disorders.

Tuberculosis and other respiratory diseases. Provides medical care and rehabilitative services to patients for whom the primary diagnosis is tuberculosis or other respiratory diseases.

Obstetrics and gynecology. Provides medical and surgical treatment to pregnant women and to mothers following delivery. Also provides diagnostic and therapeutic services to women with diseases or disorders of the reproductive organs.

Eye, ear, nose, and throat. Provides diagnosis and treatment of diseases and injuries of the eyes, ears, nose, and throat.

Rehabilitation. Provides a comprehensive array of restoration services for the disabled and all support services necessary to help them attain their maximum functional capacity.

Orthopedic. Provides corrective treatment of deformities, diseases, and ailments of the locomotive apparatus, especially affecting the limbs, bones, muscles, and joints.

Chronic disease. Provides medical and skilled nursing services to patients with long-term illnesses who are not in an acute phase, but who require an intensity of services not available in nursing homes.

Institution for the mentally retarded. Provides health-related care on a regular basis to patients with psychiatric or developmental impairment who cannot be treated in a skilled nursing unit.

Alcoholism and other chemical dependency. Provides diagnostic and therapeutic services to patients with alcoholism or other drug dependencies.

B. ORGANIZATIONAL STRUCTURE (continued)

3. c. Is the hospital part of a health care system? If yes, please provide the name, city, and state of the system headquarters: ...... YES ☐ NO ☐

   Name: ______________ City: ______________ State: ________

   d. Does the hospital itself operate subsidiary corporations? ...... YES ☐ NO ☐

   If yes, please provide a separate list of the name(s) and address(es) of your subsidiary corporations.

   e. Is the hospital contract managed? If yes, please provide the name, city, and state of the organization that manages the hospital: YES ☐ NO ☐

   Name: ______________ City: ______________ State: ________

   f. Is the hospital a participant in a network? If yes, please provide the name and telephone number of the network. If the hospital participates in more than one network, please provide the name, address, city, state, and telephone number of the network(s) on page 15, under supplemental information. . YES ☐ NO ☐

   Name: ______________ Telephone: ______________

   g. Does the hospital participate in a group purchasing arrangement? If yes, please provide the name, city, and state of the group purchasing organization: .... YES ☐ NO ☐

   Name: ______________ City: ______________ State: ________

C. FACILITIES AND SERVICES

For each service or facility listed below, please check all the categories that describe how each item is provided as of the last day of the reporting period. Check all categories that apply for an item. Leave all categories blank for a facility or service that is not provided. Column 2 refers to the systems that were identified in section B, question 3c. Column 3 refers to the networks that were identified in section B, question 3h.

***Please report # Beds that were provided within your hospital and were set up and staffed for use at the end of the reporting period.**

	(1) Owned or provided by my hospital or it's subsidiary		(2) Provided by my Health System (in my local community)	(3) Provided by my network (in my local community)	(4) Provided through formal contractual arrangement or joint venture with another provider that is not in my system or network (in my local community)
1. General medical-surgical care	☐	(# Beds:_______)	☐	☐	☐
2. Pediatric medical-surgical care	☐	(# Beds:_______)	☐	☐	☐
3. Obstetrics [Level of unit (1-3): _____]	☐	(# Beds:_______)	☐	☐	☐
4. Medical surgical intensive care	☐	(# Beds:_______)	☐	☐	☐
5. Cardiac intensive care	☐	(# Beds:_______)	☐	☐	☐
6. Neonatal intensive care	☐	(# Beds:_______)	☐	☐	☐
7. Neonatal intermediate care	☐	(# Beds:_______)	☐	☐	☐
8. Pediatric intensive care	☐	(# Beds:_______)	☐	☐	☐
9. Burn care	☐	(# Beds:_______)	☐	☐	☐
10. Other special care	☐	(# Beds:_______)	☐	☐	☐
11. Other intensive care (specify: _______) ..	☐	(# Beds:_______)	☐	☐	☐
12. Physical rehabilitation	☐	(# Beds:_______)	☐	☐	☐
13. Alcoholism-drug abuse or dependency care ..	☐	(# Beds:_______)	☐	☐	☐
14. Psychiatric care	☐	(# Beds:_______)	☐	☐	☐
15. Skilled nursing care	☐	(# Beds:_______)	☐	☐	☐
16. Intermediate nursing care	☐	(# Beds:_______)	☐	☐	☐
17. Acute long term care	☐	(# Beds:_______)	☐	☐	☐
18. Other long term care	☐	(# Beds:_______)	☐	☐	☐
19. Other care (specify: __________)....	☐	(# Beds _______)	☐	☐	☐

B. ORGANIZATIONAL STRUCTURE

3. OTHER
   b. **Osteopathic.** Osteopathic medicine is a medical practice based on a theory that diseases are due chiefly to a loss of structural integrity which can be restored by manipulation of the neuro-muscular and skeletal system, supplemented by therapeutic measures (as use of medicine or surgery).
   c. **Health care system.** A corporate body that owns, leases, religiously sponsors, and/or manages health provider facilities.
   d. **Subsidiary.** A company that is wholly controlled by another or one that is more than 50% owned by another organization.
   e. **Contract managed.** General day-to-day management of an entire organization by another organization under a formal contract. Managing organization reports directly to the board of trustees or owners of the managed organization; managed organization retains total legal responsibility and ownership of the facility's assets and liabilities.
   f. **Network.** A group of hospitals, physicians, other providers, insurers and/or community agencies that voluntarily work together to coordinate and deliver health services.
   g. **Group Purchasing Organization.** An organization whose primary function is to negotiate contracts for the purpose of purchasing for members of the group or has a central supply site for its members.

SECTION C
FACILITIES AND SERVICES
Definitions

1. **General medical-surgical care.** Provides acute care to patients in medical and surgical units on the basis of physicians' orders and approved nursing care plans.
2. **Pediatric medical-surgical care.** Provides acute care to pediatric patients on the basis of physicians' orders and approved nursing care plans.
3. **Obstetrics.** Levels should be designated: (1) unit provides services for uncomplicated maternity and newborn cases; (2) unit provides services for uncomplicated cases, the majority of complicated problems, and special neonatal services; and (3) unit provides services for all serious illnesses and abnormalities and is supervised by a full-time maternal/fetal specialist.
4. **Medical surgical intensive care.** Provides patient care of a more intensive nature than the usual medical and surgical care, on the basis of physicians' orders and approved nursing care plans. These units are staffed with specially trained nursing personnel and contain monitoring and specialized support equipment for patients who, because of shock, trauma, or other life-threatening conditions, require intensified, comprehensive observation and care. Includes mixed intensive care units.
5. **Cardiac intensive care.** Provides patient care of a more specialized nature than the usual medical and surgical care, on the basis of physicians' orders and approved nursing care plans. The unit is staffed with specially trained nursing personnel and contains monitoring and specialized support or treatment equipment for patients who, because of heart seizure, open-heart surgery, or other life-threatening conditions, require intensified, comprehensive observation and care. May include myocardial infarction, pulmonary care, and heart transplant units.
6. **Neonatal intensive care.** A unit that must be separate from the newborn nursery providing intensive care to all sick infants including those with the very lowest birth weights (less than 1500 grams). NICU has potential for providing mechanical ventilation, neonatal surgery, and special care for the sickest infants born in the hospital or transferred from another institution. A full-time neonatologist serves as director of the NICU.
7. **Neonatal intermediate care.** A unit that must be separate from the normal newborn nursery and that provides intermediate and/or recovery care and some specialized services, including immediate resuscitation, intravenous therapy, and capacity for prolonged oxygen therapy and monitoring.
8. **Pediatric intensive care**. Provides care to pediatric patients that is of a more intensive nature than that usually provided to pediatric patients. The unit is staffed with specially trained personnel and contains monitoring and specialized support equipment for treatment of patients who, because of shock, trauma, or other life-threatening conditions, require intensified, comprehensive observation and care.
9. **Burn care.** Provides care to severely burned patients. Severely burned patients are those with any of the following: (1) second-degree burns of more than 25% total body surface area for adults or 20% total body surface area for children: (2) third-degree burns of more than 10% total body surface area; (3) any severe burns of the hands, face, eyes, ears, or feet; or (4) all inhalation injuries, electrical burns, complicated burn injuries involving fractures and other major traumas, and all other poor risk factors.
10. **Other special care.** Provides care to patients requiring care more intensive than that provided in the acute area, yet not sufficiently intensive to require admission to an intensive care unit. Patients admitted to this area are usually transferred here from an intensive care unit once their condition has improved. These units are sometimes referred to as definitive observation, step-down, or progressive care units.
12. **Physical rehabilitation.** Provides care encompassing a comprehensive array of restoration services for the disabled and all support services necessary to help patients attain their maximum functional capacity.
13. **Alcoholism-drug abuse or dependency care.** Provides diagnosis and therapeutic services to patients with alcoholism or other drug dependencies. Includes care for inpatient/residential treatment for patients whose course of treatment involves more intensive care than provided in an outpatient setting or where patient requires supervised withdrawal.
14. **Psychiatric care.** Provides acute or long-term care to emotionally disturbed patients, including patients admitted for diagnosis and those admitted for treatment of psychiatric problems, on the basis of physicians' orders and approved nursing care plans. Long-term care may include intensive supervision to the chronically mentally ill, mentally disordered, or other mentally incompetent persons.
15. **Skilled nursing care.** Provides non-acute medical and skilled nursing care services, therapy, and social services under the supervision of a licensed registered nurse on a 24-hour basis.
16. **Intermediate nursing care.** Provides health-related services (skilled nursing care and social services) to residents with a variety of physical conditions or functional disabilities. These residents do not require the care provided by a hospital or skilled nursing facility, but do need supervision and support services.
17. **Acute long term care.** Provides specialized acute hospital care to medically complex patients who are critically ill, have multisystem complications and/or failure, and require hospitalization averaging 25 days, in a facility offering specialized treatment programs and therapeutic intervention on a 24 hour/7 day a week basis.
18. **Other long term care.** Provision of long term care other than skilled nursing care or intermediate care. This can include residential care-elderly housing services for those who do not require daily medical or nursing services, but may require some assistance in the activities of daily living, or sheltered care facilities for developmentally disabled.
19. **Other care.** (specify) Any type of care other than those listed above.

C. FACILITIES AND SERVICES (continued)

	(1) Owned or provided by my hospital or it's subsidiary	(2) Provided by my Health System (in my local community)	(3) Provided by my network (in my local community)	(4) Provided through a formal contractual arrangement or joint venture with another provider that is not in my system or network (in my local community)
20. Adult day care program				
21. Alcoholism-drug abuse or dependency outpatient services				
22. Ambulance services				
23. Angioplasty				
24. Arthritis treatment center				
25. Assisted living				
26. Auxiliary				
27. Birthing room - LDR room -LDRP room				
28. Breast cancer screening/mammograms				
29. Cardiac catheterization laboratory				
30. Case management				
31. Children wellness program				
32. Chiropractic services				
33. Community outreach				
34. Complementary medicine services				
35. Crisis prevention				
36. Dental services				
37. Emergency services:				
a. Emergency department				
b. Trauma center (certified) [Level of unit (1-3):]				
38. Enabling services				
39. End of life services				
a. Hospice program				
b. Pain management program				
c. Palliative care program				
40. Enrollment assistance services				
41. Extracorporeal shock wave lithotripter (ESWL)				
42. Fitness center				
43. Freestanding outpatient care center				
44. Geriatric services				
45. Health fair				
46. Health information center				
47. Health screenings				
48. Hemodialysis				
49. HIV-AIDS services				
50. Home health services				
51. Hospital-based outpatient care center-services				
52. Meals on wheels				
53. Nutrition programs				
54. Occupational health services				
55. Oncology services				
56. Open heart surgery				

C. FACILITIES AND SERVICES (continued)

20. **Adult day care program.** Program providing supervision, medical and psychological care, and social activities for older adults who live at home or in another family setting, but cannot be alone or prefer to be with others during the day. May include intake assessment, health monitoring, occupational therapy, personal care, noon meal, and transportation services.
21. **Alcoholism-drug abuse or dependency outpatient services.** Organized hospital services that provide medical care and/or rehabilitative treatment services to outpatients for whom the primary diagnosis is alcoholism or other chemical dependency.
22. **Ambulance services.** Provision of ambulance services to the ill and injured who require medical attention on a scheduled or unscheduled basis.
23. **Angioplasty.** The reconstruction or restructuring of a blood vessel by operative means or by nonsurgical techniques such as balloon dilation or laser.
24. **Arthritis treatment center.** Specifically equipped and staffed center for the diagnosis and treatment of arthritis and other joint disorders.
25. **Assisted living.** A special combination of housing, supportive services, personalized assistance and health care designed to respond to the individual needs of those who need help in activities of daily living and instrumental activities of daily living. Supportive services are available, 24 hours a day, to meet scheduled and unscheduled needs, in a way that promotes maximum independence an dignity for each resident and encourages the involvement of a resident's family, neighbor and friends.
26. **Auxiliary.** A volunteer community organization formed to assist the hospital in carrying out its purpose and to serve as a link between the institution and the community.
27. **Birthing room-LDR room-LDRP room.** A single-room type of maternity care with a more homelike setting for families than the traditional three-room unit (labor/delivery/recovery) with a separate postpartum area. A birthing room combines labor and delivery inone room. An LDR room accommodates three stages in the birthing process--labor, delivery, and recovery. An LDRP room accommodates all four stages of the birth process--labor, delivery, recovery, and postpartum.
28. **Breast cancer screening/mammograms.** Mammography screening - The use of breast x-ray to detect unsuspected breast cancer in asymptomatic women. Diagnostic mammography - The x-ray imaging of breast tissue in symptomatic women who are considered to have a substantial likelihood of having breast cancer already.
29. **Cardiac catheterization laboratory.** Facilities offering special diagnostic procedures for cardiac patients. Available procedures must include, but need not be limited to, introduction of a catheter into the interior of the heart by way of a vein or artery or by direct needle puncture. Procedures must be performed in a laboratory or a special procedure room.
30. **Case management.** A system of assessment, treatment planning, referral and follow-up that ensures the provision of comprehensive and continuous services and the coordination of payment and reimbursement for care.
31. **Children wellness program.** A program that encourages improved health status and a healthful lifestyle of children through health education, exercise, nutrition and health promotion.
32. **Chiropractic services.** An organized clinical service including spinal manipulation or adjustment and related diagnostic and therapeutic services.
33. **Community outreach.** A program that systematically interacts with the community to identify those in need of services, alerting persons and their families to the availability of services, locating needed services, and enabling persons to enter the service delivery system.
34. **Complementary medicine services.** Organized hospital services or formal arrangements to providers that provide care or treatment not based solely on traditional western allopathic medical teachings as instructed in most U.S. medical schools. Includes any of the following: acupuncture, chiropractic, homeopathy, osteopathy, diet and lifestyle changes, herbal medicine, massage therapy, etc.
35. **Crisis prevention.** Services provided in order to promote physical and mental well being and the early identification of disease and ill health prior to the onset and recognition of symptoms so as to permit early treatment.
36. **Dental Services.** An organized dental service or dentists on staff, not necessarily involving special facilities, providing dental or oral services to inpatients or outpatients.

37a. **Emergency department.** Hospital facilities for the provision of unscheduled outpatient services to patients whose conditions require immediate care.

37b. **Trauma center (certified).** A facility to provide emergency and specialized intensive care to critically ill and injured patients. **Level 1:** A regional resource trauma center, which is capable of providing total care for every aspect of injury and plays a leadership role in trauma research and education. **Level 2:** A community trauma center, which is capable of providing trauma care to all but the most severely injured patients who require highly specialized care. **Level 3:** A rural trauma hospital, which is capable of providing care to a large number of injury victims and can resuscitate and stabilize more severely injured patients so that they can be transported to level 1 or 2 facilities. Please provide explanation on page 15 if necessary.

38. **Enabling services.** A program that is designed to help the patient access health care services by offering any of the following: linguistic services, transportation services, and/or referrals to local social services agencies.
39. **End of life services.**

39a. **Hospice Program.** A recognized clinical program with specific eligibility criteria that provides palliative medical care focused on relief of pain and symptom control and other services that address the emotional, social, financial and spiritual needs of terminally ill patients and their families. Hospice care can be provided either at home, in a hospital setting, or a free-standing facility.

39b. **Pain management program.** A recognized clinical service or program providing specialized medical care, drugs or therapies for the management of acute or chronic pain and other distressing symptoms, administered by specially trained physicians and other clinicians, to patients suffering from an acute illness of diverse causes.

39c. **Palliative care program.** An organized program providing specialized medical care, drugs or therapies for the management of acute or chronic pain and/or the control of symptoms administered by specially trained physicians and other clinicians; and supportive care services, such as counseling on advanced directives, spiritual care, and social services, to patients with advanced disease and their families.

40. **Enrollment assistance services.** A program that provides enrollment assistance for patients who are potentially eligible for public health insurance programs such as Medicaid, State Children's Health Insurance, or local/state indigent care programs. The specific services offered could include explanation of benefits, assist applicants in completing the application and locating all relevant documents, conduct eligibility interviews, and/or forward applications and documentation to state/local social service or health agency.
41. **Extracorporeal shock wave lithotripter (ESWL).** A medical device used for treating stones in the kidney or urether. The device disintegrates kidney stones noninvasively through the transmission of acoustic shock waves directed at the stones.
42. **Fitness center.** Provides exercise, testing, or evaluation programs and fitness activities to the community and hospital employees.

2001 AHA ANNUAL SURVEY

C. FACILITIES AND SERVICES (continued)	(1) Owned or provided by my hospital or it's subsidiary	(2) Provided by my Health System (in my local community)	(3) Provided by my network (in my local community)	(4) Provided through a formal contractual arrangement or joint venture with another provider that is not in my system or network (in my local community)
57. Outpatient surgery	☐	☐	☐	☐
58. Patient education center	☐	☐	☐	☐
59. Patient representative services	☐	☐	☐	☐
60. Physical rehabilitation outpatient services	☐	☐	☐	☐
61. Primary care department	☐	☐	☐	☐
62. Psychiatric services:				
a. Psychiatric child-adolescent services	☐	☐	☐	☐
b. Psychiatric consultation-liaison services	☐	☐	☐	☐
c. Psychiatric education services	☐	☐	☐	☐
d. Psychiatric emergency services	☐	☐	☐	☐
e. Psychiatric geriatric services	☐	☐	☐	☐
f. Psychiatric outpatient services	☐	☐	☐	☐
g. Psychiatric partial hospitalization program	☐	☐	☐	☐
63. Radiation therapy	☐	☐	☐	☐
64. Radiology, diagnostic:				
a. CT scanner	☐	☐	☐	☐
b. Diagnostic radioisotope facility	☐	☐	☐	☐
c. Magnetic resonance imaging (MRI)	☐	☐	☐	☐
d. Positron emission tomography (PET)	☐	☐	☐	☐
e. Single photon emission computerized tomography (SPECT)	☐	☐	☐	☐
f. Ultrasound	☐	☐	☐	☐
65. Reproductive health	☐	☐	☐	☐
66. Retirement housing	☐	☐	☐	☐
67. Sleep Center	☐	☐	☐	☐
68. Social work services	☐	☐	☐	☐
69. Sports medicine	☐	☐	☐	☐
70. Support groups	☐	☐	☐	☐
71. Teen outreach services	☐	☐	☐	☐
72. Tobacco Treatment/Cessation Program	☐	☐	☐	☐
73. Transplant services	☐	☐	☐	☐
74. Transportation to health facilities	☐	☐	☐	☐
75. Urgent care center	☐	☐	☐	☐
76. Volunteer services department	☐	☐	☐	☐
77. Women's health center/services	☐	☐	☐	☐

C. FACILITIES AND SERVICES (continued)

43. **Freestanding outpatient care center.** A facility owned and operated by the hospital, but physically separate from the hospital, that provides various medical treatments on an outpatient basis only. In addition to treating minor illnesses or injuries, the center will stabilize seriously ill or injured patients before transporting them to a hospital. Laboratory and radiology services are usually available.
44. **Geriatric services.** The branch of medicine dealing with the physiology of aging and the diagnosis and treatment of disease affecting the aged. Services could include: Adult day care; Alzheimer's diagnostic-assessment services; Comprehensive geriatric assessment; Emergency response system; Geriatric acute care unit; and/or Geriatric clinics.
45. **Health fair.** Community health education events that focus on the prevention of disease and promotion of health through such activities as audiovisual exhibits and free diagnostic services.
46. **Health information center.** Education which is directed at increasing the information of individuals and populations. It is intended to increase the ability to make informed personal, family and community health decisions by providing consumers with informed choices about health matters with the objective of improving health status.
47. **Health screening.** A preliminary procedure such as a test or examination to detect the most characteristic sign or signs of a disorder that may require further investigation.
48. **Hemodialysis:** Provision of equipment and personnel for the treatment of renal insufficiency on an inpatient or outpatient basis.
49. **HIV-AIDS services** (could include). HIV-AIDS unit-Special unit or team designated and equipped specifically for diagnosis, treatment, continuing care planning, and counseling services for HIV-AIDS patients and their families. General inpatient care for HIV-AIDS-Inpatient diagnosis and treatment for human immunodeficiency virus and acquired immunodeficiency syndrome patients, but dedicated unit is not available. Specialized outpatient program for HIV-AIDS-Special outpatient program providing diagnostic, treatment, continuing care planning, and counseling for HIV-AIDS patients and their families.
50. **Home health services.** Service providing nursing, therapy, and health-related homemaker or social services in the patient's home.
51. **Hospital-based outpatient care center-services.** Organized hospital health care services offered by appointment on an ambulatory basis. Services may include outpatient surgery, examination, diagnosis, and treatment of a variety of medical conditions on a nonemergency basis, and laboratory and other diagnostic testing as ordered by staff or outside physician referral.
52. **Meals on wheels.** A hospital sponsored program which delivers meals to people, usually the elderly, who are unable to prepare their own meals. Low cost, nutritional meals are delivered to individuals' homes on a regular basis.
53. **Nutrition programs.** Those services within a health care facility which are designed to provide inexpensive, nutritionally sound meals to patients.
54. **Occupational health services.** Includes services designed to protect the safety of employees from hazards in the work environment.
55. **Oncology services.** An organized program for the treatment of cancer by the use of drugs or chemicals.
56. **Open heart surgery.** Heart surgery where the chest has been opened and the blood recirculated and oxygenated with the proper equipment and the necessary staff to perform the surgery.
57. **Outpatient surgery.** Scheduled surgical services provided to patients who do not remain in the hospital overnight. The surgery may be performed in operating suites also used for inpatient surgery, specially designated surgical suites for outpatient surgery, or procedure rooms within an outpatient care facility.
58. **Patient education center.** Written goals and objectives for the patient and/or family related to therapeutic regimens, medical procedures, and self care.
59. **Patient representative services.** Organized hospital services providing personnel through whom patients and staff can seek solutions to institutional problems affecting the delivery of high-quality care and services.
60. **Physical rehabilitation outpatient services.** Outpatient program providing medical, health-related, therapy, social, and/or vocational services to help disabled persons attain or retain their maximum functional capacity.
61. **Primary care department.** A unit or clinic within the hospital that provides primary care services (e.g. general pediatric care, general internal medicine, family practice, gynecology) through hospital-salaried medical and/or nursing staff, focusing on evaluating and diagnosing medical problems and providing medical treatment on an outpatient basis.
62. **Psychiatric services:**
    a. **Psychiatric child-adolescent services.** Provides care to emotionally disturbed children and adolescents, including those admitted for diagnosis and those admitted for treatment.
    b. **Psychiatric consultation-liaison services.** Provides organized psychiatric consultation/liaison services to nonpsychiatric hospital staff and/or departments on psychological aspects of medical care that may be generic or specific to individual patients.
    c. **Psychiatric education services**. Provides psychiatric educational services to community agencies and workers such as schools, police, courts, public health nurses, welfare agencies, clergy, and so forth. The purpose is to expand the mental health knowledge and competence of personnel not working in the mental health field and to promote good mental health through improved understanding, attitudes, and behavioral patterns.
    d. **Psychiatric emergency services**. Services of facilities available on a 24-hour basis to provide immediate unscheduled outpatient care, diagnosis, evaluation, crisis intervention, and assistance to persons suffering acute emotional or mental distress.
    e. **Psychiatric geriatric services.** Provides care to emotionally disturbed elderly patients, including those admitted for diagnosis and those admitted for treatment.
    f. **Psychiatric outpatient services.** Provides medical care, including diagnosis and treatment, of psychiatric outpatients.
    g. **Psychiatric partial hospitalization program.** Organized hospital services of intensive day/evening outpatient services of three hours of more duration, distinguished from other outpatient visits of one hour.
63. **Radiation therapy.** The branch of medicine concerned with radioactive substances and using various techniques of visualization, with the diagnosis and treatment of disease using any of the various sources of radiant energy. Services could include: megavoltage radiation therapy; radioactive implants; stereotactic radiosurgery; therapeutic radioisotope facility; X-ray radiation therapy.
64. **Radiology, diagnostic:**
    a. **CT scanner.** Computed tomographic scanner for head or whole body scans.
    b. **Diagnostic radioisotope facility.** The use of radioactive isotopes (Radiopharmaceuticals) as tracers or indicators to detect an abnormal condition or disease.
    c. **Magnetic resonance imaging (MRI).** The use of a uniform magnetic field and radio frequencies to study tissue and structure of the body. This procedure enables the visualization of biochemical activity of the cell in vivo without the use of ionizing radiation, radioisotopic substances, or high-frequency sound.
    d. **PET.** Positron emission tomography scanner is a nuclear medicine imaging technology which uses radioactive (positron emitting) isotopes created in a cyclotron or generator and computers to produce composite pictures of the brain and heart at work. PET scanning produces sectional images depicting metabolic activity or blood flow rather than anatomy.

C. FACILITIES AND SERVICES (continued)

78. Which of the following physician arrangements does your hospital or system/network participate in? Column 2 refers to the systems that were identified in section B, question 3c. Column 3 refers to the networks that were identified in section b, question 3h. For hospital level physician arrangements that are reported in column 1, please report the number of physicians involved.

	(1) My Hospital	(2) My Health System	(3) My Health Network
a. Independent Practice Association	☐	☐	☐
b. Group practice without walls	☐	☐	☐
c. Open Physician-Hospital Organization (PHO)	☐	☐	☐
d. Closed Physician-Hospital Organization (PHO)	☐	☐	☐
e. Management Service Organization (MSO)	☐	☐	☐
f. Integrated Salary Model	☐	☐	☐
g. Equity Model	☐	☐	☐
h. Foundation	☐	☐	☐

Please provide a separate list of the name(s) and address(es) of the hospital's physician arrangements reported in column 1.

79. Does your hospital, health system or health network have an equity interest in any of the following insurance products? (Check all that apply) Contractual relationships with HMOs and PPOs should not be reported here but in Question 80. Column 2 refers to the systems that were identified in section B, question 3c. Column 3 refers to the networks that were identified in section B, question 3.f.

	(1) My Hospital	(2) My Health System	(3) My Health Network	(4) Joint Venture With Insurer
a. Health Maintenance Organization	☐	☐	☐	☐
b. Preferred Provider Organization	☐	☐	☐	☐
c. Indemnity Fee For Service Plan	☐	☐	☐	☐

80. Does your hospital have a formal written contract that specifies the obligations of each party with:
   a. Health maintenance organization (HMO) ..... YES ☐ NO ☐ b. If YES, how many contracts? .... ______
   c. Preferred provider organization (PPO) ...... YES ☐ NO ☐ d. If YES, how many contracts? .... ______

81a. What percentage of the hospital's net patient revenue is paid on a capitated basis?
If the hospital does not participate in capitated arrangements, please enter "0") .... ______ %

81b. What percentage of the hospital's net patient revenue is paid on a shared risk basis? .... ______ %

82. Does your hospital contract directly with employers or a coalition of employers to provide care on a capitated, predetermined, or shared risk basis? .... YES ☐ NO ☐

83. If your hospital has arrangements to care for a specific group of enrollees in exchange for a capitated payment, how many lives are covered? .... ______

D. COMMUNITY ORIENTATION

1. Does your hospital's mission statement include a focus on community benefit? .... YES ☐ NO ☐
2. Does your hospital have a long-term plan for improving the health of its community? .... YES ☐ NO ☐
3. Does your hospital have resources for its community benefit activities? .... YES ☐ NO ☐
4. Does your hospital work with other providers, public agencies, or community representatives to conduct a health status assessment of the community? .... YES ☐ NO ☐
5. Does your hospital use health status indicators (such as rates of health problems or surveys of self-reported health) for defined populations to design new services or modify existing services? .... YES ☐ NO ☐

6a. Does your hospital work with other local providers, public agencies, or community representatives to develop a written assessment of the appropriate capacity for health services in the community? .... YES ☐ NO ☐

6b. If yes, have you used the assessment to identify unmet health needs, excess capacity, or duplicative services in the community? .... YES ☐ NO ☐

7. Does your hospital work with other providers to collect, track, and communicate clinical and health information across cooperating organizations? .... YES ☐ NO ☐
8. Does your hospital either by itself or in conjunction with others disseminate reports to the community on the quality and costs of health care services? .... YES ☐ NO ☐
9. Does your hospital self-assess against Baldrige like criteria for sustained continuous improvement? .... YES ☐ NO ☐

e. **SPECT.** Single photon emission computerized tomography is a nuclear medicine imaging technology that combines existing technology of gamma camera imaging with computed tomographic imaging technology to provide a more precise and clear image.

f. **Ultrasound.** The use of acoustic waves above the range of 20,000 cycles per second to visualize internal body structures.

65. **Reproductive health** (could include). Fertility counseling - A service that counsels and educates on infertility problems and includes laboratory and surgical workup and management for individuals having problems conceiving children. In vitro fertilization - Program providing for the induction of fertilization of a surgically removed ovum by donated sperm in a culture medium followed by a short incubation period. The embryo is then reimplanted in the womb.
66. **Retirement housing.** A facility which provides social activities to senior citizens, usually retired persons, who do not require health care but some short-term skilled nursing care may be provided. A retirement center may furnish housing and may also have acute hospital and long-term care facilities, or it may arrange for acute and long term care through affiliated institutions.
67. **Sleep Center.** Specially equipped and staffed center for the diagnosis and treatment of sleep disorders.
68. **Social work services** (could include). Organized services that are properly directed and sufficiently staffed by qualified individuals who provide assistance and counseling to patients and their families in dealing with social, emotional, and environmental problems associated with illness or disability, often in the context of financial or discharge planning coordination.
69. **Sports medicine**. Provision of diagnostic screening and assessment and clinical and rehabilitation services for the prevention and treatment of sports-related injuries.
70. **Support groups.** A hospital sponsored program which allows a group of individuals with the same or similar problems who meet periodically to share experiences, problems, and solutions in order to support each other.
71. **Teen outreach services.** A program focusing on the teenager which encourages an improved health status and a healthful lifestyle including physical, emotional, mental, social, spiritual and economic health through education, exercise, nutrition and health promotion.
72. **Tobacco Treatment/Cessation Program.** Organized hospital services with the purpose of ending tobacco-use habits of patients addicted to tobacco/nicotine.
73. **Transplant services.** The branch of medicine that transfers an organ or tissue from one person to another or from one body part to another to replace a diseased structure or to restore function or to change appearance. Services could include: Bone marrow transplant program; kidney transplant; organ transplant (other than kidney); tissue transplant.
74. **Transportation to health facilities.** A long-term care support service designed to assist the mobility of the elderly. Some programs offer improved financial access by offering reduced rates and barrier-free buses or vans with ramps and lifts to assist the elderly or handicapped; others offer subsidies for public transport systems or operate mini-bus services exclusively for use by senior citizens.
75. **Urgent care center.** A facility that provides care and treatment for problems that are not life-threatening but require attention over the short term. These units function like emergency rooms but are separate from hospitals with which they may have backup affiliation arrangements.
76. **Volunteer services department.** An organized hospital department responsible for coordinating the services of volunteers working within the institution.
77. **Women's health center/services.** An area set aside for coordinated education and treatment services specifically for and promoted to women as provided by this special unit. Services may or may not include obstetrics but include a range of services other than OB.

78a. **Independent practice association (IPA).** AN IPA is a legal entity that holds managed care contracts. The IPA then contracts with physicians, usually in solo practice, to provide care either on a fee-for-services or capitated basis. The purpose of an IPA is to assist solo physicians in obtaining managed care contracts.

78b. **Group practice without walls.** Hospital sponsors the formation of, or provides capital to physicians to establish, a "quasi" group to share administrative expenses while remaining independent practitioners.

78c. **Open physician-hospital organization (PHO).** A joint venture between the hospital and all members of the medical staff who wish to participate. The PHO can act as a unified agent in managed care contracting, own a managed care plan, own and operate ambulatory care centers or ancillary services projects, or provide administrative services to physician members.

78d. **Closed physician-hospital organization (PHO).** A PHO that restricts physician membership to those practitioners who meet criteria for cost effectiveness and/or high quality.

78e. **Management services organization (MSO)**. A corporation, owned by the hospital or a physician/hospital joint venture, that provides management services to one or more medical group practices. The MSO purchases the tangible assets of the practices and leases them back as part of a full-service management agreement, under which the MSO employs all non-physician staff and provides all supplies/administrative systems for a fee.

78f. **Integrated salary model.** Physicians are salaried by the hospital or another entity of a health system to provide medical services for primary care and specialty care.

78g. **Equity model.** Allows established practitioners to become shareholders in a professional corporation in exchange for tangible and intangible assets of their existing practices.

78h. **Foundation.** A corporation, organized either as a hospital affiliate or subsidiary, which purchases both the tangible and intangible assets of one or more medical group practices. Physicians remain in a separate corporate entity but sign a professional services agreement with the foundation.

81a. **Capitation.** An at-risk payment arrangement in which an organization receives a fixed prearranged payment and in turn guarantees to deliver or arrange all medically necessary care required by enrollers in the capitated plan. The fixed amount is specified within contractual agreements between the payor and the involved organization. The fixed payment amount is based on an actuarial assessment of the services required by enrollees and the costs of providing these services, recognizing enrollees adjustment factors such as age, sex, and family size.

81b. **Shared risk payments.** A payment arrangement in which a hospital and a managed care organization share the risk of adverse claims experience. Methods for sharing risk could include: capitation with partial refunds or supplements if billed hospital charges or costs differ from capitated payments, and service or discharge-based payments with withholds and bonus payouts that depend on expenditure targets.

D. COMMUNITY ORIENTATION

9. **Self assessment** is an evaluation of an organization's management system through achievements in areas such as: leadership, strategic planning, human resource management, information management, process management, customer focus and satisfaction, and business results.

2001 AHA ANNUAL SURVEY

E. TOTAL FACILITY BEDS, UTILIZATION, FINANCES, AND STAFFING

Please report beds, utilization, financial, and staffing data for a 12 month period that is consistent with the period reported on page 1. Report financial data for reporting period only. Include within your operations all activities that are wholly owned by the hospital, including subsidiary corporations regardless of where the activity is physically located. Please do not include within your operations distinct and separate divisions that may be owned by your hospital's parent corporation. If final figures are not available, please estimate. Round to the nearest dollar. Report full-time and part-time personnel who were on the payroll and whose payroll expenses are reported in E3f. (Please refer to specific definitions on page 12.)

> Fill out column (2) if hospital owns and operates a nursing home type unit/facility. Column (1) should be the combined total of hospital plus Nursing Home Unit/Facility.

	(1) Total Facility	(2) Nursing Home Unit/Facility
1. BEDS AND UTILIZATION		
a. Beds set up and staffed for use at the end of the reporting period (Do not report licensed beds)	______	______
b. Bassinets set up and staffed for use at the end of the reporting period	______	
c. Births (exclude fetal deaths)	______	
d. Admissions (exclude newborns, include neonatal & swing admissions)	______	______
e. Inpatient days (exclude newborns, include neonatal & swing days)	______	______
f. Emergency room visits	______	
g. Total outpatient visits (include emergency room visits & outpatient surgeries)	______	
h. Inpatient surgical operations	______	
Number of operating rooms	______	
i. Outpatient surgical operations	______	
2. MEDICARE/MEDICAID UTILIZATION (exclude newborns, include neonatal & swing days and deaths)		
a1. Total Medicare (Title XVIII) inpatient discharges (including Medicare Managed Care)	______	______
a2. How many Medicare inpatient discharges were Medicare Managed Care	______	______
b1. Total Medicare (Title XVIII) inpatient days (including Medicare Managed Care)	______	______
b2. How many Medicare inpatient days were Medicare Managed Care	______	______
c1. Total Medicaid (Title XIX) inpatient discharges (including Medicaid Managed Care)	______	______
c2. How many Medicaid inpatient discharges were Medicaid Managed Care	______	______
d1. Total Medicaid (Title XIX) inpatient days (including Medicaid Managed Care)	______	______
d2. How many Medicaid inpatient days were Medicaid Managed Care	______	______
3. FINANCIAL		
* a. Net patient revenue	.00	.00
* b. Tax appropriations	.00	
* c. Other operating revenue	.00	
* d. Nonoperating revenue	.00	
* e. TOTAL REVENUE (add 3a thru 3d)	.00	.00
f. PAYROLL EXPENSES (only)	.00	.00
g. Employee benefits	.00	.00
h. Depreciated expense (for reporting period only)	.00	
i. Interest expense	.00	
j. TOTAL EXPENSES (Payroll plus all non-payroll expenses, including bad debt)	.00	.00
***4. REVENUE BY TYPE**		
a. Total gross inpatient revenue	.00	
b. Total gross outpatient revenue	.00	
c. Total gross patient revenue	.00	
***5. UNCOMPENSATED CARE**		
a. Bad debt expense	.00	
b. Charity (Revenue forgone at full established rates. Include in gross revenue)	.00	

***These data will be treated as confidential and not released without written permission. AHA will, however, share these data with your respective state hospital association and, if requested, with your appropriate metropolitan/regional association. The state/ metropolitan/regional association may not release these data without written permission from the hospital.**

SECTION E
TOTAL FACILITY BEDS, UTILIZATION, FINANCES, AND STAFFING
Instructions and Definitions

1. For the purposes of this survey, nursing home type unit/facility provides care for the elderly and chronic care in a non-acute setting in any of the following categories: *Skilled nursing care *Intermediate care *Residential care/elderly housing (*see page 4 definitions)
The nursing home type units/facilities are to be owned an operated by the hospital. Only one legal entity may be vested with title to the physical property or operate under the authority of a duly executed lease of the physical property.

1a. Report the number of **beds** regularly available (those set up and staffed for use) at the end of the reporting period. Report only operating beds, not constructed bed capacity. Include all bed facilities that are set up and staffed for use by inpatients who have no other bed facilities, such as pediatric bassinets, isolation units, quiet rooms, and reception and observation units assigned to or reserved for them. Exclude newborn bassinets and bed facilities for patients receiving special procedures for a portion of their stay and who have other bed facilities assigned to or reserved for them. Exclude, for example, labor room, postanesthesia, or postoperative recovery room beds, psychiatric holding beds, and beds that are used only as holding facilities for patients prior to their transfer to another hospital.

b. Report the number of normal newborn **bassinets**. Do not include neonatal intensive care or intermediate care bassinets. These should be reported on page 3, C6 and C7.

c. Total **births** should exclude fetal deaths.

d. Include the number of adult and pediatric **admissions** only (exclude births). This figure should include all patients admitted during the reporting period, including neonatal and swing admissions.

e. Report the number of adult and pediatric days of care rendered during the entire reporting period. Do not include days of care rendered for normal infants born in the hospital, but do include those for their mothers. Include days of care for infants born in the hospital and transferred into a neonatal care unit. Also include swing bed inpatient days. **Inpatient day** of care (also commonly referred to as a **<u>patient day</u>** or a **<u>census day</u>**, or by some federal hospitals as an **occupied bed day**) is a period of service between the census-taking hours on two successive calendar days, the day of discharge being counted only when the patient was admitted the same day.

f. **Emergency room visits** should reflect the number of visits to the emergency unit. Emergency outpatients can be admitted to the inpatient areas of the hospital, but they are still counted as emergency visits and subsequently as inpatient admissions.

g. An **Outpatient visit** is a visit by a patient who is not lodged in the hospital while receiving medical, dental, or other services. Each appearance of an outpatient in each unit constitutes one visit regardless of the number of diagnostic and/or therapeutic treatments that the patient receives. Total outpatient visits should include all clinic visits, referred visits, observation services, outpatient surgeries, home health service visits, and emergency room visits.
Clinic visits should reflect total number of visits to each specialized medical unit that is responsible for the diagnosis and treatment of patients on an outpatient, nonemergency basis (i.e., alcoholism, dental, gynecology, etc.). Visits to the satellite clinics and primary group practices should be included if revenue is received by the hospital.
Referred visits should reflect total number of outpatient ancillary visits to each specialty unit of the hospital established for providing technical aid used in the diagnosis and treatment of patients. Examples of such units are diagnostic radiology, EKG, pharmacy, etc.
Observation services are those services furnished on a hospital's premises, including use of a bed and periodic monitoring by a hospital's nursing or other staff, which are reasonable and necessary to evaluate an outpatient's condition or determine the need for a possible admission to the hospital as an inpatient. Observation services usually do not exceed 24 hours. However, there is no hourly limit on the extent to which they may be used.
Home health service visits are visits by home health personnel to a patient's residence.
Also include the number of outpatient surgeries reported on line E1i. and the emergency room visits reported on line E1f.

h-i. Count each patient undergoing surgery as one surgical operation regardless of the number of surgical procedures that were performed while the patient was in the operating or procedure room.

i. For outpatient surgical operations, please record operations performed on patients who do not remain in the hospital overnight. Include all operations whether performed in the inpatient operating rooms or in procedure rooms located in an outpatient facility. Include an endoscopy only when used as an operative tool and not when used for diagnosis alone.

3a. **Net patient revenue.** Reported at the estimated net realizable amounts from patients, third-party payors, and others for services rendered, including estimated retroactive adjustments under reimbursement agreements with third-party payors. Retroactive adjustments are accrued on an estimated basis in the period the related services are rendered and adjusted in future periods as final settlements are determined.

c. **Other operating revenue.** Revenue from services other than health care provided to patients, as well as sales and services to nonpatients. Revenue that arises from the normal day-to-day operations from services other than health care provided to patients. Includes sales and services to nonpatients, and revenue from miscellaneous sources (rental of hospital space, sale of cafeteria meals, gift shop sales). Also include operating gains in this category.

d. **Nonoperating revenue.** Includes investment income, extraordinary gains and other nonoperating gains.

f. **Payroll expenses.** Include payroll for all personnel including medical and dental residents/interns and trainees.

g. **Employee benefits.** Includes social security, group insurance, retirement benefits, workman's compensation, unemployment insurance, etc.

j. **Total expenses.** Includes all payroll and non-payroll expenses (including bad debt) as well as any nonoperating losses (including extraordinary losses).

5a. **Bad debt expense.** The provision for actual or expected uncollectibles resulting from the extension of credit. Because bad debts are reported as an expense and not a deduction from revenue, the gross charges that result in bad debts will remain in net revenue (E3a).

b. **Charity care.** Health services that were never expected to result in cash inflows. Charity care results from a provider's policy to provide health care services free of charge to individuals who meet certain financial criteria. **<u>For purposes of this survey, charity care is measured on the basis of revenue forgone, at full established rates.</u>**

E. TOTAL FACILITY BEDS, UTILIZATION, FINANCES, AND STAFFING (continued)

*6. REVENUE BY PAYOR (report total facility gross and net figures)

			(1) Gross	(2) Net
a.	GOVERNMENT	(1) Medicare:		
		a) Routine patient revenue	.00	.00
		b) Managed care revenue	.00	.00
		c) Total (a + b)	.00	.00
		(2) Medicaid:		
		a) Routine patient revenue	.00	.00
		b) Managed care revenue	.00	.00
		c) Total (a + b)	.00	.00
		(3) Other government:	.00	.00
b.	NONGOVERNMENT	(1) Self-pay	.00	.00
		(2) Third-party payors:		
		a) Managed care (includes HMO and PPO)	.00	.00
		b) Other third-party payors	.00	.00
		c) Total third-party payors (a + b)	.00	.00
		(3) All Other nongovernment:	.00	.00
c.	TOTAL		.00	.00

(Total gross should equal 4c on page 11, total net should equal 3a on page 11.)

Are the financial data on pages 11 and 13 from your audited financial statement? YES ☐ NO ☐

7. FIXED ASSETS

a.	Property, plant and equipment at cost	.00
b.	Accumulated depreciation	.00
c.	Net property, plant and equipment (a-b)	.00

8. STAFFING

Report full-time (35 hours or more) and part-time (less than 35 hours) personnel who were on the hospital/facility **payroll at the end of your reporting period.** Include members of religious orders for whom dollar equivalents were reported. Exclude private-duty nurses, volunteers, and all personnel whose salary is financed entirely by outside research grants. Exclude physicians and dentists who are paid on a fee basis.

		(1) Full-Time (35 hr/wk or more) On Payroll	(2) Part-Time (less than 35 hr/wk) On Payroll
a.	Physicians and dentists		
b.	Medical and dental residents/interns		
c.	Other trainees		
d.	Registered nurses		
e.	Licensed practical (vocational) nurses		
f.	All other personnel		
g.	Total facility personnel (add 8a through 8f) (Should include hospital plus nursing home type unit/facility personnel)		
h.	Nursing home type unit/facility personnel (if applicable - please break out these personnel from the total facility number.)		

***These data will be treated as confidential and not released without written permission. AHA will, however, share these data with your respective state hospital association and, if requested, with your appropriate metropolitan/regional association. The state/metropolitan/regional association may not release these data without written permission from the hospital.**

SECTION E
Instructions and Definitions

7. **Fixed Assets.** Represent land and physical properties that are consumed or used in the creation of economic activity by the health care entity. The historical or acquisition costs are used in recording fixed assets. Net plant, property, and equipment represent the original costs of these items less accumulated depreciation and amortization.

8a. **Physicians and dentists.** Include only those physicians and dentists engaged in clinical practice and on the payroll. Those who hold administrative positions should be reported in "All other personnel."

c. **Other trainees**. A trainee is a person who has not completed the necessary requirements for certification or met the qualifications required for full salary under a related occupational category. Exclude medical and dental residents/interns who should be reported on line 7b.

d. **Registered nurses.** Nurses who have graduated from approved schools of nursing and who are currently registered by the state. They are responsible for the nature and quality of all nursing care that patients receive. Do not include any registered nurses more appropriately reported in other occupational categories, such as facility administrators, and therefore listed under "All other personnel."

e. **Licensed practical (vocational) nurses.** Nurses who have graduated from an approved school of practical (vocational) nursing who work under the supervision of registered nurses and/or physicians.

g. **Total facility personnel.** This line is to include the total facility personnel - hospital plus nursing home type unit/facility personnel (for those hospitals that own and operate a nursing home type unit/facility).

h. **Nursing home type unit/facility personnel.** This line should be filled out only by hospitals that own and operate a nursing home type unit/ facility, where only one legal entity is vested with title to the physical property or operates under the authority of a duly executed lease of the physical property. If nursing home type unit/facility personnel are reported on the total facility personnel line, but cannot be broken out, please write "cannot break out" on this line.

SUPPLEMENTAL INFORMATION

1. **Joint Venture.** A contractual arrangment betwen two or more parties forming an unincorporated business. The participants in the arrangement remain independent and separate outside of the venture's purpose.

2001 AHA ANNUAL SURVEY

SUPPLEMENTAL INFORMATION

1. Does your hospital participate in any joint venture arrangements? .... YES ☐ NO ☐
   If yes, please provide a separate list of the name(s) and address(es) of the arrangements.

2. Does your hospital provide services through a satellite facility(s)? .... YES ☐ NO ☐
   If yes, please provide a separate list of the name(s) and address(es) of the satellite.

3. For the titles listed below, please indicate the name and the exact title of the person who holds the position in the hospital.

	Name	Title
a. Chief Financial Officer	____________	____________
b. Chief Information Officer	____________	____________
c. Vice President, Strategic Planning	____________	____________
d. Chief of the Medical Staff	____________	____________

Use this space or an additional sheet if more space is required for comments or to elaborate on any of the information supplied on this survey. Refer to the response by page, section, and item name. Also, use this space to describe your community benefit activities.

GWUMC

P182SH

2001 AHA ANNUAL SURVEY

As declared previously, hospital specific revenue data are treated as confidential. AHA's policy is not to release these data without written permission from your institution. The AHA will however, share these data with your respective state hospital association and if requested with your appropriate metropolitan/regional association.

On occasion, the AHA is asked to provide these data to external organizations, both public and private, for their use in analyzing crucial health care policy or research issues. The AHA is requesting your permission to allow us to release your confidential data to those requests that we consider legitimate and worthwhile. In every instance of disclosure, the receiving organization will be prohibited from releasing hospital specific information.

Please indicate below whether or not you agree to these types of disclosure:

[ ] I hereby grant AHA permission to release my hospital's revenue data to external users that the AHA determines have a legitimate and worthwhile need to gain access to these data subject to the user's agreement with the AHA not to release hospital specific information.

____

Chief Executive Officer Date

[ ] I do not grant AHA permission to release my confidential data.

____

Chief Executive Officer Date

Does your hospital or health system have an Internet or Homepage address? **Yes** ☐ **No** ☐
If yes, please provide the address: http:// ______________________________

Thank you for your cooperation in completing this survey. If there are any questions about your responses to this survey, who should be contacted?

____________________		(____) __________
Name (please print)	Title	(Area Code) Telephone Number
__ __/__ __/__ __	____________________	(____) __________
Date of Completion	Chief Executive Officer	Hospital's Main Fax Number

NOTE: PLEASE PHOTOCOPY THE INFORMATION FOR YOUR HOSPITAL FILE BEFORE RETURNING THE ORIGINAL FORM TO THE AMERICAN HOSPITAL ASSOCIATION. ALSO, PLEASE FORWARD A PHOTOCOPY OF THE COMPLETED QUESTIONNAIRE TO YOUR STATE HOSPITAL ASSOCIATION. THANK YOU.